Adverse effects. A critical review of COVID vaxgenes

Karina A. Acevedo-Whitehouse

Adverse effects. A critical review of COVID vaxgenes

Karina A. Acevedo-Whitehouse

First published in Spanish by K. A. Acevedo-Whitehouse

ISBN 978-969-43-9267-7 (paperback)

First English edition: February 2024

To all that have refused trading freedom for promises of safety, and for all who surrendered their freedom but have now started to ask questions.

To Runa.

If you look for truth, you may find comfort in the end; if you look for comfort you will not get either comfort or truth only soft soap and wishful thinking to begin, and in the end, despair.

C.S. Lewis

Prologue by Dr. Roxana Bruno

Once upon a time, many years ago, there was a chemist, who was also an engineer and an inventor whose inventions destroyed many lives. But this fact has been forgotten. Year after year he is remembered as the great benefactor that allowed bestowing a prize to those whose contribution is exceptional and beneficial for humanity. The prize awarded this year, 2023, which might '*make hesitant people take the vaccine and be sure it's very efficient and safe*', recreates the paradox and becomes a stigma for awarders and awardees: everyone will be eternally remembered for what their inventions have meant for humankind.

Every instant, and every human being, is unique and unrepeatable. The moment in which you are discovering this book, as well as every life that is honoured in its pages is also unique and unrepeatable.

As if it were about innocent lab rats and not human lives, more than thirteen billion doses were injected, under duress. An unprecedented massive experiment unfolded, one that has already taken hostage three fourths of the world's population. And more are being promised. Many people feel challenged by the pandemic of mythomania that affects our planet: hand in hand with an abject and dystopic science it became possible to ingrain lives strongly to fear, disconnecting them and intentionally pushing them towards a complex crossroads.

This book offers us a guide for our journey through those dark labyrinths, opening the way towards real comprehension of what is a deliberate technology, whose effects could be predicted and whose evidence is still being denied. As a deep declaration of justice and love, Karina Alethya Acevedo Whitehouse gives voice to forbidden science and rescues the anonymous cases of destroyed life for history. With empathy and understanding she leads us to the final crossroad of the labyrinth, where she opens the door to truth and embraces the vibrant hope that joins all beings in all corners of the universe.

Prologue by Miriam García

From a seed you could learn,

that anything that wants to be born,

must begin by moving through the darkness.

From a tree you could learn,

that anyone who wishes to flourish,

must work hard on himself,

in silence and in solitude.

(Arnau de Tera)

Getting to know Karina has been a privilege. I never imagined where our phone conversation, on March 19, 2020, days after the pandemic was declared, would lead her to. She told me that she would not sit idly by and would do everything in her power to contribute with what she knew to help the community of Akasha and the university where she worked. I never imagined the reach and strength of those words, of that conviction.

Reading her book and seeing the seed of her intention and her actions crystallized after more than three years and a half, is proof that it is possible to move from darkness to the light of knowledge and make decisions that create new realities for humanity.

I confess that although I have read what she has shared during this time in the '*Akasha Comunidad*' Telegram channel, her book was not easy to read — it moved me deeply — but it was essential and I believe it will be so for the understanding of those who dare to look beyond the data, that wish to be touched by reason and by different dimensions of consciousness; for everyone to take responsibility in making decisions for their life and for future generations.

I knew that it was not easy for her to write the book, and after reading it, I understand why. It was also not easy for her to fully accept the implications of some of the things she researched and understood in order to share in the channel or during interviews and conferences. It was not easy to receive attacks, censorship and defamation. I was a witness to all of this. I saw her tiredness, her sadness for what was happening and for those that did not want to listen, I saw her touched at times by hopelessness and yet she continued with a burning desire to provide knowledge so that more and more people would understand, so that we could choose in an informed and conscious way, beyond fear, for the love of life.

During this time, how many questions have remained without truthful answers, how much desire to make sense of the chaos has been born and sustained; desire to understand what was not easy to understand, whether due to lack of training, lack of honest science-based information, or due to fear? This book is an attempt to provide answers to doubts and meaning to chaos.

I thank Karina for attempting to provide answers, for her purpose and her meaning, for transforming her worries into generous time that she dedicated to research, for offering her voice, her silence and her moments of solitude and her resilient gaze at the service of humanity, and for her brave heart who loves life and helps generate it.

...For explaining to us about the components, study phases, adverse effects, and pathophysiology of these gene therapy products, and for giving us the tools needed to learn and understand that we do not have to go through the same painful places again if we take responsibility as adults, individually and as a community.

...For helping us, by writing this book, go beyond the three pandemics that she sees: COVID, censorship and fear.

...For her ability to investigate, relate topics and shake our awareness while getting us closer to science; for expressing it bravely and truthfully. For bringing transparency where there was none and for leading us from knowing to understanding. It's not little.

...For this book that is a legacy for human history.

These pages that you will read are a journey towards understanding. When there is understanding, there is no turning back. This is a book that contains the past to learn from it, and that contains future and hope if we do our job.

I hope there is no turning back and that, from the present, we can honour those seeds of consciousness in each one, honour those who have suffered and continue to suffer adverse effects, those who left and those of us who remain...

To keep creating Life.

Acknowledgements and note to the reader

I would not have been able to write this book without the support and encouragement of '*Akasha Comunidad*' team members, that group of people who have given so much of themselves because they believe that something else is possible. To each and every one of them, whether still part of the team or not, I thank your trust, your energy and your support in what has been both difficult and enjoyable moments. In particular, I thank you for helping me remember that the act of creation can only be done from the heart, never from fear. Thank you, Miriam, for everything; thank you Lorenia, Ale, Pablo, Rita, Victoria, Fernando, Adriana, Melisa, Malika, Daria, JuanCa, Rafa, Ernesto, Erick, Jeza, Juan Carlos, Alejandra, Tanya, Susana, Sira, Faby, Gaby, Robbie, Virginia, Unai and Lumi. This would not have been possible without you. I specially thank Fausto and Guri, from my heart. Your patience, love, and absolute respect for what I have chosen to do is fuel to continue in this path.

This book was born from a wish. The wish to transmit knowledge in a way that can be understood by everyone, regardless of their professional background, and from the wish that that this knowledge should help counteract fear and help make conscious and responsible decisions that arise from the freedom to choose. In fact, I have been precisely doing that for three years and a half: trying to transmit knowledge regarding the COVID pandemic, first during invited interviews at my university, and then with videos and short informal texts that I publish in the '*Akasha Comunidad*' channel in Telegram[1], but this is the first time that I attempted to weave the issues together to form a coherent whole. It was time to do so, and I embarked on this journey happily and with a lot of love.

I cannot help thanking Dr. Teresa Forcades, whom since 2009, with her congruence and courage, helped me look beyond what I learned during my academic training and encouraged me to ask the necessary questions to start understanding in a much deeper way key processes related to what we are experiencing as humanity. I also want to thank the medical doctors and scientists who had the courage to speak up, responsibly and with solid

[1] Akasha Comunidad [Telegram channel; Spanish] Available at: https://t.me/akashacomunidad

bases, to alert others about the risks posed by vaccines that are based on gene therapy, even if doing so affected their professional careers and their personal wellbeing. Naming each of them would be a very long list, and I do not wish to accept the risk of omitting anyone due to forgetfulness, but I am filled with hope that from all corners of earth, there exist women and men that are committed to truth and to honesty, that do what they do because they love humanity. We may disagree with some points or perspectives, but while we maintain the commitment of helping from veracity and congruency, we will be walking together in the same direction.

I wish to thank my lab members and students for being patients with me. I know that the time that I have dedicated to these science communication activities and to writing the book have meant less attention from me. Please know that your patience and support have been central to finishing this task.

Finally, I thank so many people who, without knowing me, opened their hearts to share their experiences after they, or their loved ones, were vaccinated. Their testimonies and, specially, their humanity, have touched me deeply, and each one of them have been part of the motor that keeps pushing me forward. None of those deaths, of those cancerous tumours that appeared suddenly and developed disproportionately fast, none of those strokes, none of those autoimmune and neurological conditions ought to have occurred. You can be sure that your testimonies inspired each of my words.

Before you start to read this book, it seems important that you know what it is and what it is not:

It is not an academic textbook, although it explains scientific topics in a serious and referenced way, always revealing the corresponding evidence for what is said.

It is not a medical reference book, but it will be useful for doctors and their patients.

It is not a popular science book, although I tried to make it as understandable as possible for everyone.

It is not a book that strives to provoke fear; rather it seeks to offer knowledge that helps understand the facts, and that helps whoever needs help, search for it.

It does not constitute 'the truth' because in science there is no single truth, but everything it exposes contains truth.

It is a book that wants to be read by humans that are open to questioning what they think they know and eager to learn, whether they are accountants, acrobats, actors, actuaries, administrators, advisors, agronomists, alchemists, anthropologists, architects, artists, assistants, astronauts, athletes, bankers, biologists, blacksmiths, bricklayers, butlers, captains, carpenters, clowns, coffee growers, comedians, computer scientists, conductors, cooks, cowboys, couturiers, customs officers, dancers, dentists, designers, detectives, directors, doctors, doormen, doulas, drivers, employees, engineers, explorers, farmers, fishermen, firefighters, forensics, friars, gourmets, guards, gentlemen, generals, geographers, geologists, guerrillas, guards, housewives, horticulturists, inspectors, kings, lawyers, linguists, makeup artists, mathematicians, mechanics, microbiologists, midwives, mimes, ministers, monks, musicians, nutritionists, oceanologists, optometrists, pacifists, paramedics, peasants, philosophers, philologists, physical mathematicians, physiotherapists, pirates, plumbers, podiatrists, policemen, presidents, prime ministers, princes, prostitutes, psychologists, pugilists, rectors, salesmen, scavengers, scientists, secretaries, senators, shoemakers, shoe shiners, sailors, sociologists, soldiers, stewards, stylists, students, taxidermists, teachers, therapists, traffic agents, ushers, unemployed, ventriloquists, veterinarians, weightlifters, writers, zoologists... as well as every profession and occupation not named here and that is needed so that, among all of us, we can help modify the course that was charted for us three and a half years.

As many topics require the use of specialized terms and biological concepts that are not necessarily known to everyone, in each chapter I have tried to explain these as best I can. I also reference previous sections of the book where I already explained the concepts. Additionally, to make reading easier, I have included definitions of some key terms at the end of the book. If, when reading the book, there are concepts that are not clear to you, there is a good chance that in the glossary you will find definitions that will help you better understand what I have explained in each chapter.

If you find this interesting, intriguing or useful, please go ahead! The words captured on these sheets will welcome you with grateful hands and clear vowels.

Preface

We find ourselves at a critical and challenging moment in human history, one that began on March 11, 2020, when the WHO declared the COVID-19 (hereafter, COVID) pandemic. In the context of uncertainty about what seemed to be a disease associated with an emerging virus, which initially appeared to have a moderate fatality rate and for which there was little information on how to treat it, the fear that engulfed a substantial part of humanity is entirely understandable. Unfortunately, when fear prevails, it becomes complex to have rational thoughts that allow for the much-needed questioning to better understand what is being experienced. Ironically, given that fear spreads too, another pandemic began in parallel: a pandemic of fear.

From that fear, humanity was subjected, to a greater or lesser degree, to the swift decisions made by health authorities. The problem was that, due to a sense of urgency or, perhaps, other reasons, not all decisions were based on scientific evidence. This might be understandable given the state of a health emergency. What is not understandable is that throughout these 1,325 days since the pandemic was declared[2], multilateral discussions or critical reviews of the strategies taken during the pandemic were neither promoted nor allowed. That is what is unforgivable because the absence of dialogue has indirectly impacted billions of people.

One reason for this lack of dialogue and self-critique is the noticeable climate of censorship towards any argument that deviates from a single authorized narrative. Those doctors and scientists who proposed alternative narratives to understand, treat, prevent, and mitigate the impact of COVID were silenced, ridiculed, and nullified, even though they spoke from their own experiences with patients or their professional knowledge of epidemiology, immunology, virology, and evolution. It is not the first time this has happened; human history is filled with censorship against those representing a paradigm shift that threatens the *status quo*[3]. William Harvey knew this well in the 17th century when, based on his observations, he postulated that blood was pumped from the heart to the entire body, not

---

[2] The pandemic was declared on March 11 2020, and this text was written on October 26 2023.
[3] Phrase in Latin that means the state of things at a given moment.

from the liver to the left side of the body, as Galen had proposed centuries earlier. Ignaz Semmelweis knew this well in the mid-19th century when he pointed out that the lack of hygiene among doctors was allowing the spread of puerperal fever. William Coley knew this well in the early 20th century when he tried to make his colleagues understand that cancer could be defeated by stimulating the immune system. All three, and many others throughout history, faced ridicule, isolation, and rejection because their colleagues preferred to be wrong rather than question the official version.

We now know about blood circulation, practice hygiene without thinking, and accept immunotherapy to treat cancer, but it took years (sometimes centuries) to change medical and scientific paradigms. This is because, whether we like to admit it or not, the scientific and medical communities are not contrarian and do not characterize themselves by questioning paradigms. Few are those who, in the words of the legendary Marcos Mundstock, manage to *reason outside the box*, and even fewer dare to express that alternative view publicly to their colleagues and the community. The fear of rejection, ostracism, and ridicule strengthens censorship, and this is also contagious. Thus, it is easy to understand why, alongside the COVID and fear pandemics, a third pandemic occurred: the pandemic of censorship.

It is regrettable that this climate of censorship persists today, and that arguments continue to be replaced by qualifying adjectives seeking to be offensive. Fallacies of authority are still promulgated as a substitute for evidence and reasoning, and the fear of a virus that is currently associated with a clinical presentation comparable to the common cold or to a mild flu, is still being used to sustain that single narrative.

The consequences of censorship, fear, and unquestionable public health measures extend far beyond these three years of the 'new normal' (one that is anything but normal). A real and direct consequence is the impact on people's health. By censoring and establishing a single health truth that skews knowledge toward a single narrative, thousands of sick people do not receive medical attention based on a real understanding of the pathophysiology of what might be happening to them. Therefore, the role of clinical doctors has been and continues to be crucial. Clinical doctors are at the border between patients and public health decisions. If doctors do not fully understand what they recommend to their patients, and what they recommend is not a safe product, then they are co-responsible, whether they accept it or not, for what happens to their patients. I use the word co-responsible with a clear intention: to point out that patients also have the responsibility to inform themselves. And that is why it is so important that those who have the knowledge make it accessible, always based on solid evidence, to doctors and to the general public.

Considering that medical training does not usually delve deeply into the knowledge of biochemistry, molecular biology, molecular genetics, molecular immunology, and evolution, it is understandable that medical doctors, when recommending COVID genetic vaccines to their patients, did not know the difference between synthetic nucleoside-modified mRNA and cellular mRNA; they did not know the formula of polysorbate 80 and polyethylene glycol, nor the physicochemical properties that allow their passage through cell membranes; they did not know that the proteins of the recombinant adenoviral vector would activate platelets upon contact with them, thereby increasing the risk of thrombotic thrombocytopenia; they had not heard of endogenous cellular transposable elements or, much less, know of the possibility that these would be activated by the presence of synthetic mRNA in the cytoplasm of those cells that were transfected by the vaccine. As I said, it is understandable; after all, doctors specialize in other subjects, and, as the saying goes, "*a cobbler sticks to his last*". However, I cannot help but wonder how it happened that they did not feel a hint of curiosity to at least superficially understand the foundations of this genetic technology that had not been used before, outside of clinical trials, to immunize the population? After all, of the 15 COVID vaccines listed to date by the WHO for emergency use, eight were made with gene therapy technologies. How is it that they did not want to inquire about what was known about their safety and what was not known? How is it that they felt confident recommending them to everyone, patients, friends, family, as if it were a simple drink of water?

I understand that questioning COVID vaccines is almost forbidden. But the point is that those who used their experience or knowledge of routine vaccines commonly used against poliovirus or rotavirus to argue that

COVID vaccines based on gene therapy platforms were safe, simply did not want to investigate anything. Let's say they chose to remain ignorant. The problem is that ignorance has consequences when it is present in those who have influence over others.

The emergency authorization of COVID vaccines, developed at an unprecedented breakneck speed, could not be based on compelling scientific evidence of their safety because it was not possible to consider evidence that, at least at that time, did not exist. Specifically, at the time of authorization, there were no accurate data on their short, medium, and long-term safety, and not a single study had been conducted on their potential genotoxicity, carcinogenicity, teratogenicity, interaction with cellular nucleic acids, or possible drug interactions. It was also unknown whether they could affect the health of people who already suffered from autoimmune or chronic degenerative diseases or those who had already generated immune responses against SARS-CoV-2 by being infected during 2020. In addition, the manufacture of billions of doses in a short time frame affected the standards of quality that would be expected for vaccines. This could help explain the presence of undeclared components in the vials, as well as the marked heterogeneity among vaccine batch numbers in terms of their associated adverse events. Regrettably, the health authorities of each country did not conduct their own analyses of the vial components, nor did they perform safety tests independently before conferring emergency use authorization of these vaccines and injecting them into their citizens.

The fact that they authorized and promoted these vaccines despite having no knowledge of the potential molecular and cellular interactions of their components in humans, nor of the adverse effects that they could cause, might lead us to reason that, at the very least, there would be a willingness to recognize and study adverse effects in a systematic and impartial way. This has not happened. Instead of this, in all countries, people, or their loved ones, that had health problems after receiving the vaccine were systematically ignored, underestimated or stigmatized, both in mass media as in social networks. This selective blindness is not only a deep lack of respect to those that chose to be vaccinated; it is also not the best way to win or maintain trust of the public towards health institutions and science. I find it ironic that it can cause an erosion of trust that *increases* generalized vaccine hesitancy.

When I was writing this book, I wished to include original art that graphically represented what has been and still is this three-pronged pandemic. I wanted an image that was based on the engravings of Hidari Jongoro in the sacred precinct of Tōshō-gū in Japan. Hidari Jingoro used monkeys to represent Confucius' 'code of conduct': Mizaru (see no evil), Iwazaru (speak no evil) and Kikazaru (hear no evil). The problem is that if we close our eyes, ears and mouth when faced with evil, we are likely to allow atrocities to be committed. History is filled with examples in which this has happened. Mizaru, represented by doctors (and some dentists), Iwazaru, represented by reporters, Kikazaru, represented by governments, and in turn, all three represented by every single person that chose not to see, not to talk and not to listen. I wanted the drawing to show these three characters grown in a Petri dish: an ideal culture media to propagate fear and to foster blind, deaf and mute obedience. I explained my idea to the artist, Miguel Ángel Rodríguez Feregrino, and he captured perfectly what I wished to express. I wanted this image to be the book's cover, but I understand that it is a strong and challenging image, one that could cause rejection in some if its intention is not fully understood. This is why I decided to include it here, after I had had a chance to explain it.

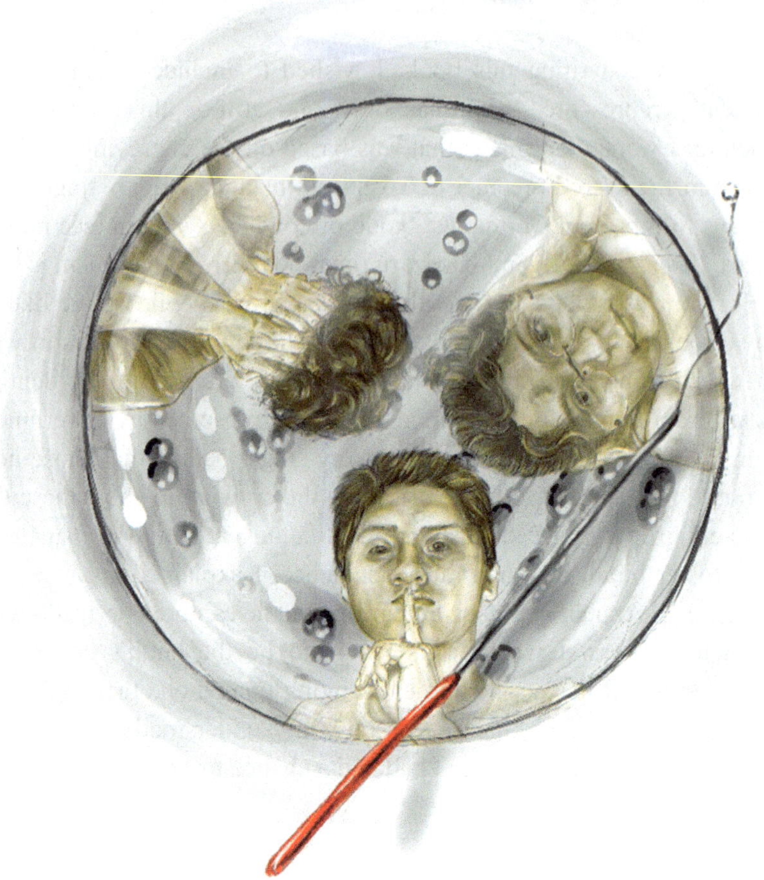

Throughout these three simultaneous pandemics, I have had Schopenhauer's words in my mind: "*All truth passes through three stages: First, it is ridiculed; second, it is violently opposed; and third, it is accepted as self-evident*". I remember his words because they imply that the paradigm shift will not be spontaneous or autonomous. It needs, first, prepared, conscious, and brave people; next, dissemination of knowledge, and last, a critical mass that has understood this knowledge. It is only from this critical mass that the perception of the crowd can change, and along with that change, so will the paradigm shift. We still need a long way to go, but I am certain, some changes are already occurring.

Table of contents

Introduction

In the context of the COVID pandemic, various types of vaccines and gene therapy-based immunizations were developed at an unprecedented speed. As of October 12, 2023, according to the World Health Organization (WHO)[4], 13,500,000,000 doses of COVID vaccines have been administered worldwide, and 70.49% of the global population has received at least one dose. Vaccination coverage varies significantly between countries and regions (Figure 1), with Cuba having the highest vaccination coverage (94.06% of the population receiving at least one dose) and Burundi having the lowest coverage (0.32% of the population receiving at least one dose), while Eritrea has not administered any COVID vaccine to its population[4].

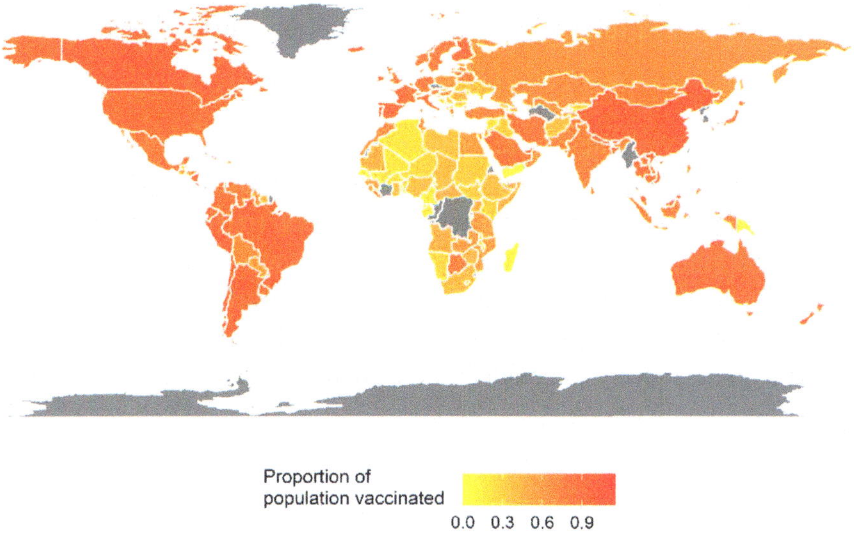

Figure 1. *Proportion of the population that has received at least one dose of COVID vaccines. The colour scale indicates the proportion. Countries shown with grey stripes lack updated information. Image created based on data from the Coronavirus Research Center*[5].

[4] Our world in Health [Internet]. Data updated to September 15, 2023; accessed September 16, 2023. Available at: https://ourworldindata.org/explorers/coronavirus-data-explorer

[5] Coronavirus Research Center, Johns Hopkins University [Internet]. Accessed October 16, 2023. Available at: https://coronavirus.jhu.edu/vaccines/international

To develop and authorize these products for emergency use in record time, a significant amount of work was undoubtedly required from international institutions and companies. Unprecedented actions in vaccinology were taken, such as simultaneously conducting different phases of clinical trials, authorizing them despite having data collected over a few months on their safety in trial volunteers, and removing the double-blind condition in several clinical trials by offering the vaccine to volunteers who had received a placebo[6].

These facts are particularly important because among the 15 COVID vaccines authorized for emergency use and listed by the WHO, eight were based on technological platforms that had not been used in humans outside of clinical trials (Table 1). It should be noted that, according to the vaccine definition used until 2021[7], products based on these technologies cannot be considered as vaccines, and given their mechanism of action (explained in section 1.3), I will refer to them as vaxgenes (for genetic vaccines) from now on.

The eight vaxgenes were manufactured based on two types of technology: one based on recombinant adenoviruses (AdV) as DNA vectors and another based on synthetic messenger RNA (mRNA) covered with small lipid molecules. Additionally, two vaxgenes against COVID based on recombinant AdV (Sputnik V and Sputnik Light, developed by the Russian pharmaceutical company Gamaleya) were authorized by 81 and 74 countries, respectively, although they are not recognized by the WHO at the time of writing this book.

---

[6] Statnews [Internet]. Accessed September 16, 2023. Available at: https://www.statnews.com/2020/11/12/pfizer-says-placebo-patients-will-eventually-get-its-COVID-vaccine-the-question-of-when-is-complicated/

[7] The definition of vaccine in Merriam-Webster's dictionary in 2013 was: "a preparation of killed microorganisms, living attenuated organisms, or living fully virulent organisms that is administered to produce or artificially increase immunity to a particular disease. [Internet]. Available at: https://web.archive.org/web/20211106075217/http://web.archive.org/web/20061017150031/https://www.merriam-webster.com/dictionary/vaccine In 2021, the definition was modified to include gene therapy, and the concept of "immunity" was changed for "stimulation of immune responses" (see: https://web.archive.org/web/20211214040643/https://www.merriam-webster.com/dictionary/vaccine).

Table 1. *COVID vaccines and vaxgenes that are currently endorsed by the WHO for emergency use, and number of countries that authorized their use. Bold font shows the common names by which they are known.*

Name(s)	Pharmaceutical company	Type	Countries
COMIRNATY® Tozinameran	**Pfizer**–BioNTech	Synthetic mRNA	149
Tozinameran + BA.1 **Bivalente**	Pfizer-BioNTech	Synthetic mRNA	92
Tozinameran + famtozinameran **Bivalente 2**	Pfizer–BioNTech	Synthetic mRNA	33
SPIKEVAX Elasomeran	**Moderna**	Synthetic mRNA	88
Elasomeran + Imelasomeran **Bivalente**	**Moderna**	Synthetic mRNA	42
VAXZEVRIA	**AstraZeneca**	Recombinant AdV	149
JCOVDEN	**Janssen**–Cilag International	Recombinant AdV	113
COVISHIELD™	Serum Institute of India	Recombinant AdV	49
CONVIDECIA	**CanSino** Biologics	Recombinant AdV	10
NUVAXOVID™	**Novavax**	Protein based	40
COVOVAX™	Serum Institute of India	Protein based	6
SKYCovione™ (GBP510)	SK Bioscience	Protein based	1
CoronaVac	**Sinovac**	Inactivated	42
COVAXIN®	Bharat Biotech	Inactivated	14
BIBP-CorV **Sinopharm** Covilo	Beijing Institute of Biological Products	Inactivated	18

Source: WHO COVID19 vaccine tracker. Accessed October 12, 2023. Available at: https://covid19.trackvaccines.org/agency/who/

As seen in Table 1, vaccine names do not always correspond to the colloquial names by which people know them. This can hinder understanding, as some individuals who received "the Pfizer vaccine" might believe it is different from those who received BNT162b2 when it is the same product. For practicality and to avoid confusion, from now onwards I will use the colloquial names when referring to specific products.

The use of technologies that had never been authorized for general population immunization is relevant, considering the short time available for clinical trials. There was no certainty about their medium-term and long-term safety, nor could it be assured that they would be safe when administered to individuals with comorbidities, predispositions to certain diseases, or physiological states such as pregnancy. At the time of their general authorization for the adult population, none of the clinical trials[8], had included volunteers with these traits (Baden et al., 2021; Falsey et al., 2021; Logunov et al., 2021; Sadoff et al., 2021; Polack et al., 2020).

Almost three years after being authorized for the general adult population and 16 months after being authorized for children aged five and older, it is justified, valid, and pertinent to question whether COVID vaxgenes have been safe. It is imperative to question this, given the number of adverse events possibly associated with COVID vaxgenes recorded in national and international monitoring systems. These events have been reported at a monthly rate that is 22 to 80 times higher than that observed for all other vaccines combined, according to adverse event reports recorded in the monitoring systems VAERS, Eudravigilance, and Vigiaccess (see Chapter 3).

It is in this context that I decided to write this book. My intention is for it to be a serious and systematic review of scientific studies on COVID vaxgenes and of the mechanisms through which severe adverse events occurring at unusual rates can be explained. However, it is a rapidly changing field of science, where studies and clinical cases are published at a dizzying pace. Therefore, it is necessary to clarify that the conclusions I present, that refer to information presented in scientific articles published to date and cited in the book, could change if the evidence published later also changes. That is the only way scientific knowledge advances, and the only way in which we will be able to increase our understanding of the events we currently face.

---

[8] Clinical trial registration numbers NCT04368728, NCT04470427, NCT04516746, NCT04526990, NCT04505722, NCT04530396 in https://clinicaltrials.gov Accessed September 8, 2023.

Chapter 1. Components and mechanism of action of COVID vaxgenes

Names and properties should accommodate to the essence of things and not the essence to the names, as things came first, and names came later.

Galileo Galilei

It might be that I am being somewhat paranoid, but I would think that when we are asked to accept being injected with a new drug, one that uses technology that had not previously been used for that purpose, it is not unreasonable to take some time to investigate what the drug contains.

If before you accepted the vaxgene, or before you recommended it, you did not have any knowledge of its content beyond what was said on TV, maybe it would be a good idea to start examining the information that the pharmaceutical companies offered regarding the components of their vaxgenes. Certainly, better late than never. In this chapter I will describe the listed components as well as those that were not listed but present, and the mechanism of action of the main components.

1.1 Declared components

According to the pharmaceutical company Pfizer, its original vaxgene (known as Tozinameran and Comirnaty®) contains BNT162b2, ALC-0315 [(4-hydroxybutyl) azanediol) bis (hexane-6,1-diol) bis], ALC-0159 [(PEG[9] -2000)-N-N-ditetradecylacetamide], cholesterol, 1,2-distearoyl-sn-glycero-3-phosphocholine (DSPC), potassium chloride, potassium dihydrogen phosphate (KH_2PO_4), sodium chloride, disodium hydrogen phosphate dihydrate, sucrose, and water. Pfizer's bivalent vaxgene contains BNT162b2 + omicron BA.1, ALC-0315, ALC-0159, DSPC, cholesterol, tromethamine, hydrochloric acid tromethamine, potassium chloride, potassium dihydrogen phosphate, sodium chloride, KH_2PO_4, sucrose, and water. Pfizer's second bivalent vaxgene contains BNT162b2 + omicron BA.4/BA.5, ALC-0315, ALC-0159, DSPC, cholesterol, tromethamine,

[9] Polyethylene glycol

hydrochloric acid tromethamine, potassium chloride, potassium dihydrogen phosphate, sodium chloride, KH_2PO_4, sucrose, and water.

According to the pharmaceutical company Moderna, its original vaxgene (known as Elasomeran and Spikevax) contains mRNA-1273, SM-102 (9-heptadecanyl 8-{(2-hydroxyethyl) [6-oxo-6-(undecyloxy)hexyl]amino}octanoate), polyethylene glycol, 1,2-dimyristoyl-rac-glycerol (DMG), DSPC, cholesterol, tromethamine, hydrochloric acid tromethamine, acetic acid, sodium acetate trihydrate, sucrose, and water. Moderna's bivalent vaxgene contains mRNA-1273, mRNA-1273.222, SM-102, PEG-DMG, DSPC, cholesterol, tromethamine, hydrochloric acid tromethamine, acetic acid, sodium acetate trihydrate, sucrose, and water.

According to the pharmaceutical company AstraZeneca, its vaxgene (named Vaxzevria) contains ChAdOx1, polysorbate 80, L-histidine, magnesium chloride hexahydrate, ethanol, sucrose, sodium chloride, sodium edetate dihydrate, and water.

According to Janssen–Cilag International, its vaxgene (named Janssen) contains AdV26, polysorbate 80, 2-hydroxypropyl-β-cyclodextrin, monohydrate citric acid, ethanol, hydrochloric acid, sodium chloride, sodium hydroxide, trisodium citrate dihydrate, and water.

According to the Serum Institute of India, its vaxgene (named Covishield) contains ChAdOx1, polysorbate 80, L-histidine, magnesium chloride hexahydrate, ethanol, sucrose, sodium chloride, sodium edetate dihydrate, and water.

According to CanSino Biologics, its vaxgene (named Convidecia) contains AdV5, polysorbate 80, mannitol, sucrose, sodium chloride, magnesium chloride, glycerine, N-(2-hydroxyethyl) piperazine-N'-(2-ethanesulfonic acid (HEPES), and water.

According to the Gamaleya Institute, its vaxgene (named Sputnik) contains AdV26 and AdV5, polysorbate 80, tris aminomethane, sodium chloride, magnesium chloride hexahydrate, EDTA disodium, sucrose, ethanol, and water. Its Sputnik light vaxgene contains AdV5, polysorbate 80, tris aminomethane, sodium chloride, magnesium chloride hexahydrate, EDTA disodium, sucrose, ethanol, and water.

It's likely that reading this list of components of COVID vaxgenes may not have been necessarily very informative or even understandable. To make sense of the list and to help make it useful, it's essential to first distinguish between the active compound and excipients, and to have at least some understanding of each component to identify the reasons for which they were added to the vaxgenes.

1.2 Function of different types of components

Excipients are defined as any substance that is not the active compound of a drug and is added to stabilize the drug. In other words, excipients are added to help maintain the physicochemical properties of compounds and ensure their biopharmaceutical properties in the body of the person receiving the drug. They can be inorganic salts, solvents, surfactants, and lipids.

I will begin by mentioning inorganic salts (potassium chloride, sodium chloride, magnesium chloride, sodium edetate dihydrate, potassium phosphate, etc.) that were added as excipients to the vaxgenes. These inorganic salts maintain isotonicity, meaning they make the concentration of solutes in the vaxgene equal to the concentration of solutes inside a cell.

According to the evaluation reports of Pfizer's vaxgene sent to the European Medicines Agency (EMA; EMA/707383/2020[10]), the added inorganic salts are *"controlled according to the corresponding European pharmacological monograph"*. At this point, we must take their word for it, as, at the time of preparing this chapter, it was not possible to access any source showing the precise amount of each inorganic salt contained in each dose of the vaxgene. However, it is reasonable to assume that they are present at a much lower concentration than the established toxic dose for

---

[10] European Medicines Agency. Assessment Report Comirnaty EMA/707383/2020 Corr.1*1 [Internet]. Available at: https://www.ema.europa.eu/en/documents/assessment-report/comirnaty-epar-public-assessment-report_en.pdf

each, as this dose is so high that it would require more milligrams of each salt than the physical space available in a vial.

Other excipients include solvents and buffers. Most COVID vaxgenes use water as a solvent, although some pharmaceutical companies added ethanol or even tromethamine (an aliphatic[11] amino alcohol used as a biological buffer) and hydrochloric acid tromethamine. Sucrose (the chemical name for common sugar) is also added because it reduces pain at the administration site (Kassab et al., 2020) and improves the thermal stability of a vaccine (Pelliccia et al., 2016).

From the perspective of their biological action, both in terms of generating an immune response and explaining adverse events (see Chapter 4), it is much more relevant to understand the lipid excipients and surfactants and the active compounds of the vaxgenes, which I will describe next.

In synthetic mRNA COVID vaxgenes, lipid excipients form nanoparticles (LNP) around synthetic mRNA (Fig. 2). This stabilizes synthetic mRNA inside the vial, and once injected into a person's arm, it prevents the degradation of synthetic mRNA in the extracellular space by plasma enzymes that have precisely that function (Eder et al., 1991), in addition to helping the synthetic mRNA be transported into the cell.

The lipid molecules added to generate LNP vary in their characteristics and polarity; some are ionizable cationic[12] lipids, others are neutral lipids, others are cell membrane-like lipids, and others are PEGylated lipids. All lipid molecules are very stable, and once formed as LNP, they can remain viable and unchanged in their conformation for more than a week at room temperature, and up to a month at 4°C (Roesler et al., 2009).

The ionizable cationic and neutral lipids, ALC-0315 and ALC-0159, used in Pfizer's vaxgenes (including Pfizer bivalent products) are new

[11] Chemical compound whose molecular structure is characterized by having an open chain.
[12] Characterized by having a molecular region that is compatible with water – that is, hydrophilic – and another region that repels water – that is, hydrophobic.

excipients that had not been used in any approved pharmaceutical product[13]. They have proprietary licensing from the biotechnology company Acuitas Therapeutics (Thorn et al., 2022), which focuses on LNP-based technology[14]. One of the lipids (ALC-0159) contains PEG, which is also found in Moderna's vaxgene. Also, this vaxgene contains SM-102, a patented ionizable synthetic amino lipid (WO2017049245A2)[15] that, like ALC-0315 and ALC-0159, had not been used in any pharmaceutical product prior to the emergency authorization of the COVID vaxgene. Moderna's vaxgene also contains polysorbate 80 (see section 4.1 to read about the potential of polysorbate 80 to cause anaphylaxis) and DMG, a synthetic lipid formed by PEGylation of myristyl myristate[16] diglyceride.

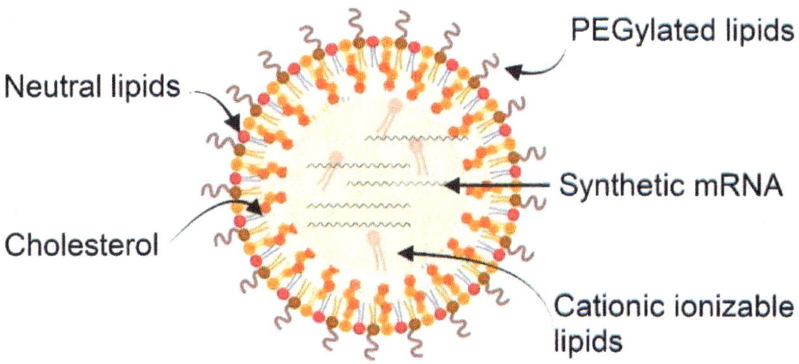

Figure 2. *Drawing of a lipid nanoparticle of a synthetic mRNA vaxgene. Drawn using BioRender.com*

According to the safety data sheet for DMG, it "*does not produce toxic effects or significant organic disease when exposure is kept under*

[13] European Medicines Agency. Assessment Report Comirnaty EMA/707383/2020 Corr.1*1 [Internet]. Available at: https://www.ema.europa.eu/en/documents/assessment-report/comirnaty-epar-public-assessment-report_en.pdf
[14] Acuitas Therapeutics [Internet]. Accessed September 6, 2023. Available at: https://acuitastx.com
[15] Google Patents. "Compounds and compositions for intracellular delivery of therapeutic agents" [Internet]. Available at: https://patents.google.com/patent/WO2017049245A2/en
[16] $C_{14}H_28O_2$

reasonable control" [17], although the toxic dose for intramuscular administration is not specified. Additionally, the technical report submitted by Moderna to regulatory agencies to request emergency authorization for its vaxgene does not indicate the amount of DMG present in each dose; it only ensures that there are 1.93 mg of total lipids per dose[18].

Synthetic mRNA vaxgenes (Pfizer, Pfizer bivalent, Pfizer bivalent 2, Moderna, and Moderna bivalent) contain DSPC, a phospholipid used for the preparation of liposomes (lipid vesicles). Its use in vaccines is indicated by regulatory agencies in their evaluation as a "*non-pharmacopeial excipient sufficiently controlled by an internal specification*" [19]. If your eyes are bulging, do not despair; in pharmacological jargon, this means that DSPC is not related to any official compendium on compounds used in pharmacology, so its use in injectable products has not been registered or evaluated by anyone to date.

The active compound in synthetic mRNA vaxgenes is the synthetic mRNA. The copies of these sequences, measuring just under 4,300 nucleotides, correspond to the complete S gene of SARS-CoV-2; that is, they contain instructions to manufacture the Spike protein of SARS-CoV-2. Once synthetic mRNA molecules enter the cell's cytoplasm, they are read by ribosomes, initiating the translation process (Fig. 3), meaning the generation of a chain of amino acids that will form proteins (Xia et al., 2011).

---

[17] Santa Cruz Biotechnology [Internet]. Accessed September 6, 2023. Available at: https://datasheets.scbt.com/sc-220511.pdf

[18] European Medicines Agency. Assessment Report Spikevax EMEA/H/C/005791/0000 [Document]. Available at: https://www.ema.europa.eu/en/documents/assessment-report/spikevax-previously-COVID-vaccine-moderna-epar-public-assessment-report_en.pdf

[19] Technical Report EMA/707383/2020 Corr.1*1. Page 29 [Document]. Available at: https://www.ema.europa.eu/en/documents/assessment-report/comirnaty-epar-public-assessment-report_en.pdf

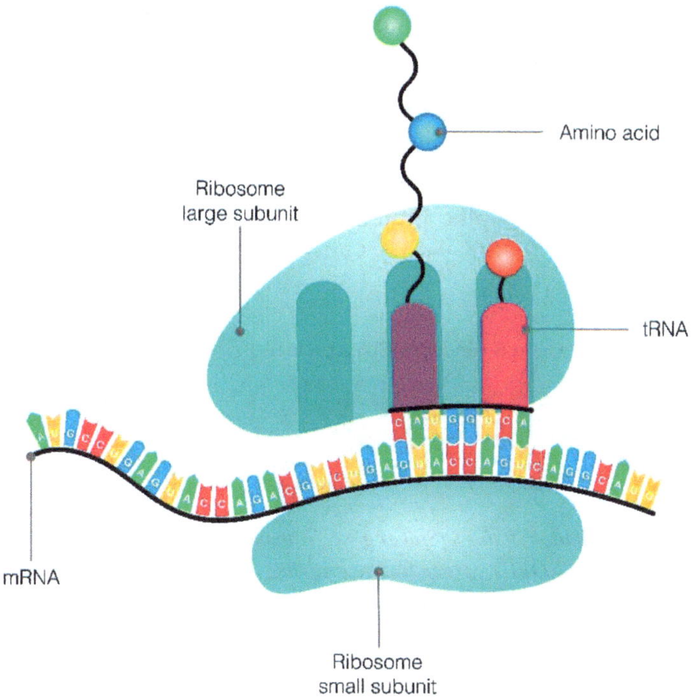

Figure 3. *Cellular or synthetic mRNA translation occurs in the ribosomes. The drawing shows the nucleotides of the mRNA sequence and how the amino acid chain is formed in the large ribosomal subunit helped by transfer RNA (tRNA). The amino acid chain is what will form the protein.*

To better understand this, it might help to think of ribosomes as protein production factories that only understand instructions when written "in RNA". The synthetic mRNA sequences of vaxgenes have a cap[20] at one end and a polyadenylated tail at the other end (Fig. 4). This means they have everything ribosomes need to recognize and decode their message and start producing copies of the protein. In that sense, but only in that sense, synthetic mRNA is like cellular mRNA: its instructions are read in ribosomes, and specific proteins are manufactured. However, the similarity ends there because what the Pfizer, Pfizer bivalent, Moderna, and Moderna bivalent vaxgenes contain are multiple copies of mRNA synthesized *in vitro* from the complete DNA sequence of the Spike gene of SARS-CoV-2. However, the sequence of the Spike gene in mRNA vaxgenes is not exactly

[20] A cap is a methylated guanine nucleotide that joins to the mRNA using a triphosphate bond in the 5' end; it is a 7-methylguanilate cap or m7G.

like that of the virus; it has been modified and contains two mutations[21] (see Fig. 4). These mutations were made with two specific intentions: one, to ensure that the resulting Spike protein has a prefusion conformation (i.e., the Spike protein remains in the state it has in the virus before it can fuse with the cell membrane and enter the cell), and two, to optimize the production rate of the Spike protein (Corbett et al., 2020; Wrapp et al., 2020).

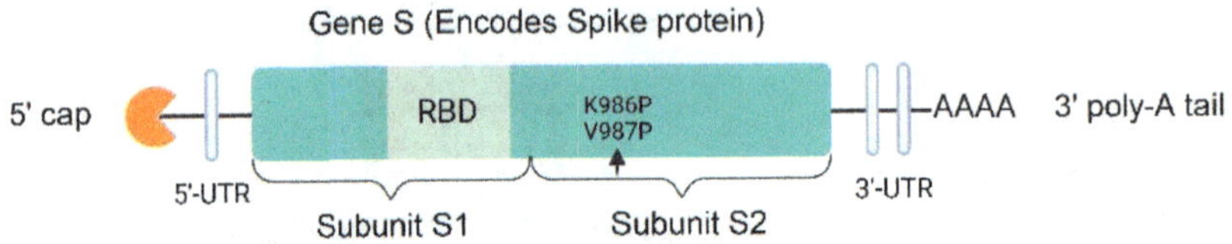

Figure 4. *Representation of the S (Spike) gene sequence which is the active compound of Pfizer and Moderna COVID vaxgenes. The drawing shows the elements that it contains and that allow it to be read by the cellular ribosomes to produce Spike protein. Both proline mutations are in the subunit S2.*

In addition to the two mutations that differentiate the Spike protein of SARS-CoV-2 from the Spike protein generated by Pfizer and Moderna's vaxgenes, the synthetic mRNA sequence of these products undergoes other modifications. Specifically, it contains N1-methylpseudouridine (N1-m1Ψ) nucleoside modifications. To understand this, it's essential to remember that RNA is composed of four nucleoside bases: adenosine, guanosine, cytidine, and uridine. When a phosphate group is added, they become nucleotides (now called adenine, guanine, cytosine, and uracil). What the manufacturers of synthetic mRNA vaxgenes did was first include pseudo uridine (Ψ) instead of uridine in the sequences (pseudo uridines use carbon-carbon bonds instead of nitrogen-carbon bonds), and then, they methylated the pseudo uridines (Morais et al., 2021). So, m1Ψ has a different chemical conformation than the uridine that forms the RNA sequences in our cells (Fig. 5).

[21] Two proline (P) mutations, one in the position 986 and one in the position 987 (see Fig. 4).

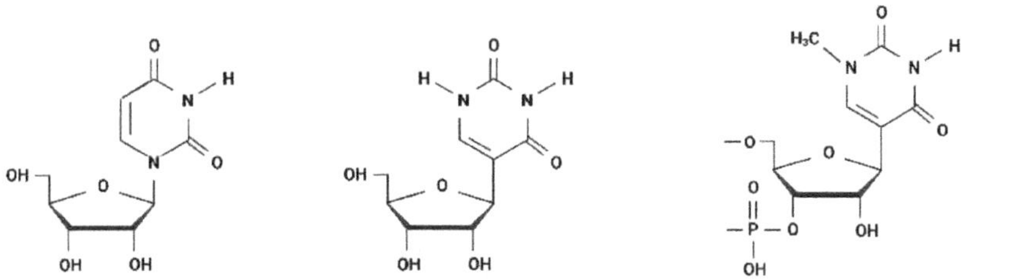

Figure 5. *Structure of uridine, pseudo uridine (Ψ) and N1-methyl pseudo uridine (m¹Ψ).*

It's important to clarify that natural Ψ uridine does exist, representing less than 0.6% of the uridine content in human cells (see Halma et al., 2023a), but not N1-m1Ψ, which has only been detected in archaea to date (Czekay and Koth, 2021). Therefore, we lack information about all the implications of its presence in human cells. What we do know is that modifying a sequence by incorporating N1-m1Ψ provides more stability to synthetic mRNA inside the cell and greater resistance to degradation by enzymes that degrade mRNA when its function is complete (Karikó et al., 2008). It also aims to reduce innate immune responses within the cell, allowing for greater and more prolonged production of the modified Spike protein (Nance and Meier, 2021; Suzuki and Ishihara, 2021).

This is why it's not accurate to think of these vaxgenes as if they were mRNA vaccines. They are made of *synthetic* mRNA, and for the sake of precision, of *synthetic nucleoside-modified* mRNA (Pardi et al., 2018a). This means it is a very different molecule from cellular mRNA, not only in terms of its components, but also in its stability inside the cell. Synthetic mRNA remains in the cytoplasm much longer than cellular mRNA, as will be discussed later.

Understanding the differences between cellular mRNA and synthetic mRNA is crucial to comprehend how the active compound of vaxgenes interacts with molecules inside cells, as well as its impact on tissues, organs, and health (see section 5.3).

It's worth mentioning that the synthetic mRNA sequences of Pfizer's and Moderna's COVID vaxgenes differ in terms of codon optimization (Table 2), as well as in the secondary structures they form (Xia, 2021). Before looking at the table, I recommend getting familiar with the concepts of codons and codon redundancy. A codon consists of three mRNA nucleotides identifying a specific amino acid. This is how mRNA sequences (both synthetic and cellular) are read in ribosomes, and transfer RNA (tRNA) adds the corresponding amino acid. Codon redundancy means that some amino acids are identified by different codons (Fig. 6).

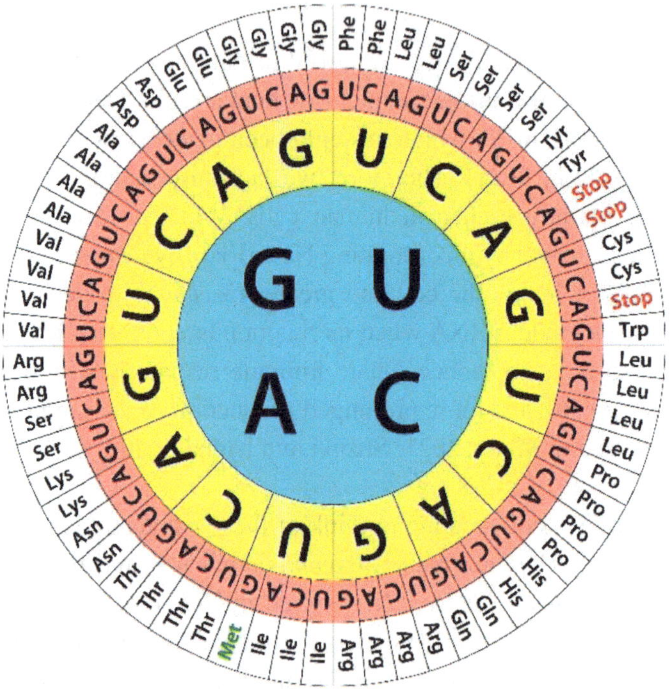

Figure 6. *Amino acid genetic code. The figure shows the codons that code for each amino acid. Methionine (Met) is only coded as AUG and is the starring codon for all proteins. Some amino acids have code redundancies. For instance, glycine (Gly) is GGG, GGA, GGC and GGU, and valine (Val) is GUG, GUA, GUC and GUU.*

Table 2. *Codon family optimization in the synthetic mRNA sequences that encode for Spike protein in Pfizer's (BNT-162b2) and Moderna's (mRNA-1273) vaxgenes in relation to the SARS-CoV-2 Spike gene sequence. Data from Xia 2021.*

Amino acid	Codon	Spike SARS CoV-2*	Spike BNT162b2	Spike ARNm-1273
Arginine	AGA	20	21	0
Arginine	AGG	10	1	2
Arginine	CGC	1	1	0
Arginine	CGG	2	19	39
Arginine	CGU	9	0	1
Leucine	CUA	9	0	1
Leucine	CUC	12	3	2
Leucine	CUG	3	105	103
Leucine	CUU	36	0	1
Leucine	UUA	28	0	1
Leucine	UUG	20	0	0
Serine	AGC	5	64	96
Serine	AGU	17	0	0
Serine	UCA	26	0	2
Serine	UCC	12	22	1
Serine	UCG	2	0	0
Serine	UCU	37	13	0

* Spike protein gene in SARS-CoV-2 reference genome (NC_045512).

The amount of synthetic mRNA per dose indicated by pharmaceutical companies to regulatory agencies for emergency use authorization also varies between brands:

- Pfizer: BNT162b2 – 30 µg per dose.
- Pfizer bivalent 1 & 2: BNT162b2 + omicron BA.1 or BA.4/BA.5 – 15 µg of each sequence, per dose.
- Moderna: mRNA-1273 – 50 µg per dose.
- Moderna bivalent – 50 µg per dose (25 µg per dose for children aged 6 months to 11 years).

However, this is not necessarily the amount received by a vaccinated individual. The reason is that the quantity of synthetic mRNA molecules encapsulated in the nanolipids is not standardized. For this reason, on July 19, 2023, McGill University in Canada initiated a study funded by Moderna to characterize and assess the quality control of LNPs. According to the university's press release, this study will be conducted "*to characterize lipid nanoparticles so that their specific size and charge distribution* [the synthetic mRNA] *can be better understood*" as "*standard techniques cannot simultaneously quantify the size and charge of LNPs, and therefore, only averages are often measured, masking individual variation*"[22]. In other words, after 33 months since emergency authorization and with billions of doses administered to citizens in 172 countries, a study began on something essential to know before administration: the quantity of synthetic mRNA contained in each LNP of each dose of the vaxgene.

On the other hand, in addition to the variation in the amount of synthetic mRNA, some reports and articles have detected the presence of degraded or double-stranded RNA (Tinari, 2021; Thacker, 2021) in synthetic mRNA-COVID vaxgenes. This could be due to errors or quality failures during the manufacturing process (Baiersdörfer et al., 2019; Karikó et al., 2011). Together, variations in the amount of synthetic mRNA per dose, as well as in its viability, plausibly may explain differences in immunogenicity, effectiveness, and the likelihood of adverse events according to vaccine batches (see Chapter 3).

If reading about synthetic mRNA has become a bit tiresome, don't despair. It's time to talk about the active compound of vaxgenes based on adenoviral vectors, such as AstraZeneca, Covishield, Janssen, Sputnik, and CanSino. This compound is an adenovirus (AdV) from humans or a chimpanzee. AdVs are considered ideal for use as vectors for gene therapy because they are thermo-stable, non-enveloped particles, easy to cultivate in vitro (Crystal, 2014), and have a broad tropism for entering different types of cells, making them strong inducers of systemic immune responses (Barry, 2018). Their genome is large (between 34,000 and 43,000 base pairs) and is composed of double-stranded DNA (Chavda et al., 2023), making it easy to genetically manipulate. AdV replication occurs within the nucleus, but it is infrequent, although not impossible (Zheng et al., 2000; Stephen et al., 2010), for the AdV genome to integrate into the cell genome,

[22] McGill University [Internet] Available at: https://www.mcgill.ca/newsroom/channels/news/mcgill-university-and-moderna-expand-collaborations-new-projects-lipid-nanoparticle-research-349107

so in general, the possibility of genotoxicity[23] due to chromosomal integration is considered low (Lukashev et al., 2016).

Now, wild-type AdVs (those freely circulating in the host population) are not used but rather recombinant AdVs. This means they were genetically modified to contain a gene that is not their own (in the case of COVID vaxgenes, it's the gene from SARS-CoV-2 that contains the information to produce the Spike protein). Recombinant AdVs used as vectors undergo other genetic modifications, such as the removal of the E1 gene from their genome so they cannot complete the viral replication cycle (i.e., they are modified to be incompetent or replication deficient) once they have entered the cell (Ledgerwood et al., 2010). The E3 gene can also be removed, so they cannot evade cell immune responses (McSharry et al., 2008). The elimination of both genes from the AdV genome allows more free space to insert the gene of interest.

It's important to clarify that, sometimes, recombinant "replication deficient" AdVs are not actually deficient. This occurs when the E1 gene was not adequately eliminated during the generation of recombinant AdVs, and they can replicate normally. This is what happened with Sputnik's COVID vaxgene, leading to Brazil litigating with the Gamaleya Institute for sending them vaccines that did not correspond to what they had indicated and could pose a security problem for their citizens, in addition to lower effectiveness against subsequent vaccinations (Moutinho and Wadman, 2021), because immune responses against the adenoviral vector would be triggered.

All COVID vaxgenes[24] based on recombinant adenoviral vectors were cultivated (the vectors) in permissive[25] cells, such as HEK293 cells (Chavda et al., 2023; Heinz and Stiasny, 2021). These are immortalized human embryonic renal cells (Graham et al., 1977) modified to express the adenovirus E1 gene that was eliminated (E1) to make them 'deficient for

---

[23] Processes that alter the structure, information or segregation of DNA, that are not necessarily due to mutations.

[24] Including Sputnik and Sputnik light vectorized COVID vaxgenes, that have not been recommended by the WHO but are used in many countries.

[25] These are cells that have all the elements that are needed by a specific virus to be able to complete their replication cycle.

replication.' This modification of the cells allows them to be used to produce many copies of defective replication adenoviruses (Almuqrin et al., 2021). I clarify that this does not mean that vaccines made this way *contain* remnants of human embryos, but rather that their vectors were *cultivated* in human embryo cells. The distinction is important.

If proper purification is performed after the cultivation of recombinant AdVs in HEK293 cells, there should not be even traces of those cells in the vial. However, if not adequately purified, their genetic material or proteins may be present in the vials (see section 1.4). Beyond any ethical or religious reasons for the presence of human embryo cell remnants, there is a serious biological problem: there could be DNA from HEK293 cells, and this has oncogenic[26] potential because these cells contain a functional oncogene[27] (Stepanenko and Dmitrenko, 2015). In other words, this HEK293 gene can induce cancerous transformation of normal tissue[28]. On the other hand, the presence of HEK293 cell proteins carries the risk of causing autoimmunity as they are human proteins (see section 5.7). It's a low risk, but it should not be ignored, given the large scale of vaccine production, leading to inaccuracies in the quality control of the COVID vaxgenes manufacturing process (Krutzke et al., 2022).

Each dose of COVID vaxgenes based on recombinant adenoviral vectors should contain 5×10^{10} AdV particles (Heinz and Stiasny, 2021; Voysey et al., 2021). However, as occurs with the variable amount of synthetic mRNA contained in each NPL, it is very difficult to standardize the quantity of AdV virions[29] present in each dose (Arand, 2021). In fact, the percentage of viable AdV virions in the vaccine can vary by up to two orders of magnitude, meaning the number of virions per vial can be 10 to 100 times different from each other (Tatsis et al., 2006). This means it is not possible to know how many AdV virions the vials of vectorized COVID vaxgenes contain, and this, in turn, can cause variations in responses

---

[26] That they can lead to malignant tumours.

[27] Gene that when expressed leads to continuous cell division.

[28] BioProcess International [Internet]. Available at: https://bioprocessintl.com/manufacturing/cell-therapies/quantitative-risk-assessment-of-limits-for-residual-host-cell-dna-ensuring-patient-safety-for-in-vitro-gene-therapies-produced-using-human-derived-cell-lines/ Accessed September 9 2023.

[29] A virion is the individual of a specific virus. The most useful analogy to understand the concept seems to be that virus is to a human what a virion is to a person.

(desired and undesired) to the vaxgenes. This problem has been known for over a decade, as it was experimentally demonstrated that the immune response to vectorized vaxgenes significantly varies depending on the quantity of viable virions they contain (Dicks et al., 2012).

The COVID vaxgenes based on adenoviral vectors do not contain LNP (lipid nanoparticles) like synthetic mRNA vaxgenes. This is because if the recombinant AdVs (adenoviruses) were enveloped in nanolipid covers, they would not be able to interact directly with the cell, which is necessary for them to enter and deliver their modified genetic material to the nucleus. The excipient present in all vectorized vaxgenes is polysorbate 80, a non-ionic detergent that functions to solubilize proteins, aiding the vaxgene components in crossing biological membranes (Cortés et al., 2020). When administered intravenously, polysorbate 80 alters the function of transporter channels in the cell membrane that forms the blood-brain barrier, allowing it to pass into the brain. This is why it has been useful for various pharmacological applications (Rocha et al., 2013). However, it implies that if they reach the bloodstream (Merchant, 2022), the components of these vaxgenes can cross the blood-brain barrier[30], and the recombinant AdVs can reach the brain, where cells express the receptor it uses to infect (Zhang and Bergelson, 2005).

1.3 Principles of action of vaxgenes

It is not my goal to talk about traditional vaccines in this book (it would end up being a much larger book!). However, the argument commonly put forward by doctors and scientists to declare that COVID vaxgenes are safe products is that '*vaccines against polio, measles, tetanus, rotavirus, etc., which have been applied since the mid-20th century, they are safe*'. This argument is incorrect and misleading to use as evidence of its safety, because COVID vaxgenes are not the same nor do they work the same as 'childhood' vaccines. It is essential that the differences in their mechanism of action be understood if we wish to begin studying their safety problems.

[30] It is not unreasonable to think that this could have happened to some vaccinated people if we consider that one of the recommendations of the WHO was to avoid back-aspirating the syringe when injecting into the muscle (Herraiz-Adillo et al., 2022).

Without a doubt, the mechanism of action of vaxgenes, both synthetic mRNA and vectorized ones, is radically different from the mechanism of action of vaccines used before December 2020. It is necessary to remember that the use of vaxgenes is precisely based on providing 'information' to the cells of the vaccinated person so that they produce the protein against which an immune response is sought. In that sense, they do not fit the definition of vaccine used before the pandemic (see footnote 7). When using vaccines, what is administered is the complete microorganism (either virus or bacteria) inactivated or attenuated. All childhood vaccines and most adult vaccines used before the pandemic were based on inactivated and attenuated platforms, although more recently, some vaccines have been manufactured from proteins (protein subunits) of the microorganism (Karch and Burkhard, 2016) instead of including the complete microorganism.

As indicated in the introduction, I will use the term 'vaxgene' throughout the book to avoid using other terms that may confuse the reader. What matters to me is that it is understood that, conceptually, they are not *vaccines* but, rather, somatic gene therapy[31] (Banoun, 2023; Kowalski et al., 2019). If what I just wrote seems exaggerated or incorrect, and even raises some scepticism, you might be interested to know that the FDA itself indicates that '*Human gene therapy seeks to modify or manipulate the expression of a gene or to alter the biological properties of living cells for therapeutic use.*' and that the '*FDA generally considers human gene therapy products to include all products that mediate their effects by transcription or translation of transferred genetic material or by specifically altering host (human) genetic sequences. Some examples of gene therapy products include nucleic acids (e.g., plasmids, in vitro transcribed ribonucleic acid (RNA)), genetically modified microorganisms (e.g., viruses, bacteria, fungi), engineered site-specific nucleases used for human genome editing (Ref. 2), and ex vivo genetically modified human*

[31] Gene therapy can be done in somatic cells (that is, any nucleated cell of the body, except for ovules and sperm cells) or in the germ cells (specifically, ovules and sperm cells).

cells.][32]. So, by the FDA's own admission, Pfizer, Moderna, AstraZeneca, Janssen, CanSino, and Sputnik 'vaccines' *are* gene therapy.

Attenuated or inactivated vaccines are based on exposing the vaccinated person to a specific microorganism with the aim of triggering a protective, specific immune response that induces robust and long-lasting memory. Obviously, the idea is to induce an immune response without causing the disease that is sought to be prevented or any harm (that's why the microorganisms in traditional vaccines are attenuated or inactivated). However, vaxgenes don't do that. Instead, they contain information that transforms the cells of the vaccinated person into a 'heterologous expression system'. The phrase sounds grandiose and complex, but its meaning is very simple: after the instructions (i.e., synthetic mRNA or DNA from adenoviral vectors) enter the cells of a vaccinated person, these cells become 'factories' that produce the desired protein, in this case, the Spike protein of SARS-CoV-2. Since it is not a human protein , its presence triggers specific immune responses against its antigens (an antigen is a small part of a molecule – almost always a protein – that the immune system recognizes and generates a response against, such as producing antibodies, among other responses).

So, there are differences in the mechanism, but also in the immunity these vaxgenes generate. This is because vaxgenes only generate immune responses against a specific protein, whereas the response to an infection or the response to inactivated or attenuated vaccines generates immune responses against many different antigens. It makes sense that vaxgenes offer less protection, since viruses have many different proteins, not just one.

Having clarity about the difference between a 'mono antigenic stimulus' and a 'poly-antigenic stimulus' is very important to understand why vaxgenes, compared to natural immunity from an infection, are not inclined to confer effective neutralizing immunity that prevents new infections or disease. It's also crucial to understand why issues of immune suppression

[32] Chemistry, Manufacturing, and Control (CMC) Information for Human Gene Therapy Investigational New Drug Applications (INDs) [Internet] (Pages 1-2). Available at: https://www.fda.gov/media/113760/download

and immune fatigue or exhaustion can occur, mechanisms I will explain in Chapter 5. Simply put, when infected by SARS-CoV-2, a person generates immune responses against 33 antigens from at least six viral proteins, including those of the Spike protein, as well as antigens from other proteins such as nucleocapsid, matrix, envelope, and polymerase proteins (Montes-Grajales and Olivero-Verbel, 2021; Anand et al., 2020). In contrast, first-generation[33] COVID vaxgenes are mono antigenic because they induce a specific and exclusive immune response against a single antigen: a region of the receptor-binding domain (RBD) of the Spike protein of SARS-CoV-2 (Lu et al., 2021). In fact, a response against the Spike protein antigen is generated, but only against the antigen of the first variant of the virus, which has not circulated on the planet since March 2020, as it was displaced by variants that emerged through mutations and that had more advantages to be transmitted and survive (Carabelli et al., 2023). Perhaps now it is easier to understand why the immunity conferred by vaxgenes practically does not provide protection against other variants of SARS-CoV-2, while immunity generated naturally from an infection does offer broader protection (Shrestha et al., 2022). Simply ask yourselves if, despite having the 'complete vaccination schedule' plus one, two, or three boosters, you have been infected with SARS-CoV-2 or suffered from COVID. Can you remember any other vaccine, including childhood vaccines, with which this has happened to you?

1.4 Undeclared components that are present in the vials

Before closing this chapter on the composition of COVID vaxgenes, it is necessary to mention that, after their authorization and the start of the global vaccination campaign, reports and scientific publications have emerged about the presence of undisclosed components in the list of ingredients. Some of these could be due to improper storage of vaxgenes, such as the presence of degraded RNA in synthetic mRNA vaxgenes (Tinari, 2021; Thacker, 2021), or errors and lack of quality control during the manufacturing process, such as the presence of double-stranded RNA

[33] I am referring to the original vaxgenes of Pfizer, Moderna and the vectorized vaxgenes, not to the bivalent vaxgenes that were authorized later in the pandemic. These las tones are bi-antigenic: they create immune responses against the same antigen but from two different SARS-CoV-2 variants, none of which is circulating widely at the time of writing this book.

(Baiersdörfer et al., 2019; Karikó et al., 2011), bacterial plasmid DNA (McKernan et al., 2023), or cellular debris (Krutzke et al., 2022), depending on the type of vaxgene in question

The interest in studying the content of COVID vaxgenes arose after a cyberattack on the EMA that took place in late 2020[34]. As a result of the attack, private documents and correspondence between Pfizer and the European Medicines Agency (EMA) were leaked. The leaked documents were anonymously sent to various agencies and to a medical journal, The British Medical Journal, which took an interest in the matter and conducted investigative journalism on it (Tinari, 2021). Specifically, the leaked documents revealed that some batches of Pfizer's vaxgene had high levels of degraded mRNA as well as truncated RNA sequences. The documents demonstrated that the EMA was aware of this fact, at least since November 2020, and that it was concerned about finding that the percentage of intact RNA varied significantly between batches used in clinical trials and batches administered to the general population (see section 2.2).

Beyond objecting to and demanding an explanation from the pharmaceutical company regarding the discrepancies in the quality of their vaxgenes, there were no major consequences. In the leaked emails, EMA regulators stated that they were not aware of the cause of the discrepancy in RNA quality between batches. This is surprising because, as you will see in the next chapter, the cause of the discrepancy is very clear and was outlined in the interim assessment report of Pfizer's vaxgene, which the EMA itself prepared and published online on December 9, 2020. Specifically, the evaluation report indicates that the batches of vaxgenes used for the clinical trials were manufactured differently from those used for the general population after the vaccines were authorized (the same happened for Moderna, as I will explain in Chapter 2). I suppose the regulator's concern expressed in the leaked emails was not excessive because on December 21, 2020, the EMA authorized Pfizer's vaxgene and ruled that its quality "*was considered sufficiently consistent and*

[34] European Medicines Agency. Cyberattack on the European Medicines Agency [Internet]. Available at: https://www.ema.europa.eu/en/news/cyberattack-european-medicines-agency Accessed October 12 2023.

acceptable"[35]. One reason they may have overlooked the fact that degraded RNA was detected in the vials is that there are no specific guidelines for determining the minimum percentage of intact RNA that mRNA vaxgenes should contain, as openly acknowledged by the UK Medicines and Healthcare products Regulatory Agency (Tinari, 2021).

A few months after the leak of the aforementioned documents, two young men in Japan died suddenly days after receiving Moderna's vaxgene[36]. The investigation by Japanese authorities identified metallic contaminants in the vials, leading to the suspension of the use of three batches of Moderna's vaxgene (equivalent to 1.63 million doses)[37]. In the European Union, contamination with metallic particles in some batches of Moderna's vaxgene was also investigated as a precaution[38]. Shortly afterward, Japanese authorities found contaminants in Pfizer's vaxgene vials, specifically white particulate matter in some vials[39]. However, beyond press releases on the subject, I could not find official reports from the Japanese government about what they found during their investigations.

Given that information access requests in different countries to obtain quality control analyses and ingredient composition determinations for vaxgenes were met with refusals or evasive responses (Fig. 7), it's understandable that some scientists have taken it upon themselves to investigate the composition of COVID vaxgenes. However, the challenge in conducting these investigations is that legally acquiring vaxgene vials has been complex and, in some countries, impossible. This hinders the publication of any results obtained in reputable scientific journals. Therefore, with the exceptions of a few peer-reviewed articles that I'll describe below, reports on undisclosed components in COVID vaxgenes are based on the examination of unsealed vials obtained unofficially,

---

[35] European Medicines Agency. Assessment Report Comirnaty EMA/707383/2020 Corr.1*1 [Internet]. Available at: https://www.ema.europa.eu/en/documents/assessment-report/comirnaty-epar-public-assessment-report_en.pdf

[36] Forbes [Internet]. Available at: https://www.forbes.com/sites/graisondangor/2021/08/28/two-men-in-japan-die-after-COVID-shots-from-supply-suspected-of-contamination/?sh=6ad49ddf75e4

[37] Reuters [Internet]. Available at: https://www.reuters.com/business/healthcare-pharmaceuticals/japan-finds-stainless-steel-particles-suspended-doses-moderna-vaccine-2021-09-01/

[38] Reuters [Internet]. Available at: https://www.reuters.com/business/healthcare-pharmaceuticals/contaminant-moderna-vaccines-suspected-be-metallic-powder-nhk-2021-08-27/

[39] The Japan Times [Internet]. Available at: https://www.japantimes.co.jp/news/2021/09/15/national/contaminants-pfizer-tokyo-osaka/ 3

without maintaining the chain of custody or cold storage. This, on its own, often invalidates the observed results. However, I will mention the findings from the most serious reports because they were prepared by researchers with expertise in the field and using analytical methods. If their results are systematically confirmed and the detected elements are quantified, it will be necessary to consider that they might be playing a direct or indirect role in the pathophysiology of adverse events.

I'll begin by discussing the undisclosed nucleic acids detected in COVID vaxgenes. Official information already indicated that synthetic mRNA vaxgenes contained variable high levels of degraded RNA (Tinari, 2021), along with double-stranded RNA (at a concentration less than or equal to 0.001 mg/g) and DNA (at a concentration less than or equal to 0.33 mg/g) [40]. The presence of DNA in these vaxgenes could be bacterial DNA, a result of an inadequate purification process during vaccine manufacturing.

To investigate the presence, quantity, and origin of DNA in Pfizer's and Moderna's vaxgenes, an independent research team analysed samples from two vials of different batches from each brand. They found variable amounts of double-stranded DNA, and their analyses conclusively showed that it was bacterial plasmid DNA (McKernan et al., 2023), used as part of the commercial mRNA vaxgene manufacturing process (Nance and Meier, 2021).

In case you haven't come across the term 'plasmid' before, it is simply circular double-stranded DNA. Bacteria normally exchange plasmids among themselves — a phenomenon known as 'bacterial sex' because it allows them to exchange genetic information. A plasmid is distinct from a bacterial chromosome, which is circular genetic material that comes from the bacterial lineage (similar to our chromosomes). In contrast, a plasmid is extrachromosomal DNA (i.e., not part of the bacterial chromosome). Their advantage lies in containing genes beneficial to bacteria, such as genes

---

[40] European Medicines Agency. Assessment Report Spikevax EMEA/H/C/005791/0000 [Document]. Available at: https://www.ema.europa.eu/en/documents/assessment-report/spikevax-previously-COVID-vaccine-moderna-epar-public-assessment-report_en.pdf

conferring antibiotic resistance or genes that enable them to colonize new environments.

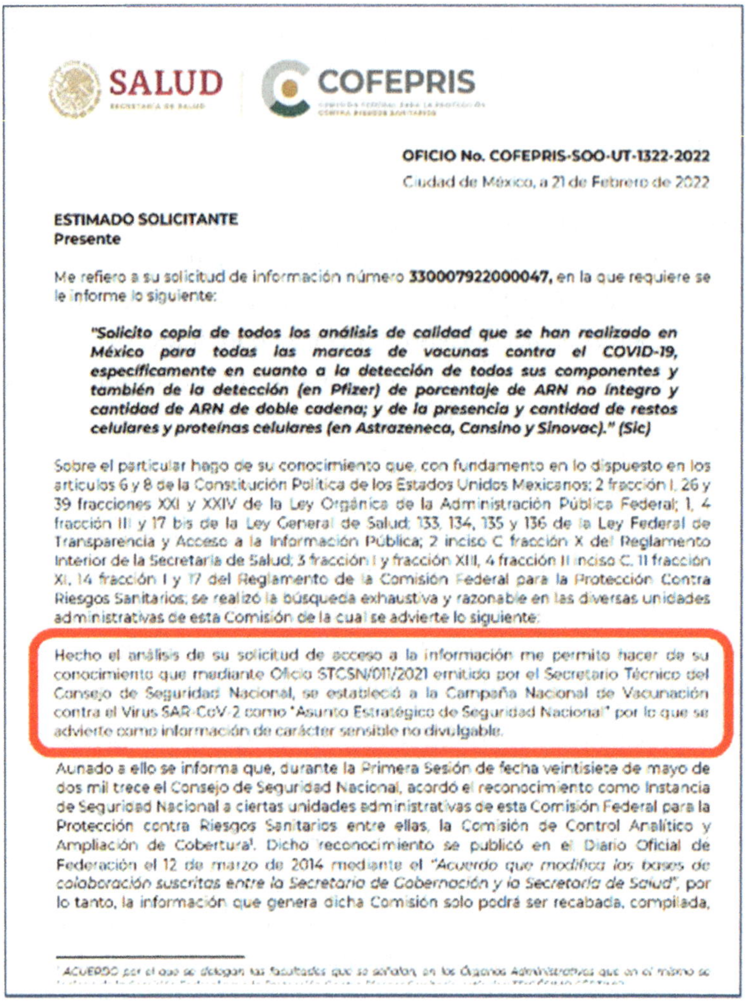

SALUD
SECRETARÍA DE SALUD

COFEPRIS
COMISIÓN FEDERAL PARA LA PROTECCIÓN CONTRA RIESGOS SANITARIOS

OFICIO No. COFEPRIS-SOO-UT-1322-2022
Ciudad de México, a 21 de Febrero de 2022

ESTIMADO SOLICITANTE
Presente

Me refiero a su solicitud de información número **330007922000047,** en la que requiere se le informe lo siguiente:

> ***"Solicito copia de todos los análisis de calidad que se han realizado en México para todas las marcas de vacunas contra el COVID-19, específicamente en cuanto a la detección de todos sus componentes y también de la detección (en Pfizer) de porcentaje de ARN no íntegro y cantidad de ARN de doble cadena; y de la presencia y cantidad de restos celulares y proteínas celulares (en Astrazeneca, Cansino y Sinovac)." (Sic)***

Sobre el particular hago de su conocimiento que, con fundamento en lo dispuesto en los artículos 6 y 8 de la Constitución Política de los Estados Unidos Mexicanos; 2 fracción I, 26 y 39 fracciones XXI y XXIV de la Ley Orgánica de la Administración Pública Federal; 1, 4 fracción III y 17 bis de la Ley General de Salud; 133, 134, 135 y 136 de la Ley Federal de Transparencia y Acceso a la Información Pública; 2 inciso C fracción X del Reglamento Interior de la Secretaría de Salud; 3 fracción I y fracción XIII, 4 fracción II inciso C, 11 fracción XI, 14 fracción I y 17 del Reglamento de la Comisión Federal para la Protección Contra Riesgos Sanitarios; se realizó la búsqueda exhaustiva y razonable en las diversas unidades administrativas de esta Comisión de la cual se advierte lo siguiente:

Hecho el análisis de su solicitud de acceso a la información me permito hacer de su conocimiento que mediante Oficio STCSN/011/2021 emitido por el Secretario Técnico del Consejo de Seguridad Nacional, se estableció a la Campaña Nacional de Vacunación contra el Virus SAR-CoV-2 como "Asunto Estratégico de Seguridad Nacional" por lo que se advierte como información de carácter sensible no divulgable.

Aunado a ello se informa que, durante la Primera Sesión de fecha veintisiete de mayo de dos mil trece el Consejo de Seguridad Nacional, acordó el reconocimiento como Instancia de Seguridad Nacional a ciertas unidades administrativas de esta Comisión Federal para la Protección contra Riesgos Sanitarios entre ellas, la Comisión de Control Analítico y Ampliación de Cobertura[1]. Dicho reconocimiento se publicó en el Diario Oficial de Federación el 12 de marzo de 2014 mediante el *"Acuerdo que modifica las bases de colaboración suscritas entre la Secretaría de Gobernación y la Secretaría de Salud"*, por lo tanto, la información que genera dicha Comisión solo podrá ser recabada, compilada,

[1] ACUERDO por el que se delegan las facultades que se señalan, en los Órganos Administrativos que en el mismo se

Figure 7. *Response (COFEPRIS-SOO-UT-1322-2022) to a freedom of information request (33000792000047) made to the Federal Commission against the Prevention of Sanitary Risks (COFEPRIS) in Mexico regarding information about the quality control analyses of COVID vaxgenes made to determine their ingredients and the amount of degraded RNA, double stranded RNA, cellular debris and cellular proteins. The red box marks the part of their response where they indicate that the information cannot be shared given that it is sensitive non-communicable information that is considered a "Strategic topic for National Security". This response is similar to what colleagues from other countries have been sent from their own health and regulatory agencies.*

Scientists recognized the potential of plasmids, and as they can be synthetically constructed, they have been used for biotechnological applications for decades. This is because when transfected[41] into bacteria, plasmids will be copied every time the bacteria divide, allowing for the rapid and cost-effective generation of billions of copies. In other words, bacteria are utilized as factories for specific genetic sequences.

There are two types of plasmids, cloning and expression plasmids, used according to specific needs. Cloning plasmids are employed to produce numerous copies of a desired gene or sequence, while expression plasmids are used to generate many copies of the product of a gene (i.e., mRNA or protein). Both types of plasmids vary in the genetic elements they contain (Tolmachov, 2009). A cloning plasmid requires an origin site, known as 'ori' that marks the origin of replication (copying) of genetic material and has sites known as 'restriction sites', which are specific sites that endonuclease enzymes identify and cut, allowing the circular DNA to be cut and generate a linear stretch of DNA. An expression plasmid contains everything a cloning plasmid does, along with other genetic regions known as promoters, enhancers, initiation sequence, termination sequence, and a stop codon (the last three bases of a gene). Briefly, promoters are genetic regions with a site for the bacterial polymerase enzyme to initiate transcription (i.e., the process of transcribing a sequence from DNA to RNA) of the gene that follows the promoter. In contrast, enhancers are genetic regions that increase the transcription rate of a gene and do not have to be near that gene.

Through different analytical methods[42], McKernan et al. (2023) detected and quantified the presence of 7.5 to 11.3 ng/μl of double-stranded DNA in the vials. This amount exceeded by several orders of magnitude the maximum limits allowed by the EMA and FDA[43] (Sheng-Fowler et al., 2009). These recommendations on the maximum allowed amount are not arbitrary; they are justified. Residual DNA can induce the synthesis of type

[41] Process that involves introducing foreign genetic material in a cell.
[42] Illumina RNA seq and sequencing with the addition of RNAse, qPCR, RT-qPCR, Fluorometry Qubit™ 3 and Agilent Tape Station™.
[43] The EMA has established the maximum permissible limit to be 330 ng of DNA per mg of RNA in the vaxgene, and the FDA has established the maximum permissible limit to be 10 ng of DNA per injected dose. The volume that is injected per dose for Pfizer's vaxgene is 300 μl, and for Moderna's vaxgene it is 500 μl.

I interferon, a molecule that triggers severe inflammatory responses, and it also poses a risk of integration into the cells' genome (Ulrich-Lewis et al., 2022). Having confirmed, after two different sequencing techniques, the presence of copies of bacterial plasmids in Pfizer's vaxgene (sequence registered in GenBank: OR134577.1)[44] and Moderna's vaxgene (sequence registered in GenBank: OR134578.1)[45] undoubtedly means that they are remnants of the manufacturing process, which has serious implications for the safety of synthetic mRNA vaxgenes, as I will explain in Section 4.6.

It is important to note that McKernan and colleagues (2023) acknowledge not knowing the origin of the vaxgene vials they analysed, given that they were sent to them anonymously by mail (and without refrigeration). In addition, four of the 12 vials were open, and the closed ones had expired. However, rather than underestimating the findings due to this fact, several considerations should be considered: unlike RNA, DNA is very stable to changes in temperature, and the results from different DNA sequencing techniques allowed the detection of any errors that could result from degradation. Moreover, the expiration date of the vials is not relevant to the analytical methods used since the presence of plasmid DNA does not depend on the expiration date. For this reason, although these vials may not have been under ideal conditions for systematic research, the analyses conducted were appropriate, and the results are valid, so it would be incorrect and unjustified to dismiss them. We can be confident that the detected and sequenced plasmids in the study by McKernan et al. (2023) are not a spurious finding but a real result resulting from the manufacturing process. In particular, the results are so important that they should prompt similar studies on vials from different sealed batches that are within the product's shelf life.

Beyond the fact of finding evidence of errors in the purification process of Pfizer's and Moderna's vaxgenes, which should concern regulatory agencies in all countries where emergency use authorizations or outright approvals were granted, it is important to clarify that the plasmid sequences

---

[44] National Center for Biotechnology Information, NCBI GenBank [Internet]. Available at: https://ncbi.nlm.nih.gov/nuccore/OR134577.1

[45] National Center for Biotechnology Information, NCBI GenBank [Internet]. Available at: https://ncbi.nlm.nih.gov/nuccore/OR134578.1

found in Pfizer's vaxgene vials contain a promoter from the simian virus 40 (SV40), including a 72 bp fragment that is, in turn, an enhancer of that promoter. This promoter was not found in the plasmids analysed from Moderna's vaxgene vials (Fig. 8). These plasmids contain two promoters expected in a bacterial expression vector: T7, as the promoter for the Spike gene, and AmpR, as the promoter for a kanamycin resistance gene, both expected when using expression plasmids to transform *Escherichia coli* (Nakano et al., 2017; Wigs et al., 1979), which is precisely what Pfizer and Moderna stated they did in their commercial production processes. I will explain more about this topic in Sections 2.2 and 4.6. In addition to the SV40 promoter, Pfizer's vaxgene plasmid contains a sequence known as the 'poly-A signal of the thymidine kinase of the herpes simplex virus' (HSV TK). Together, the presence of the SV40 promoter and the HSV TK signal indicates that Pfizer vaxgene used an expression plasmid designed to transfect mammalian cells (like ours) and not bacterial cells (Gorman, 1985).

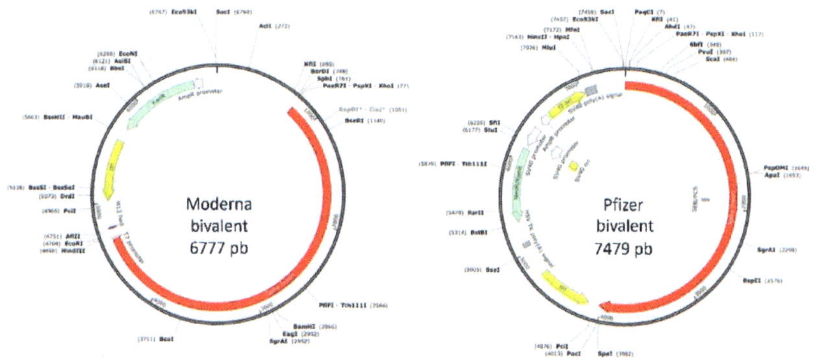

Figure 8. *Genetic map of the plasmids detected in the COVID vaxgenes of Moderna and Pfizer. To the left is Moderna's vaxgene plasmid, with the Spike gene in red, the kanamycin resistance gene in green and two promoters of bacterial transcription (AmpR and T7). To the right is Pfizer's vaxgene plasmid, with the Spike gene in red, the neomycin/kanamycin resistance gene in green and in white the promoter of mammalian transcription of SV40. Image from McKernan and colleagues (2023).*

The FDA recommends that pharmaceutical companies producing products based on gene technology for use in the United States should conduct tests "*to ensure the identity, purity, potency, and safety of the final product*" [46]. For drugs manufactured using a plasmid, the tests include determinations of "*sterility, endotoxins, and purity (including the percentage of supercoiled and residual forms of cellular DNA, RNA, and protein levels)*". This aligns with the position of the EMA in its guidance document on the quality and non-clinical and clinical aspects of gene therapy medicinal products (EMA/CAT/80183/2014)[47], stating that "*Impurities related to the products* [...] *must be identified and their levels quantified. The possibility of foreign DNA sequences co-packaged with the vector must be explored*". In this sense, it is difficult to understand why regulatory agencies did not request any evidence from pharmaceutical companies to demonstrate compliance with these recommendations, especially considering that most countries chose these vaxgenes for their citizens. In the European Union alone, Pfizer's and Moderna's vaxgenes accounted for 90% of all doses administered since the start of the COVID immunization campaign (Fig. 9), corresponding to 809,870,000 doses of these products applied.

In Latin America, the situation is different, as other types of COVID vaccines were more favoured (Fig. 10). For example, of the total doses administered, Pfizer's and Moderna's vaxgenes account for 33% in Argentina, 44% in Uruguay, and 68% in Chile[48], while in Mexico[49], these vaxgenes represent 26% of the doses received until March 9, 2022.

---

[46] FDA Chemistry, Manufacturing, and Control (CMC) Information for Human Gene Therapy Investigational New Drug Applications (INDs) [Internet]. (Page 27) Available at: https://www.fda.gov/media/113760/download

[47] Guideline on the quality, non-clinical and clinical aspects of gene therapy medicinal products. EMA/CAT/80183/2014. Page 16 [Document]. Available at: https://www.ema.europa.eu/en/documents/scientific-guideline/guideline-quality-non-clinical-clinical-aspects-gene-therapy-medicinal-products_en.pdf Downloaded October 13 2023. [48] Official data collated by Our World in Data. Data updated to October 15 2023. [Internet]. Available at:

[48] Official data collated by Our World in Data. Data updated to October 15 2023. [Internet]. Available at: https://ourworldindata.org/covid-vaccinations

[49] Secretaría de Relaciones Exteriores (Foreign affairs Secretariat, Mexico). Transparency. Data updated to March 9 2022. [Internet; Spanish]. Available at: https://portales.sre.gob.mx/transparencia/gestion-diplomatica-vacunas-covid

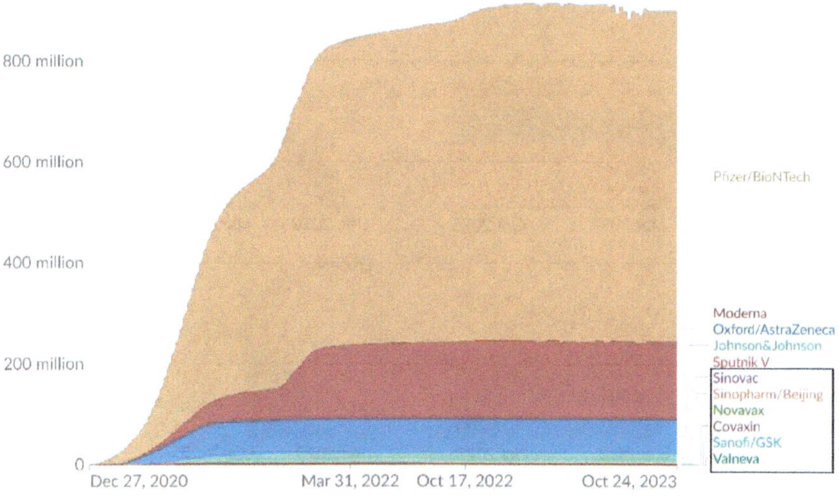

Figure 9. *Doses of COVID vaccines and vaxgenes administered in the European Union. The rectangle shows the inactivated or protein-based vaccines. Data updated to October 12 2023. Source: Our World in Data (ourworldindata.org/covid-vaccinations). Mathieu et al., 2020.*

After the findings by McKernan and colleagues (2023) were disclosed, other research groups have analysed vials, providing evidence, through various methods, that they indeed contain plasmid DNA used to transform bacteria during the manufacturing process of mRNA vaxgenes. In the case of Pfizer, this plasmid indeed contains the SV40 promoter. One of these studies has been submitted to a scientific repository and, at the time of writing this book, is under peer review (Speicher et al., 2023). Specifically, this study analysed 27 vials of synthetic mRNA vaxgenes (19 from Moderna and eight from Pfizer) belonging to 12 different batches. Plasmid DNA was detected in all of them, confirming that Pfizer's vaxgenes contain the SV40 promoter as well as the HSV TK signal (Speicher et al., 2023). Given the medical and legal relevance and implications, it is important to note that replicability is being observed across studies, which is crucial for understanding that a phenomenon truly occurs and is not a spurious finding.

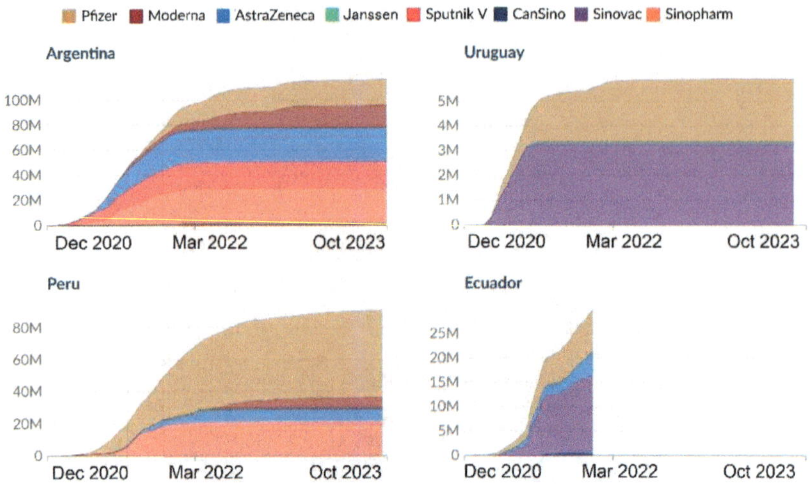

Figure 10. *Doses of COVID vaccines and vaxgenes administered in Argentina, Peru, Uruguay and Ecuador. Data updated to October 15 2023. Source: Our World in Data (ourworldindata.org/covid-vaccinations). Mathieu et al., 2020.*

In an interesting turn, it seems that the Ministry of Health of Canada, in an interview with The Epoch Times, has acknowledged that the pharmaceutical company Pfizer did not indicate that the plasmid they used for process 2 contained the SV40 promoter sequence, and they confirmed the presence of the enhancer based on the plasmid sequence. In other words, if this news is genuine, it means that a government agency has acknowledged that the plasmid containing a eukaryotic promoter is present in the vaxgenes[50].

Now I will mention the contaminating proteins detected in analysed vials of vectorized vaxgenes: A published study demonstrated that AstraZeneca's vaxgene contained high levels of human cellular proteins and free viral proteins (i.e., not part of the adenoviral vectors) (Krutzke et al., 2022). The authors identified protein impurities in four batches of AstraZeneca[51] by using sodium dodecyl sulphate-polyacrylamide gel

[50] The Epoch Times [Internet]. Available at: https://www.theepochtimes.com/world/exclusive-health-canada-confirms-undisclosed-presence-of-dna-sequence-in-pfizer-shot-5513277

[51] Batch numbers ABV4678, ABV5811, ABV7764 and ABV9317.

electrophoresis (SDS-PAGE[52]) and silver staining. They observed a very different banding pattern from the three analysed vials compared to a control (a purified AdV culture), where bands corresponding to adenovirus capsid-associated proteins hexon, penton base, III1, and fibre were clearly visible.

The second step of their analysis was the identification and quantification of proteins in the vials using biochemical methods and mass spectrometry. They found many human cellular proteins (HCP) derived from the used HEK293 cells. Among the most abundant HCP were two heat shock proteins (HSP), various cytoskeleton proteins, epsilon 14-3-3 protein (YWHAE), vimentin, endoplasmin, galectin-binding protein, and nuclear autoantigenic sperm protein (NASP)[53]. The concentrations of these proteins were 25 times higher than the maximum dose allowed by the EMA (≤ 0.4 μg of HCP per dose), and hundreds of times higher than what AstraZeneca had indicated (≤ 0.05 μg of HCP per dose). Of the total proteins detected in each vial, between 44% and 71% corresponded to HCP (Krutzke et al., 2022). The marked variation in detected proteins among the four analysed batches suggests that the purification process of AstraZeneca's vaxgenes was inadequate. I will explain the relevance of finding these cell proteins in AstraZeneca's vaxgene vials later (see section 4.7).

Let's continue with other undisclosed elements found in COVID vaxgenes. A group of researchers from Germany published a technical report[54] on the analysis of more than 10 vials[55] of Pfizer, Moderna, AstraZeneca, and Janssen vaxgenes. In all vials, without exception, there were elements not declared in the pharmaceutical companies' ingredient lists. These elements were visible under dark-field microscopy. Using X-ray dispersion spectroscopy (EDX), mass spectroscopy (MS), and

[52] Protein identification technique. Briefly, proteins are extracted from a sample and run on an acrylamide gel. As proteins are negatively charged, electricity makes them move towards the positive electrode. Proteins have a different molecular weight, so we can see them as "bands" of a specific molecular weight for each different protein.
[53] List of proteins detected by mass spectrometry in three AstraZeneca vaxgene lots. Supplementary material in Krutzke et al., 2022. Available at: https://cdn.elifesciences.org/articles/78513/elife-78513-fig2-data1-v2.xlsx
[54] Summary of preliminary findings. Working group for COVID vaccine analysis. [Document]. Available at: https://drtrozzi.org/wp-content/uploads/2022/09/report-from-working-group-of-vaccine-analysis-in-germany.pdf.
[55] The total number of vials analysed for each method.

inductively coupled plasma analysis (ICP)[56], they detected elements, mostly metallic. Specifically, in samples from Pfizer, Moderna, and AstraZeneca[57] vials, they detected alkali metals (caesium and potassium), alkaline earth metals (calcium and barium), transition metals (cobalt, iron, chromium, and titanium), rare metals (cerium and gadolinium), mining metals (aluminium), as well as silicon and sulphur. In the vial of Moderna's vaxgene, they found the same metallic elements plus antimony. Most of the metallic elements found were at toxic concentrations according to international medical and toxicological guidelines. It's worth mentioning that the report indicates that all analysed vials were already opened, and the samples "*came from unused residues of vials that could no longer be used for inoculation or in which the cold chain had been interrupted*"[58].

Finally, in November 2021, a technical report commissioned specifically to investigate the presence of graphene in COVID vaxgenes was published (Campra Madrid, 2021). Like the report on the presence of metallic elements, Campra Madrid's report (2021) was not peer-reviewed or published in a scientific journal. Using microscopy coupled with Raman spectroscopy to detect graphene signals, the report aimed to verify the structure and identity of objects present in seven vials of COVID vaxgenes (four Pfizer vials, one AstraZeneca vial, one Moderna vial, and one Janssen vial; the last two were unsealed)[59]. The cited report indicated the presence of 110 objects that upon initial inspection had a "*translucent or opaque carbonaceous lamellar typology*", and 28 of the 110 objects had a "*spectral pattern compatible with graphene*". The report itself clarifies that due to limitations of the employed technique, it is not possible to confirm or rule out the presence of graphene structures in many of the 110 objects, proposing the use of other analytical techniques, which, as of writing this book, have not been carried out. Of the 28 objects whose identity could be graphene, eight presented spectral patterns similar to what is expected for graphene oxide."

---

[56] See the glossary at the end of the book.
[57] Batch numbers analysed: Pfizer FE7011, FE8045 and 1F1010A, Moderna 3004217, AstraZeneca 210101 and 1423474.
[58] Page 36 of the report.
[59] Lot numbers analysed: Pfizer EY3014, FD8271, F69428 and FE4721, Moderna 3002183, AstraZeneca ABW0411, Janssen: there was no information provided about the lot number analysed.

A second technical report on the same topic[60], commissioned to an association called "Global Humanitarian Crisis Response and Prevention Unit" in the UK, indicated finding signals compatible with graphene, as well as iron oxide and carbon derivatives in four vials of COVID vaxgenes (two from Moderna, one from Pfizer, and one from AstraZeneca)[61]. The report mentioned that the spectroscopic signals of the analytical technique used (microscopy coupled with Raman spectroscopy) were difficult to separate to unequivocally determine their identity.

Neither of the two reports could determine how much graphene was present in the vials. This data is essential to know in order to compare it with the sub-toxic, toxic, and lethal concentrations already determined for human cells and for animals in general. In other words, as Paracelsus said more than 500 years ago, "*the dose makes the poison*". If graphene oxide is a component of COVID vaxgenes and is present in equal or greater amounts than the toxicity threshold[62], then its presence would undoubtedly be a problem. However, if graphene were present in amounts below the toxicity threshold, its potential impact would be different. Of course, I am not saying that its presence should be underestimated, because even at low concentrations, it could have synergistic and additive effects with other components of the vaxgenes.

If the presence of metallic elements and graphene compounds in COVID vaxgenes were systematically confirmed, it could be explained in two ways:

1) That manufacturing processes did not have the expected quality control. We already know this with the findings of bacterial plasmid DNA and PEG reported in the previously cited studies (McKernan et al., 2023, and Krutzke et al., 2022), so this is a coherent possibility. The explanation for their presence offered by both the authors of the report detecting metallic elements and Dr. Campra Madrid in his report is that they could be remnants

---

[60] Project CUNIT-2-112Y6580. Qualitative Evaluation of Inclusions In Moderna, AstraZeneca and Pfizer COVID vaccines. Available at: http://ukcitizen2021.org/Case_Briefing_Document_and_lab_report_Ref_AUC_101_Report%20.pdf Downloaded October 9 2023.

[61] Batch numbers analysed: Pfizer FC9001, Moderna 3004731 and 3004737, AstraZeneca PW40167.

[62] That is found at higher concentrations than those that are toxic for humans, determined to be more than 20 μg/mL (Wang et al., 2011).

from the manufacturing process. If this were the case, they would be contaminants that were not purified or were inadvertently deposited during manufacturing, packaging, or distribution (Luisetto et al., 2023).

2) That their presence in the vaxgene vials is intentional. In the specific case of graphene, they could be part (not disclosed) of nanomolecules such as ALC-0315, ALC-0159, and SM-102, which, for patent protection reasons, have not been described in detail by pharmaceutical companies. Considering that there are already patents for COVID vaccines (for example, CN112220919A[63] and CN113069541A[64]) that openly indicate containing graphene oxide and that its use as a biotransporter in vaccines has been proposed before the pandemic (for example, Cao et al., 2020; Xu et al., 2016), this scenario is plausible.

How can we aspire to differentiate between both explanations for the possible presence of metallic elements and graphene compounds? Well, if it were the first option, we would expect the quantity present to vary between batches, with some containing little or none, and others containing more material. If it were the second option, we would expect these elements to be present at the same concentration in all batches.

If it were demonstrated that COVID vaxgenes contain graphene and metals at toxic concentrations, we would have to consider their potential role in the pathophysiology of adverse events related to vaxgenes. This is because graphene compounds can interact harmfully with cells and impact organisms. For example, it is known that graphene oxide promotes blood vessel formation (angiogenesis) and cell division (known as mitosis) and can negatively affect reproduction (Rhazouani et al., 2021). In addition, studies conducted in mice suggest that graphene oxide administered at high concentrations can accumulate in the liver, spleen, and lungs and persist for up to six months (Wen et al., 2015). However, as I mentioned before, without information on the quantity that may be present in the vials of COVID vaxgenes and without these studies being systematically conducted

---

[63] Google Patents. "Application CN202011031367.1A events" [Internet]. Available at: https://patents.google.com/patent/CN112220919A/

[64] Google Patents. "Application CN202110381548.5A events" [Internet]. Available at: https://patents.google.com/patent/CN113069541A/

on different sealed vials obtained officially and with certainty of the chain of custody, it would not be ethical to speculate without serious scientific evidence that graphene oxide, other graphene compounds, and metallic elements are responsible for the pathophysiology leading to the observed adverse events.

If there's anything we've seen during the pandemic, it's the ease with which knowledge is manipulated, and half-truths, unsupported interpretations, or outright lies are disseminated. The only way to help more people make informed decisions and understand the situations that arise is to communicate science with truthfulness and the utmost rigor possible. As this book is based on scientific knowledge, not speculations, I will only share what has solid and substantiated evidence. For this reason, even though I am aware that such missing evidence may be published sometime after I finish writing this book, given the current lack of evidence of consistency in the presence of metallic elements and graphene compounds among vaxgene batches and the unknown quantity of graphene present per vial, I will not mention these elements again in the following sections of the book.

Chapter 2. Preclinical and clinical trials of COVID vaxgenes

Life gives you what you settle for.

James Serengia

COVID vaxgenes were developed, tested and issued emergency authorization after only 10 months. This has no precedent in the history of public health and drug regulation. Normally, the entire process, from the initial development to the approval of any new drug or vaccine, takes more than 10 years (Van Norman, 2016). Of course, it could be argued that the accelerated timeframe was justified because a health emergency had been declared. However, if hurried, some stages of development and authorization of a drug or vaccine could be a problem for the safety of those who will use it.

2.1 Brief history of drug regulation

The use of drugs is neither new nor modern and attempts to regulate their use have historical roots. For instance, records indicate that in 120 BC, King Mithridates VI of Pontus (Anatolia), also known as Eupator Dionysius, concocted a compound with 41 herbs called “mitridatium” (Rägo and Santoso, 2008). This remedy was believed to be a cure-all for almost every ailment, without any regulation. It wasn't until 1540 AD that an attempt was made to bring some order to the preparation of mitridatium and other drugs. Under the legal framework of the Apothecaries' Wares, Drugs, and Stuffs[65] Act of England, drug preparation was regulated (Griffin, 2004). However, this act was not the inception of drug regulation. It seems to trace back to the 13th century in Sicily when the Medical Edict of Salerno was proclaimed, obliging apothecaries to prepare their medicines in a standardized manner (Rägo and Santoso, 2008). Since then, throughout history, there have been endeavours to regulate drugs, often with the

[65] This is not a joke. That was the name of the act.

intention of preventing short, medium, and long-term adverse events and health problems in those who use them.

Despite regulations existing, they don't always work effectively. A well-known example is thalidomide (trade names: Thalidomide, Contergan, Imidan, Varian), which was used in almost 50 countries since the 1950s. Originally developed in Germany as a tranquilizer, the drug was approved by the UK Medicines and Healthcare products Regulatory Agency (MHRA) in 1958, although its use shifted to being a treatment for pregnancy-related nausea (Vargesson and Stephens, 2021). Unfortunately, thalidomide turned out to be teratogenic[66], and by 1961, it was estimated to have caused congenital deformities in 10,000 to 20,000 babies, earning it the title of "*the biggest iatrogenic[67] disaster in history*" (Vargesson, 2015) [68]. Another, more recent example is rofecoxib (trade name: Vioxx), approved by the Food and Drug Administration (FDA) for use as a non-steroidal anti-inflammatory drug in 1999, which had to be withdrawn from the market five years later due to an increased risk of strokes and heart attacks. Kudos to the FDA for this action! Unfortunately, it came after rofecoxib had been prescribed to 80 million people[69]. It is estimated to have caused up to 140,000 heart attacks[70], resulting in the deaths of nearly 90,000 people, in the United States alone.

So, regulatory agencies can certainly make mistakes in evaluating the safety of authorized medications. The reasons for these and similar errors are diverse but may, to some extent, reflect the lack of studies on various aspects of drug safety before granting approval. It's not just about considering the results of adverse events observable in volunteers immediately after the drug or vaccine is administered, nor what happens seven days, 30 days, or two months later. Adverse effects can occur over a

---

[66] Something that causes foetal malformations.
[67] Medical error.
[68] It is possible that your thoughts about what has been the biggest iatrogenic disaster in history is different once you finish reading this book.
[69] National Public Radio (NPR). Merck Pulls Arthritis Drug Vioxx from Market [Internet]. Available at: https://web.archive.org/web/20101111103315/http://www.npr.org/templates/story/story.php?storyId=4054991
[70] New Scientist. Up to 140,000 heart attacks linked to Vioxx [Internet]. Available at: https://www.newscientist.com/article/dn6918-up-to-140000-heart-attacks-linked-to-vioxx/

much longer period. For example, rofecoxib caused cardiac or vascular damage after being used for 18 months (Garner et al., 2005). A safety study that only evaluates what happens to those using rofecoxib within two months of taking it could not detect that effect. Unfortunately, given the time required for studies to determine the occurrence of long-term adverse events, they are rarely analysed before a drug is approved.

It could also be the case that a drug, like thalidomide, causes transgenerational adverse effects if administered to pregnant women or if distributed to ovules or sperm (Yohn et al., 2015). If this possibility is not studied during clinical trials, there is no way to know what constitutes a risk, let alone to warn the patient about that risk. The use of model organisms in which such effects can be observed (e.g., Srinivasan et al., 2023; Zhou et al., 2020) allows for the preclinical study of potential long-term adverse effects, but such studies are also rarely conducted for an extended period.

One might argue that the lack of these studies is not as problematic when it comes to drugs used sporadically and in few patients. If serious safety issues arise that were previously unknown, pharmacovigilance systems are designed to withdraw the previously approved drug temporarily or permanently from the market, as happened with the antibiotic alatrofloxacin, which was withdrawn from the market due to liver damage it caused (Qureshi et al., 2011), or amoproxan, which causes serious adverse effects in the eyes and skin (Fung et al., 2001). However, when it comes to a product like a vaccine (or a vaxgene) intended for the majority of the population, starting from six months of age[71], caution and extensive knowledge are required before mass administration.

Back to the history of shaping the legal framework for the regulation of new pharmaceutical products, it began in the United States in 1902 with the publication of the Biologics Control Act (Darrow et al., 2020). Over the decades following its publication, many new regulations were implemented

---

[71] US Food and Drug Administration. FDA News. Coronavirus (COVID) Update: FDA Authorizes Moderna and Pfizer-BioNTech COVID Vaccines for Children Down to 6 Months of Age [Internet]. Available at: https://www.fda.gov/news-events/press-announcements/coronavirus-COVID-update-fda-authorizes-moderna-and-pfizer-biontech-COVID-vaccines-children

by the FDA, all aimed at ensuring greater certainty about the safety of products. However, in the late 1980s, during the AIDS epidemic, a new regulation called *"fast track"* was implemented to expedite the authorization process for new drugs (Darrow et al., 2020). This, along with another amendment to the law in 1992, allowed pharmaceutical companies to pay fees for faster product reviews, significantly reducing the FDA's review times for drug authorization[72]. Since then, the average review time was reduced to 12 months, then 10 months, and for new drugs considered "priority drugs", the time was further reduced to six months[73]. This is not the space to discuss what these changes have meant in economic terms for the pharmaceutical industry and the FDA, but if you are interested in these details, I recommend reading Darrow et al. (2020).

Regardless of these reductions in the review times for a new product, the development times of the product, which must necessarily occur *before* the review, are usually long because they require preclinical studies and clinical trials of phase 1, phase 2, and phase 3[74] before seeking authorization (Piantadosi, 1997).

If you choose, you can read in detail about the differences and details of the clinical phases in any Pharmacology or Epidemiology textbook. Still, since they are essential to understanding what happened during the emergency authorization process of the COVID vaxgenes, I will describe some generalities of each phase that must be completed before authorization.

Preclinical studies: These studies are conducted during the development of a drug or vaccine using laboratory animals to investigate the product's biosafety, pharmacokinetics, and pharmacodynamics. They offer the opportunity to conduct various trials in a short period (Huang W. et al., 2020).

---

[72] Prescription Drug User Fee Act of 1992, Pub L No. 102–571, 106 Stat 4491.
[73] Food and Drug Administration Modernization Act of 1997, Pub L No. 105-115, 111 Stat 2296.
[74] Institute of Medicine (US) Committee on Strategies for Small-Number-Participant Clinical Research Trials; Evans CH Jr., Ildstad ST, editors. Small Clinical Trials: Issues and Challenges. Washington (DC): National Academies Press (US); 2001. 2, Design of Small Clinical Trials. [Internet]. Available at: https://www.ncbi.nlm.nih.gov/books/NBK223329/

Phase 1 clinical trials: These studies involve humans, where a small number of people (typically 20 to 80 healthy volunteers) are recruited to gather information on the pharmacokinetics[75] and pharmacodynamics[76] of a vaccine or drug. This helps establish the appropriate dosage, for example. Sometimes, if a control group is included, the study results provide a preliminary idea of the product's efficacy.

Phase 2 clinical trials: These studies focus on evaluating adverse effects and efficacy in hundreds of volunteers. For drugs, participants typically have the condition that would be treated with that drug. For vaccines, healthy participants, susceptible to the microorganism against which the vaccine is designed, are recruited. These trials can be "blinded" and randomized.

Phase 3 clinical trials: These studies recruit thousands of participants and are often multinational, meaning the trials take place in different geographical locations. These trials aim to compare the efficacy[77] of the drug or vaccine between groups, usually in terms of improving health, increasing survival, or preventing an infection or disease. Participants must be randomly assigned to each group (randomization) and should not know which of the two experimental groups they have been assigned to (blinded study). As part of the evaluation in these trials, the safety of the drug or vaccine is also assessed. Safety is measured as the difference in the incidence of expected and unexpected adverse effects in each group during a period defined by the researchers. Ideally, doctors and researchers should also be unaware of which group each participant has been assigned to, avoiding biases in interpretations.

In some cases, regulatory agencies may request ***phase 4 clinical trials*** after granting emergency authorization or approval for a new product. These are considered part of post-marketing surveillance, allowing additional data to be obtained on the risks and benefits of using the product

---

[75] Study of the absorption, distribution, metabolism and excretion of a drug.
[76] Study of the biochemical and physiological effects of a drug in a living organism.
[77] It means the reduction in the relative risk between the group that receives the drug and the group that receives a placebo (non-active substance).

in the population. They also help determine the long-term effects of using the drug or vaccine.

2.2 Authorization process of COVID vaxgenes

The authorization process for a new vaccine, before the pandemic, took more than a decade because preclinical studies and each phase of clinical trials had to be conducted separately. This means that preclinical studies are done first, and if there are no alarming signals (such as the majority of animals vaccinated with the new vaccine dying), the first phase of the clinical trial proceeds. If everything goes well, and there is no need for adjustments, such as the dosage of the product, then the second phase begins. After completing the second phase, if the results were promising, the third phase is initiated. Each phase requires ethical approval from the institution conducting it and registration in each country's Clinical Trials Registry. Time is needed to announce the trial, recruit participants, filter them according to inclusion and exclusion criteria, explain the study's objective, duration, as well as the risks and benefits of participation (in other words, informed consent). Of course, each trial will take as long as necessary. If, for example, you want to see the protection provided by a vaccine against a particular disease for at least six months, there is no way to accelerate that time; six months are six months, regardless of the cutting-edge technology used for the vaccine! It is understandable, therefore, that it takes more than a decade to gather all the information on pharmacokinetics, pharmacodynamics, efficacy, and, above all, safety before requesting regulatory agencies to review and, if applicable, approve the vaccine.

In the case of the COVID vaxgenes, the process was radically different. Why and how was it different? Well, let's start with the history of their development:

In the context of the health emergency declared by the WHO on January 30, 2020 (37 days before its pandemic declaration[78]), various COVID

[78] World Health Organization. Archived: WHO Timeline - COVID [Internet]. Available at: https://www.who.int/news/item/27-04-2020-who-timeline---COVID

vaccines and vaxgenes began to be developed rapidly. At the time of the health emergency declaration, there were 7,828 cases and 177 deaths worldwide, according to WHO data[79]. However, the "*pandemic-speed*" (Lurie et al., 2020) development of several vaccine candidates began immediately. I'm not exaggerating! The clinical trial for the Moderna vaxgene started on March 16, 2020[80], just *five days* after the pandemic was announced. Moreover, the phases did not start consecutively for each vaxgene; instead, in most cases, they were conducted simultaneously. For example, Pfizer simultaneously conducted phases 1, 2, and 3, both in the United States[81] and Europe[82]. CanSino simultaneously conducted phases 1 and 2[83], as did Janssen[84], and there was also an overlap between phases 1 and 2[85] and phases 2 and 3[86] for AstraZeneca. While researchers working for or with pharmaceutical companies justified these alterations to the process due to the urgency caused by the pandemic and the significant technological advances available (Bok et al., 2021; Lurie et al., 2020; Sreepadmanabh et al., 2020), as I mentioned earlier, there are things that cannot and should not be rushed, regardless of the urgency and the available technology.

On the other hand, time was also "saved" in the development process of the COVID vaccines and vaxgenes as they were largely based on preclinical studies of vaccine candidates against SARS (the beta coronavirus associated with Severe Acute Respiratory Syndrome, SARS, detected in 2002). These vaccine candidates had been developed, but since the SARS

---

[79] Our World In Data. Estimated cumulative excess deaths per 100,000 people during COVID, Oct 17, 2023 [Internet]. Available at: https://ourworldindata.org/explorers/coronavirus-data-explorer.

[80] NIH National Library of Medicine. Clinical Trials [Internet]. Available at: https://clinicaltrials.gov/study/NCT04283461

[81] NIH National Library of Medicine. Clinical Trials [Internet]. Available at: https://clinicaltrials.gov/study/NCT04368728

[82] NIH National Library of Medicine. Clinical Trials [Internet]. Available at: https://media.tghn.org/medialibrary/2020/11/C4591001_Clinical_Protocol_Nov2020_Pfizer_BioNTech.pdf

[83] NIH National Library of Medicine. Clinical Trials [Internet]. Available at: https://clinicaltrials.gov/study/NCT04398147

[84] NIH National Library of Medicine. Clinical Trials [Internet]. Available at: https://clinicaltrials.gov/study/NCT04436276

[85] NIH National Library of Medicine. Clinical Trials [Internet]. Available at: https://clinicaltrials.gov/study/NCT04324606

[86] NIH National Library of Medicine. Clinical Trials [Internet]. Available at: https://clinicaltrials.gov/study/NCT04400838

epidemic was declared over a few months after it started, there was no need to continue developing these SARS vaccines after 2003.

It was precisely these preclinical studies of vaccines against SARS that made it clear that their use increased the risk of Vaccine-Associated Enhanced Disease (V-ADE) if vaccinated animals were infected later. This process is characterized by an increased risk of severe disease if the vaccinated individual is subsequently infected with the virus (the topic will be explained in detail in section 5.7). The phenomenon of V-ADE has been well known since 1969 after clinical trials of the vaccine against respiratory syncytial virus, in which 80% of the vaccinated individuals who became infected required hospitalization (Kim, 1969), and it has also occurred with the dengue vaccine (Halstead, 2016) and the feline coronavirus vaccine (Takano et al., 2019). Since V-ADE after vaccination against the SARS virus was observed in eight independent preclinical studies, regardless of the vaccine platform used, there was uncertainty about whether this could occur with vaccines and vaxgenes designed against SARS-CoV-2 (Lambert et al., 2020).

What is interesting, and frankly concerning, is that despite the Coalition for Epidemic Preparedness Innovations (CEPI) and the Brighton Collaboration's Platform Safety Platform for Emergency Vaccines (SPEAC) having identified the V-ADE syndrome as a potential risk for vaccinees in early 2020, the development of COVID vaccines and vaxgenes continued (Lambert et al., 2020). This recommendation was made despite calls to focus on safety (Zellweger et al., 2020). Even CEPI and SPEAC stated that "*Experts agreed that these models and others under development should be utilized to evaluate vaccine candidates for any evidence of disease enhancement as specified in later sections.*" (Lambert et al., 2020). Specifically, their recommendations were as follows:

- Data is required to understand if decreasing vaccine antibody levels increases the risk of COVID exacerbation when vaccinated individuals are exposed to the virus in the long term.

- Animal studies should provide information on the type of immune response generated by COVID vaccines.

- Post-vaccination challenges in non-human primates, with a careful assessment of damage induced by immune responses, are needed.

- Safety studies of COVID vaccines in hamsters, ferrets, and mice would be important.

- When possible, controlled experiments on immunopathology should be conducted.

- For vaccine platforms inducing immune responses that may exacerbate the disease, the group's consensus was that "*while Phase 1 studies are cautiously proceeding with careful review of safety data, animal studies run in parallel could provide useful information for the further clinical development*" of vaccines.

- The presence of suggestive safety data in animal models should not prevent the clinical development of vaccines, and "*potential risk should be thoroughly evaluated by developers and regulators on a vaccine product-specific basis*".

Ironically, despite identifying the need for preclinical studies, the few "preclinical"[87] studies of COVID vaccines and vaxgenes began *after* the start of clinical trials. At the time of publishing their assessment of the potential risks of COVID vaccines and vaxgenes (based on what was known about vaccines and vaxgenes designed against the first SARS virus), no animal studies had been initiated to assess the wider biological effects or potential harm of these products.

So, summarizing, the development of COVID vaxgenes was markedly different from the development of any new vaccine before the pandemic (Fig. 11). Never in human history had any new vaccine been authorized for mass use in the population the way it was done for COVID.

[87] I place it between quotation marks because, by definition, these trials should be done *before* the clinical trials, and in the case of the COVID vaxgenes, this was not the case.

In the registration pages of phase 3 clinical trials of COVID vaxgenes, you can see which events were studied, and for how long, to assess the safety of the vaccine products. These were the data taken into account for the authorization of COVID vaxgenes by regulatory agencies in each country. It is important to understand this because the public and the medical community might have had the idea that vaxgene safety was extensively evaluated, but that does not correspond to reality. Below are key safety aspects evaluated in the clinical trials of each COVID vaxgene:

Pfizer (Initiation of phases 1/2/3: April 29, 2020; end of phase 3: February 10, 2023)[88]:

- Haematology and blood chemistry values altered up to seven days after receiving the first dose and up to seven days after the second dose.
- Pain at the injection site, redness, and swelling occurring within seven days of receiving a dose.
- Solicited systemic adverse events (fever, fatigue, headache[89], chills, vomiting, diarrhoea, new or worsened muscle pain[90], new or worsened joint pain) occurring within seven days of receiving the first or second dose.
- Non-severe adverse events occurring between the first dose and up to one month after the last dose.
- Severe adverse events occurring between the first dose and up to six months after the last dose[91].

Moderna (Initiation of phase 3: July 27, 2020; end of phase 3: December 29, 2022)[92]:

[88] NIH National Library of Medicine. Clinical Trials [Internet]. Available at: https://classic.clinicaltrials.gov/ct2/show/NCT04368728
[89] Known as cephalalgia.
[90] Known as myalgia.
[91] It must be considered that six months the from first dose had not yet passed when these vaxgenes were authorized.
[92] NIH National Library of Medicine. Clinical Trials [Internet]. Available at: https://classic.clinicaltrials.gov/ct2/show/NCT04470427

- Events requiring medical attention that led to the suspension of participation in the trial up to 759 days after receiving the second dose.
- Solicited local and systemic adverse events up to seven days and up to 35 days after receiving the first dose (seven days after the second dose).
- Unsolicited adverse events occurring within 28 days after each dose.
- Severe adverse events occurring within 759 days (two years after the second dose).

AstraZeneca (Initiation of phase 3: August 28, 2020; end of phase 3: February 10, 2023)[93]:

- Adverse events occurring within 28 days after receiving the second dose (57 days from the first dose).
- Severe adverse events requiring medical attention or considered of special interest occurring between the first day of vaccination and March 5, 2021, or the date of discontinuation, unmasking, or receipt of a non-study COVID vaccine or vaxgene, up to a maximum of 27 weeks.
- Predefined local or systemic adverse events up to seven days after each dose.

Janssen (Initiation of phase 3: August 10, 2020; end of phase 3: May 6, 2023)[94]:

- Solicited local adverse events (specifically erythema and pain) occurring seven days after receiving a booster.
- Solicited systemic adverse events (specifically, fever, fatigue, headache, nausea, muscle pain) occurring up to seven days after receiving a booster.
- Unsolicited adverse events up to 28 days after receiving the dose.

---

[93] NIH National Library of Medicine. Clinical Trials [Internet]. Available at: https://classic.clinicaltrials.gov/ct2/show/NCT04516746

[94] NIH National Library of Medicine. Clinical Trials [Internet]. Available at: https://classic.clinicaltrials.gov/ct2/show/NCT04505722

- Severe adverse events occurring until the end of the trial.
- Adverse events of special interest occurring until the end of the study.
- Severe adverse events up to 35 weeks after receiving a dose.
- Severe adverse events of special interest up to 35 weeks after receiving a dose.
- Adverse events requiring medical attention within six months of receiving the first dose.
- Adverse events requiring medical attention leading to the suspension of participation in the study (within 35 weeks of receiving the first dose).
- Solicited local adverse events within seven days of receiving the vaxgene.
- Solicited systemic adverse events within seven days after vaccination.
- Unsolicited adverse events within 28 days after vaccination.

CanSino (Initiation of phase 3: September 15, 2020; end of phase 3: October 21, 2022)[95]:

- Severe adverse events occurring within 12 months of receiving the vaxgene.
- Solicited adverse events occurring between the day of vaccination and 28 days post-vaccination.

Sputnik (Initiation of phase 3: September 7, 2020; end of phase 3: May 1, 2021)[96]:

- Adverse events occurring during the study (180 days).

- Severe adverse events occurring during the study (180 days).

---

[95] NIH National Library of Medicine. Clinical Trials [Internet]. Available at: https://classic.clinicaltrials.gov/ct2/show/NCT04526990
[96] NIH National Library of Medicine. Clinical Trials [Internet]. Available at: https://classic.clinicaltrials.gov/ct2/show/NCT04530396

It is also important to understand the definition of each type of adverse event considered in the clinical trials. According to the U.S. clinical trials registry system, these definitions are as follows:

- *Severe adverse event*: any medical occurrence that may result in death, is life-threatening, requires hospitalization, or prolongs an existing hospitalization, results in persistent disability or incapacity, or is a congenital anomaly or birth defect.

- *Adverse event of special interest*: adverse events considered of special interest due to their clinical significance, or to their known or suspected effect. They can be serious or not serious.

- *Adverse event requiring medical attention*: adverse events requiring a visit to the doctor, including hospital, emergency room, or any healthcare provider visit for any reason.

- *Solicited local adverse event*: events occurring at the injection site and reported by participants. It includes pain, tenderness, erythema, and swelling that occurs on the day of vaccination and persists for up to seven days.

- *Solicited systemic adverse event*: any event not localized at the injection site that participants are asked to report daily. It includes fever, fatigue, headache, nausea, myalgia (muscle pain).

- *Unsolicited systemic adverse event*: all events not localized at the injection site that may occur and that were not explicitly mentioned to the participant.

These events were recorded, and regulatory agencies relied on them when presenting preliminary results in an interim report two months after the start of phase 2 trials to grant emergency use authorization.

Another fundamental difference between the development process of all pre-COVID vaccines and COVID vaxgenes was that participants who had received placebo injections (i.e., the study controls) were offered the vaccines after the FDA and EMA issued emergency use authorization, which occurred six months after initiation, and well before the completion of the clinical trials (Michels et al., 2023; see Fig. 11). This unprecedented action in the history of vaccinology is concerning, as it does not allow for any further comparative analyses of efficacy or safety between the vaccinated and control groups.

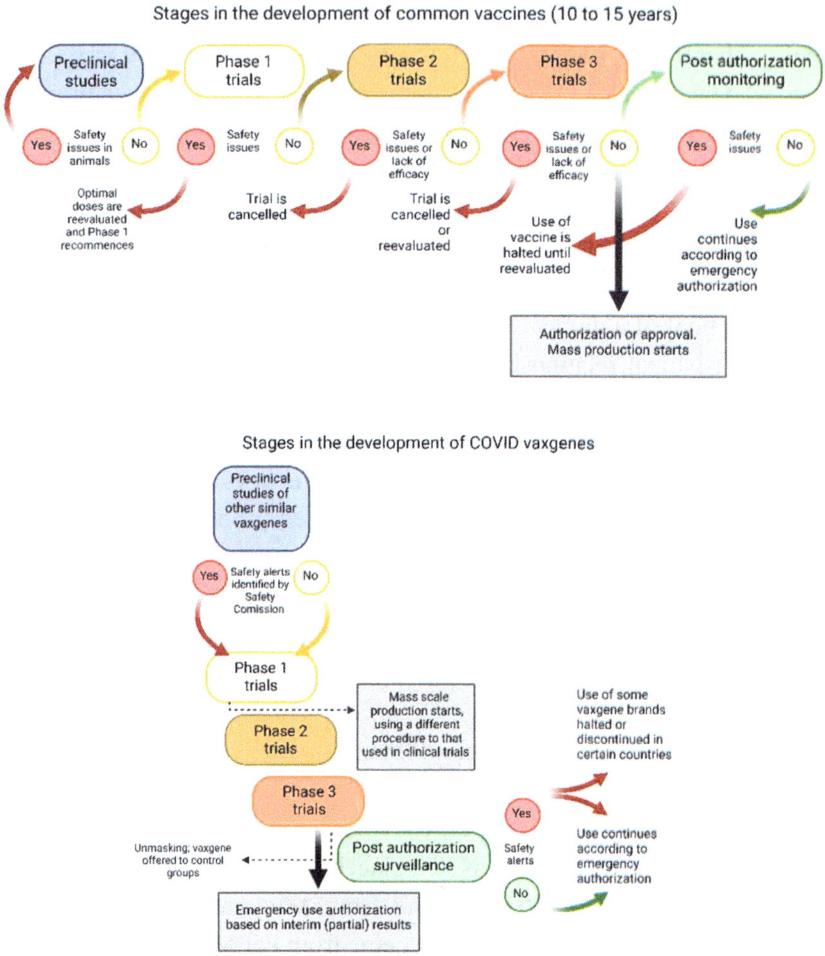

Figure 11. *Comparison of the development of new vaccines prior to the pandemic and development of COVID vaccines. Figure made using BioRender.*

This unprecedented event occurred because, in 2020, the FDA published recommendations on how to proceed if it was found that COVID vaxgenes were effective. Specifically, they indicated that if it was judged that an COVID vaxgene was safe and effective, "*a discussion may be necessary to address the ethical arguments of unblinding the trial and offering the* [genetic] *vaccine to participants who received placebo*" (Wendler et al., 2020). Based on this recommendation, some argued that it was unethical to continue the clinical trials of those COVID vaxgenes that had shown high efficacy and safety during the interim evaluation of their preliminary results. Therefore, it was considered a moral duty to offer the vaxgene to those who had received a placebo in the clinical trials. Some even proposed that it would be unethical for future vaccines and vaxgenes to conduct clinical trials with control groups (Maggioni and Andreotti, 2021; Ortiz-Millán 2021; Stoehr et al., 2021). They argued that vaccinating controls (or conducting clinical trials without participants in the control group) would protect participants from excessive risks. However, this view seems to ignore the goal of a clinical trial, which is entirely different from the goal of a doctor-patient relationship (Hey et al., 2017). It also ignores the fact that maintaining masking in the study groups and blinding in the trial, as well as keeping the control groups unvaccinated during the entire duration of the trial, is essential to conduct independent reviews and minimize safety risks to the population receiving the authorized product (Wendler et al., 2020). Participants in a clinical trial agree to participate in the study and must have been informed of the risks. This is the ethics of a clinical trial, not potentially endangering billions by deciding to unmask the study groups and offer a vaccine or vaxgene to participants in the control group.

Beyond ethical arguments, the problem of unmasking and vaccinating participants who had received placebos is that it becomes impossible to make comparisons between the efficacy and safety of those who received the vaxgene and those who received a placebo. For example, in the Phase 3 clinical trial of the COVID vaxgene from Moderna, participants who received a placebo were offered the vaccine from February 1, 2021[97], a year and 10 months before the trial concluded. This means that there was only a

[97] NIH National Library of Medicine. Clinical Trials [Internet]. Available at: https://www.youtube.com/watch?v=wXJ4yc74PEc

six-month period of safety data. If specific health problems were to arise in volunteers who were vaccinated beyond those six months, it would be impossible to conduct a comparative study to see if that problem is due to chance, other factors, or to the vaxgene itself.

Another point that needs to be known is that the manufacturing of synthetic mRNA COVID vaxgenes was different for clinical trials than for mass production for general population use (Guetzkow, 2023). Yes, just as you read it: the manufacturing process of the vaxgenes used in clinical trials was different from the manufacturing process of the vaxgenes used for the general population. Specifically, what happened was as follows:

For the clinical trials, a process (referred to as Process 1 for Pfizer[98] and Scale A for Moderna[99]) was used to obtain mRNA from an *in vitro* process based on using polymerase chain reaction (PCR)[100] to generate billions of copies of the 4,280 nucleotides that make up the complete genetic sequence encoding the Spike protein. These sequences were then transcribed into mRNA through an *in vitro* reaction using the RNA polymerase enzyme (RNA pol II). The mRNA was purified, filtered, and a "cap" was added to the 5' end through enzymatic processes (see Introduction). It was then purified and filtered again, and voilà! This method allows for the generation of high-quality mRNA without the need for using any organism to produce it. It's excellent as far as biotechnology processes go, but very expensive.

As this process was not (as) profitable for pharmaceutical companies due to its cost (Kis et al., 2021), Pfizer and Moderna used a second manufacturing process (referred to in the interim clinical trial evaluation report as 'Process 2' for Pfizer and 'Scale B' for Moderna) for the mass production of their vaxgenes (Warne et al., 2023). This second process is the same one that is still used, to date, to produce the vaxgenes (including the bivalent vaxgenes). According to the interim evaluation report by the

---

[98] European Medicines Agency. Assessment Report Comirnaty EMA/707383/2020 Corr.1*1 [Internet]. Page 18. Available at: https://www.ema.europa.eu/en/documents/assessment-report/comirnaty-epar-public-assessment-report_en.pdf

[99] European Medicines Agency. Assessment Report Moderna EMA/15689/2021 Corr.1*1 [Internet]. Page 19. Available at: https://www.ema.europa.eu/en/documents/assessment-report/spikevax-previously-COVID-vaccine-moderna-epar-public-assessment-report_en.pdf

[100] The polymerase chain reaction (PCR) is an *in vitro* technique that is based on making millions of copies of a fragment of a known genetic sequence within a sample.

EMA[97,98], for this second process, a plasmid (see section 1.4 for the definition of plasmid) containing the complete sequence of the Spike gene is used, which is transfected (i.e., introduced) into bacterial cells (specifically, *Escherichia coli* cells that are competent to receive foreign genetic material). The *E. coli* bacteria, now containing the plasmid, are grown in bioreactors, and thus, they produce billions of copies of the plasmid and, consequently, copy the Spike gene billions of times. All they need are the right nutrients and conditions for growth. Once the bacterial colonies have grown, they are lysed by chemical or mechanical means, and the billions of copies of the plasmid in the bacterial culture are extracted. These copies are then cut with enzymes to generate linear sequences that are transcribed into RNA with a polymerase enzyme, in the presence of modified uridines ($m^1\Psi$, see Section 1.2). This results in the DNA sequence that was the target of the vaxgene (the Spike gene) now being present as modified synthetic mRNA molecules (Nance and Meier, 2021; Yu and Meier, 2014). Finally, bacterial proteins, bacterial DNA and plasmid DNA are removed through enzyme processes, and the product is purified (Schmeer et al., 2017). In other words, instead of having to buy expensive PCR enzymes when producing billions of copies of the desired sequence, the cost of this part of manufacturing is reduced by using bacteria that copy the desired sequence themselves (Whitley et al., 2022).

'*And?*' - you might think – '*What does it matter if they use a different process to make the vaxgenes used in the clinical trials than to make the vaxgenes given to all people?*' Well, it does matter, and it matters a lot. To start with, the second manufacturing process was not the one used to produce the vaxgenes used in the clinical trials. Therefore, in reality, regulatory agencies granted emergency use authorization for products that were not the ones they evaluated. Pfizer made a modification to the Phase 3 clinical trial protocol (C4591001), indicating that almost all doses used in the trial come from batches produced by Process 1 (Polack et al., 2020). Approximately 250 participants in the clinical trial would receive vaxgenes from two batches produced by Process 2 (after the cut-off date for emergency authorization). Investigators stated that they would do this to conduct comparative safety studies between the two processes. However, at the time of writing of this book, there is no report or published article showing the results of the safety profile comparison of the vaxgenes between the two processes used (Guetzkow, 2023).

Based on documents obtained through Freedom of Information Act requests to the FDA, it was possible to learn about the number of batches generated by Process 2 that had been administered to a group of volunteers in the clinical trial after unblinding[101]. It's important to note that these doses were offered starting in late November 2020 to control group volunteers (those who had received a placebo) when the Phase 3 clinical trial had not yet concluded (see page 60 of this section). The Pfizer vaxgene lots manufactured by Process 2 (lot numbers EE8493Z and EJ0553Z) administered to 250 control group volunteers, as well as to the general public after authorization, have high numbers of associated adverse events (658 adverse events for EE8493Z and 491 for EJ0553Z), including 21 deaths associated with EJ0553Z and two associated with EE8493Z (Guetzkow, 2023). In the six-month update to the provisional report of the Phase 3 clinical trial results for Pfizer (post-authorization evaluation), it is stated that the risk of having any adverse event and at least one serious adverse event for participants who originally received a placebo and later received the vaxgene is higher than for participants who originally received the vaxgene (manufactured through Process 1) [102].

The high number of adverse events associated with vaxgene lots generated by Process 2 may reflect contamination or quality control issues. If DNA is not properly eliminated through purification after extracting the plasmid from the bacterial culture, vials can be contaminated with fragments of bacterial DNA (see section 1.3) or plasmid DNA. If this were to happen, even in small amounts, it would pose a serious risk to the health of those receiving these contaminated products (Sun et al., 2020). I specifically refer to the risk that this contaminating DNA could enter cells and enter the cell nucleus. Since synthetic mRNA vaxgenes contain LNP

[101] Public Health and Medical Professionals for Transparency [Document]. Available at: https://phmpt.org/wp-content/uploads/2022/06/125742_S1_M5_5351_c4591001-fa-interim-patient-batches.pdf and https://phmpt.org/wp-content/uploads/2022/06/125742_S1_M5_5351_c4591001-interim-mth6-patient-batches.pdf

[102] Public Health and Medical Professionals for Transparency [Document]. Available at: https://phmpt.org/wp-content/uploads/2023/04/125742_S1_M5_5351_c4591001-interim-mth6-report-body.pdf

that interact with nucleic acids (i.e., not only with mRNA molecules but also with DNA molecules that may be present in the vial), DNA plasmids would be covered by the LNP and could easily enter the cell through a process called endocytosis. Plasmids and fragments of bacterial DNA would be free in the cytoplasm and could even reach the nucleus, with the risk of causing 'genetic chaos' due to insertional mutagenesis (Langer et al., 2013), a process that will be explained in section 5.6.

I understand that some might roll their eyes and exclaim – '*It's pure speculation!*' – '*We don't even know if they contain those plasmids*'. I understand, but it would mean that those who roll their eyes did not read the previous chapter of this book. We now know that at least some batches of synthetic mRNA vaxgenes contain plasmids. In April 2023, more than two years after the authorization of these vaxgenes, a group of independent researchers found plasmid DNA in various vials of Pfizer and Moderna vaxgenes (McKernan et al., 2023) [103]. Their results were recently confirmed in 27 vials from different batches (Speicher et al., 2023)[102]. This in itself is worrying, but even more worrying is that the plasmid used by Pfizer contains an SV40 promoter, which is normally used in vectors for gene therapy because it contains a nuclear localization signal (Vacik et al., 1999) that helps the plasmid's genetic material enter the cell nucleus and integrate into the genome (see section 1.4).

Before proceeding, I need to make something very clear: when plasmids are constructed with the intention of introducing them into cells to make copies of that genetic material or to express a specific gene found in the plasmid, promoters and enhancers compatible with those cells must be included. There are promoters that only allow the transcription of a gene in bacteria, and there are promoters that only allow the transcription of a gene in eukaryotic cells (i.e., cells with a nucleus, like ours). Even within eukaryotic cells, there are promoters more suitable for use in mammals, in plants, in yeast, etc. The SV40 promoter detected in Pfizer's vaxgene only allows the expression of a gene (in this case, the Spike gene) if the plasmid enters the nucleus of mammalian cells. Period. Inside a bacterium, that promoter along with its 72 base pairs that act as an enhancer can only be

---

[103] This study has not been peer-reviewed at the time of writing this chapter.

copied millions of times in the bacterial culture that contains these sequences; but they cannot be transcribed to mRNA or be expressed as proteins. However, if not properly purified in the vaxgene, they can be transcribed and expressed in human cells. Therefore, there is no biological or technical justification for including a mammalian genetic promoter when the method reported for Process 2 used a plasmid for the bacterial vector to copy the genetic material, according to what Pfizer told regulatory agencies was its Process 2. If they wanted to save on the use of the RNA pol II enzyme and instead have the bacteria generate copies of the Spike gene mRNA, and not copies of the plasmid (in other words, have the bacteria transcribe the Spike gene from the plasmid), then they should have used a plasmid containing a bacterial genetic promoter (Tolmachov, 2009), as Moderna apparently did (see section 1.4), instead of including a mammalian genetic promoter, such as the SV40 promoter (after all, SV40 infects mammals, not bacteria).

It is important to mention that, given the relevance of the findings by McKernan and colleagues (2023), Dr. Phillip Buckhaults, a Molecular Biologist and Cancer Geneticist who is a professor at the University of South Carolina, USA, was called to testify before the South Carolina Senate to explain the relevance of the presence of bacterial plasmid DNA and, above all, the SV40 promoter found in synthetic mRNA vaxgenes[104]. This fact alone demonstrates that the results of the aforementioned study were considered sufficiently valid. The scientific and medical community should be concerned and question the reasons for including an SV40 promoter in the vaxgene. This is because:

1) They are incompatible with the technology that the pharmaceutical company claims to use to manufacture its vaxgenes. The inclusion of an SV40 promoter and enhancer in a synthetic mRNA vaxgene would be scientifically unjustified because these genetic elements are incompatible with bacteria and the mechanism of action of the vaxgenes.

[104] Appearance before the *Ad hoc* Committee on Medical Affairs of the Senate of South Carolina (US) on September 13 2023 [Internet] Available at: https://odysee.com/@akashacomunidad:0/DrPhillipBuckhaultsSenado2023:3

2) Their presence implies a potential risk to the safety of that product. The safety of vaccines and vaxgenes must be evaluated during clinical trials, and regulatory agencies are responsible for authorizing products if they consider that they have met safety parameters. Any unexplained and unauthorized change in the composition or manufacturing method of the vaccine or vaxgene would be of great concern and a violation of national and international health laws, which should have legal consequences.

3) Transparency and informed consent are essential when a new product is administered to the population, especially when made with technology that had not been used before for the purpose of immunization, and when the product has not been licensed but, instead, authorized for emergency use when starting widespread use. Any breach of trust, such as vaccines and vaxgenes containing undisclosed components or being produced by methods different from those authorized, could erode public trust in regulatory agencies, and in health institutions in general.

4) The disclosure that they contain these undeclared elements, which can have serious implications for the health of those who received them (see section 5.6), should lead to a thorough investigation, without conflicts of interest, into how and why these elements were included in synthetic mRNA vaxgenes. Violating health regulation laws should not go unpunished, and legal responsibility must be established for those found responsible.

COVID vaxgenes based on adenoviral vectors also used a different process to produce batches used in clinical trials compared to those applied to the general population. Specifically, AstraZeneca reported using Processes 1, 2, and 3 for clinical trials and Process 4 for commercial production of its vaxgene. The interim evaluation conducted by the EMA on the safety and efficacy of AstraZeneca's vaxgene, published on January 29, 2021, when granting emergency use authorization, states on page 18[105]:

---

[105] European Medicines Agency. Committee for Medicinal Products for Human Use (CHMP) for AstraZeneca. Assessment Report Comirnaty EMA/94907/2021 [Internet]. Available at:

"*Regarding the commercial AS*[106] *manufacturing sites, from the pre-PPQ/PPQ*[107] *data submitted degradation rates are comparable to Process 3. The applicant states that all available lot release, characterisation and stability test results from the AS comparability studies meet the pre-defined comparability assessment criteria and demonstrate that AZD1222 Process 4 AS is comparable to Process 1, 2, 3 AS. This conclusion had not been fully supported during initial assessment since it could not be concluded that AZD1222 Process 4 AS is comparable to Process 1, 2, 3 AS for all three AS sites until further results were evaluated. This was considered a Major Objection*" [108]. The WHO was also aware of this, as on page 4 of its recommendation for emergency use of AstraZeneca's vaxgene, issued in February 2021[109], it states: "*Through the pharmaceutical development of the vaccine, AZ used 4 processes that evolved from Process 1 to Process 4. Processes 1, 2 and 3 were used for manufacture of clinical batches used in studies COV001, COV002, COV003 and COV005 and Process 4 is used for commercial scale production*". The document also indicates that the pharmaceutical company has until February 25 to provide the results of analytical comparability of commercial batches with those used in clinical trials (Page 12)[110]. On the same page, it is stated that the pharmaceutical company should update the product insert to specify that the vaxgene should be discarded within six hours of opening the vial or at the end of the immunization session, whichever comes first, and that vials should be kept between 2° and 8°C during immunization. It appears that the pharmaceutical company did not comply with the WHO's

---

https://www.ema.europa.eu/en/documents/assessment-report/vaxzevria-previously-COVID-vaccine-astrazeneca-epar-public-assessment-report_en.pdf

[106] AS: Active substance.

[107] PPQ: Process performance qualification.

[108] I reckon that the objection was not so serious, given that they extended the emergency use authorization for Europe in January 2021.

[109] World Health Organization. Recommendation for an emergency use listing of AZD1222 submitted by AstraZeneca AB and manufactured by SK Bioscience Co Ltd.
[Internet] Available at:
https://extranet.who.int/prequal/sites/default/files/document_files/AZD1222_TAG_REPORT_EUL%20vaccine_FEB2021_v2.pdf

[110] I was unable to find any evidence that AstraZeneca delivered the results to the WHO.

recommendations, as the insert for AstraZeneca's vaxgene, at least in Canada[111], states the following:

"*After first opening, use the vial within:*

- *6 hours when stored at room temperature (up to 30°C), or*

- *48 hours when stored in a refrigerator (2 to 8°C).*

The vial can be re-refrigerated, but the cumulative storage time at room temperature must not exceed 6 hours, and the total cumulative storage time must not exceed 48 hours. After this time, the vial must be discarded."

In Peru, the insert for AstraZeneca's vaxgene contains almost identical information on page 5[112]: "*From the moment of vial opening (the first needle puncture), use it within 6 hours if kept at a temperature of up to 30°C. After this time, the vial must be discarded. Do not return it to the refrigerator. Alternatively, an open vial can be stored in a refrigerator (2°C–8°C) for a maximum of 48 hours if immediately returned to the refrigerator after each puncture*". Therefore, it is reasonable to assume that in all countries where emergency use authorization was granted for this vaxgene, similar information was included in the product insert.

As far as I know, there is a difference of 22°C between 8°C and 30°C, although in these post-truth times, perhaps some might consider it to be the same temperature. Setting aside the *post-truth reasoning*, it seems that AstraZeneca cared little about the WHO's recommendation. In section 5.7, I will explain why this 22°C storage difference during immunization matters, given the presence of contaminating cell debris in the vaxgene vials (see section 1.4).

---

[111] Product monograph including patient medication information. AstraZeneca COVID vaccine [Internet]. Available at: https://www.azCOVID.com/content/dam/azcovid/pdf/canada/ca-pm-azd1222-en.pdf

[112] Medical Department of AstraZeneca Peru. Vaxzevria Information for the Patient (ChAdOx1-S [recombinant* Injectable solution) [Internet]. Available at: https://www.azCOVID.com/content/dam/azcovid/pdf/peru/pr-epil-Vacuna-AstraZeneca-COVID.pdf

Despite these unprecedented peculiarities in the development, clinical trials, mass production, and authorization of COVID vaxgenes, and despite evidence of quality control issues, most of the scientific and medical community applauded and praised them at the time of their authorization. They did so even with the scarcity of information regarding the safety of vaxgenes prior to their authorization. A review of scientific literature published on the PubMed platform indicates that before January 2020, only 82 articles on mRNA vaxgenes were published, including 24 reviews, and only four articles correspond to phase 1 or 2 clinical trials of vaxgenes. The first of these articles describes the phase 1 clinical trial of a synthetic mRNA vaxgene against lung cancer in oncology patients[113], which would compare adverse effects associated with radiotherapy occurring within 61 days between vaccinated and non-vaccinated patients (Sebastian et al., 2014). The second article published the results of that same clinical trial (Sebastian et al., 2019). The third and fourth articles are phase 1 and 2 clinical trials conducted by the same research group, evaluating the immune response and safety (determined as solicited local and systemic adverse events) of a synthetic mRNA vaxgene against melanoma. Of these, one (Weide et al., 2008) was based on 15 patients and stated that no conclusions could be drawn about safety. The other (Weide et al., 2009) was conducted in 21 patients and did not include any control group, making it impossible to determine if the frequency of adverse events was a cause for concern; also, since seven of the 21 patients in the study had died before 18 weeks of receiving the vaxgene, and an additional five patients died before 36 weeks, it was not possible to draw any conclusions regarding its medium-term safety.

As you can gather from what I explained above, before the COVID pandemic, not a single study had been published presenting the results of a clinical trial with a synthetic mRNA vaxgenes against any infectious disease, and none of the four studies mentioned above used synthetic mRNA with the modifications found in COVID vaxgenes, nor did they use LNP.

---

[113] NIH National Library of Medicine. Clinical Trials [Internet]. Available at: https://clinicaltrials.gov/study/NCT01915524

However, despite this lack of safety evidence for COVID synthetic mRNA vaxgenes, a review article published in the prestigious scientific journal Nature on January 12, 2018, stated the following[114]: "*The use of mRNA has several beneficial features over subunit, killed and live attenuated virus, as well as DNA-based vaccines. First, safety: as mRNA is a non-infectious, non-integrating platform, there is no potential risk of infection or insertional mutagenesis. Additionally, mRNA is degraded by normal cellular processes, and its in vivo half-life can be regulated through the use of various modifications and delivery methods*[9,10,11,12]. *The inherent immunogenicity of the mRNA can be down-modulated to further increase the safety profile*[9,12,13]. *Second, efficacy: various modifications make mRNA more stable and highly translatable*[9,12,13]. *Efficient in vivo delivery can be achieved by formulating mRNA into carrier molecules, allowing rapid uptake and expression in the cytoplasm (reviewed in Refs*[10,11]*). mRNA is the minimal genetic vector; therefore, anti-vector immunity is avoided, and mRNA vaccines can be administered repeatedly. Third, production: mRNA vaccines have the potential for rapid, inexpensive and scalable manufacturing, mainly owing to the high yields of in vitro transcription reactions.*" (Pardi et al., 2018b, page 261).

This article was one of the most cited by other studies discussing the safety of COVID vaxgenes based on synthetic mRNA. The issue is that we can see the authors don't cite any references for their assertion that there is "*no risk of insertional mutagenesis*", and they also don't cite any reference to support their claim that synthetic mRNA vaxgenes can be administered repeatedly. Additionally, the citations they used to support the claim that the lower immunogenicity of synthetic mRNA can further increase its safety profile did not establish that fact conclusively. The first of the cited articles (Reference 9 in Pardi et al., 2018b) was a study reporting that modifying the nucleosides in the sequence of synthetic mRNA, specifically incorporating pseudo uridine instead of uridine (see section 1.1), allows for greater translation capacity (i.e., production of the target protein). They reported that this modification resulted in a lower quantity of two pro-inflammatory molecules than synthetic mRNA without modification. This

[114] Textual quotation of Pardi et al., 2018b, including the references that he mentions in the paper. Available at: https://www.nature.com/articles/nrd.2017.243

was determined by performing an *in vitro* experiment on four mouse fibroblast cultures and an *in vivo* experiment on five mice (Karikó et al., 2008). The second cited article also observed that the injected animals produced a higher amount of the target protein when the synthetic mRNA had this modification. They measured the quantity of three pro-inflammatory molecules in four mice, three pigs, and four cynomolgus monkeys (*Macaca fascicularis*) six hours after injection (Thess et al., 2015).

Regarding vaxgenes using adenoviral vectors, before 2020, fewer than 20 articles had been published reporting the results of phase 2 and 2 clinical trials of recombinant AdV-vectored vaxgenes against six infectious agents (HIV, respiratory syncytial virus, influenza virus, hepatitis B virus, *Mycobacterium tuberculosis*, and *Plasmodium falciparum*). Of these, only one clinical trial assessed safety over an extended period of 2 years.

I don't know about you, but I find it perplexing that before authorizing COVID vaxgenes based on adenoviral vectors, there wasn't widespread discussion about the fact that since 2010, based on the results of two clinical trials of a human adenoviral vector (Ad5) vaxgene against HIV, it was known that these products were not effective in preventing infection. On the contrary, they increased the risk of HIV infections in vaccinated, uncircumcised men compared to the placebo group (Gray et al., 2010; Gray et al., 2011; Duerr et al., 2012; Richie and Villasante, 2013). This fact led to the publication of an article at the end of 2020, urging caution in using vaxgenes based on human adenovirus[115] for the COVID immunization strategy (Buchbinder et al., 2020).

Looking at the number of doses of vaxgenes based on adenoviral vectors that have been administered worldwide[116], we must conclude that little attention was given to that call for caution. Unfortunately, nearly three years after starting to administer these vaxgenes to millions of people, there is

[115] Specifically, they were referring to the vaxgenes made with human adenovirus 5, such as Janssen, CanSino and Sputnik.

[116] According to the WHO, up to October 9 2023: 67.16 million doses of AstraZeneca, 18.70 million doses of Janssen and 1.85 doses of Sputnik (data on CanSino are not available). Source: https://ourworldindata.org/covid-vaccinations

beginning to be some evidence that the warning was not mere alarmism (see section 5.6).

It is also perplexing to realize that it was known, at least since 2016, that the hexon protein of the AdV capsid could induce thrombocytopenia[117] (Raddi et al., 2016). This happens because the hexon protein interacts with platelets, promoting the release of platelet factor 4, also called platelet-activating factor 4 (PF4), which attracts more platelets and neutrophils (Greinacher et al., 2021). This interaction triggers a cascade of events that can culminate, in susceptible individuals, in the formation of blood clots that can impact various organs and tissues. In section 5.4, I will explain in more detail this aspect of the pathophysiology of adenoviral vectors. However, despite this known risk, there was no mention of it in the document produced by CEPI and SPEAC regarding safety concerns with COVID AdV-vectorized vaxgenes (Lambert et al., 2020). It's challenging to comprehend the reason for this omission, particularly because cases of thrombotic thrombocytopenia in people who received AstraZeneca's COVID vaxgenes began to occur within weeks of starting mass vaccinations. This led to the suspension of their use or their restriction to certain age groups[118] in several European countries (Wise, 2021).

Below, I list the studies conducted before the emergency authorization of COVID vaxgenes, which would have been essential to determine their safety, especially before administering them massively to the population.

2.3 Biodistribution studies

As part of the interim reports that Pfizer[119] and Moderna[120] submitted to regulatory agencies to request emergency authorization for their vaxgenes,

---

[117] A reduction in the number of platelets in the blood.

[118] The New York Times. European Countries Suspend Use of AstraZeneca Shots Over Worries About Blood Clots [Internet]. Available at: https://www.nytimes.com/2021/03/11/business/astrazeneca-vaccine-denmark-blood-clots.html

[119] European Medicines Agency. Assessment Report Comirnaty EMA/707383/2020 Corr.1*1 [Document]. Available at: https://www.ema.europa.eu/en/documents/assessment-report/comirnaty-epar-public-assessment-report_en.pdf

[120] European Medicines Agency. Assessment Report Spikevax EMEA/H/C/005791/0000 [Document]. Available at: https://www.ema.europa.eu/en/documents/assessment-report/spikevax-previously-COVID-vaccine-moderna-epar-public-assessment-report_en.pdf

data on the biodistribution (see section 5.2) of lipid nanoparticles (LNP) coupled with synthetic mRNA in mice and rats were included. In the case of COVID vaxgenes based on adenoviral vectors (AstraZeneca and Janssen), data on the biodistribution (also known as pharmacokinetics) of recombinant AdV virions in vaccinated mice were also presented.

For none of the COVID vaxgenes were any studies conducted (or at least not published as scientific articles or technical reports) on biodistribution in humans or any other primates before their authorization. At the writing of this book, not a single biodistribution study of any COVID vaxgenes in humans or any primate species had been published yet.

Studies on the possibility of excretion of the components of vaxgenes, as well as their end product (Spike protein), in faeces, urine, semen, saliva, or breast milk were also not conducted (see section 5.9).

2.4 Pharmacodynamics studies

Pharmacodynamics is the study of the response that various organs and tissues have to a drug. The organs chosen for study are based on pharmacokinetic studies of the active compounds of a drug being studied before its authorization or approval. In the case of COVID vaxgenes, no pharmacodynamics studies were conducted, or they were not published, before their authorization, and as of the writing of this book, they have not been conducted yet.

2.5 Studies on drug interactions

No studies were conducted, or they were not published, on possible drug interactions between the components of COVID vaxgenes and common drugs before their authorization, and as of the writing of this book, no such studies have been conducted.

2.6 Studies on the risk of vaccine-driven disease enhancement (V-ADE)

Preclinical studies conducted with animal models to investigate the risk of vaccine-associated enhanced disease (V-ADE) associated with vaccines against the first SARS virus found evidence of immunopathology[121] in vaccinated animals subsequently exposed to the virus (see studies in Lambert et al., 2020). However, before their emergency authorization, no studies were conducted to assess the medium- and long-term risk of V-ADE for COVID vaxgenes. Of the few studies conducted to investigate this risk in laboratory animals, the risk was only examined for COVID inactivated vaccines (reviewed by Gartlan et al., 2022), and only two studies assessed the occurrence of V-ADE in animals injected with synthetic mRNA vaxgenes but they did not examine the risk beyond seven weeks post-vaccination. Additionally, in no case were the animals exposed to SARS-CoV-2 variants different from the variant on which the vaxgenes were based (DiPiazza et al., 2021; Vogel et al., 2021).

2.7 Studies on genotoxicity

Not a single study of genotoxicity was performed prior to the authorization of the COVID vaxgenes, and at the time or writing this book none has been conducted.

2.8 Studies on carcinogenicity

Not a single study of carcinogenicity[122] was performed prior to the authorization of the COVID vaxgenes, and at the time or writing this book none has been conducted.

---

[121] Damage caused by exaggerated immune responses.

[122] A carcinogen is a physical, chemical or biological agent that can cause cancer in a healthy organism.

2.9 Studies on teratogenicity

Not a single study of teratogenicity[123] was performed prior to the authorization of the COVID vaxgenes, and at the time or writing this book none has been conducted.

2.10 Studies on transgenerational effects

Not a single study of transgenerational effects[124] was performed prior to the authorization of the COVID vaxgenes, and at the time or writing this book none has been conducted.

2.11 Studies on the safety of using different vaxgene types

No study was performed prior to starting the use of different vaxgene types on the same individual, and at the time or writing this book not all vaxgene combinations have been conducted.

2.12 Studies on the safety of receiving boosters

No study was performed prior to the authorization of COVID vaxgene boosters.

2.13 Studies on vaxgene safety in children

No study had been completed prior to the authorization of COVID vaxgenes for this age group.

---

[123] Ability of a physical, chemical or biological agent of causing foetal malformations or anomalies.
[124] A physical, chemical or biological agent that could cause adverse effects in the offspring of the person that was exposed to that agent.

2.14 Studies on vaxgene safety during pregnancy and breastfeeding

No study regarding safety of vaxgenes for pregnant women, for their foetus and for babies that are breast-feeding had been completed prior to their authorization in pregnant and lactating women.

Based on what has been presented here, it is reasonable to ask the following question: "*If those studies were not conducted, exactly what did pharmaceutical companies, regulatory agencies, and health authorities rely on to assure the public that COVID vaxgenes were safe for everyone?*"

2.15 Adverse effects registered in phase 3 clinical trials

In early December 2020, most of the world's population celebrated that regulatory agencies in their countries had authorized or were about to authorize COVID vaccines and vaxgenes. The review of the partial results of clinical trials (interim evaluation) was interpreted as a sign that these were safe products. For example, in their reviews of serious adverse events (see section 2.2 to recall the definition of a serious adverse event) contained in the reports of Pfizer's[125] and Moderna's[126] vaxgenes, the FDA concluded that those recorded within the first two months of Phase 3 did not vary significantly between those who received the vaxgene and those who received the placebo (the control group), indicating that they did not find safety signals that concerned them.

However, this might not necessarily reflect the reality. If the data on adverse events from Pfizer's and Moderna's vaxgenes are reanalysed according to the prioritized list of potential relevant adverse events prepared by the Brighton Collaboration[127] and endorsed by the WHO, the safety

---

[125] Food and Drug Administration. Emergency Use Authorization for Pfizer-BioNTech COVID-19 Vaccine Review Memo [Internet]. Available at: https://www.fda.gov/media/144416/download

[126] Food and Drug Administration. Moderna COVID-19 Vaccine EUA FDA review memorandum [Internet]. Available at: https://www.fda.gov/media/144673/download

[127] The interdisciplinary group of specialists in vaccine safety that I mentioned in section 2.2 of this book.

scenario of these vaxgenes does not appear to be so encouraging. This analysis is precisely what Fraiman and colleagues did (2022).

Before explaining what Fraiman and colleagues found, it should be clarified that the first list of adverse events of special interest proposed on September 9, 2020, by the Brighton Collaboration[128], based on knowledge about vaccines against SARS and the pathogenesis of the SARS-CoV-2 Spike protein, included the following events:

- Anaphylaxis
- Multisystem inflammatory syndrome in children
- Acute respiratory distress syndrome
- Cardiovascular damage (myocarditis, pericarditis, arrhythmias, heart failure, infarctions)
- Thrombocytopenia
- Coagulation disorders (coagulopathies, thrombosis, thromboembolism, internal and external bleeding, strokes)
- Acute kidney damage
- Acute liver damage
- Guillain-Barré syndrome
- Acute disseminated encephalomyelitis
- Aseptic meningitis
- Meningoencephalitis
- Generalized seizures
- Facial nerve paralysis

[128] Law B. SO2-D2.1.3 Priority List of COVID Adverse events of special interest [Document]. Available at: https://brightoncollaboration.us/wp-content/uploads/2023/06/SPEAC_SO1_2.2_2.3-SO2-D2.0_Addendum_AESI-Priority-Tiers-Aug2020-v1.2.pdf Last updated document Available at: https://brightoncollaboration.us/wp-content/uploads/2023/08/Updated-COVID-AESI-list_Oct2022-1.pdf

- Deafness
- Anosmia and ageusia
- Optic neuritis
- Loss of visual acuity and blindness (including uveitis and retinitis)
- Perniosis-like skin lesions (Chilblain)
- Cutaneous vasculitis
- Erythema multiforme
- Alopecia

These adverse events were supposed to be thoroughly investigated and reported during clinical trials. Unfortunately, despite the Brighton Collaboration being considered a global authority on vaccine safety, the list was not considered by regulatory agencies to assess the safety of vaxgenes.

What Fraiman and colleagues (2023) found, upon reanalysing the data presented in the preliminary reports of Pfizer's and Moderna's vaxgenes (adverse events recorded in participants of Phase 3 clinical trials between the trial start date and November 16 and 25, 2020, for Pfizer and Moderna, respectively, which was when the interim assessment by regulatory agencies was conducted)[129], is that synthetic mRNA vaxgenes were associated with an excess risk of special adverse events of 10.1 and 15.1 per 10,000 vaccinated individuals, compared to the baseline observed in those who received a placebo. Concerning serious adverse events, Pfizer's vaxgenes showed a higher risk, with a 36% increase in the vaccinated group (18 serious adverse events per 10,000 vaccinated) compared to the control group, while Moderna's vaxgene exhibited a 6% increase in the risk of serious adverse events (Fraiman et al., 2023).

[129] It was not possible to include data that exceeded that time frame as participants that had been in the control group were unmasked and many of them were vaccinated. This means that it is no longer possible to compare between groups.

By using the list of serious adverse events of special interest described above, Fraiman and colleagues (2023) found 52 events in Pfizer's vaxgene clinical trial (meaning a rate of 27.7 per 10,000 vaccinated) in the group that received the vaxgene and 33 (meaning a rate of 17.6 per 10,000 volunteers who received the placebo) in the control group. This represents a 57% increase in the risk of serious adverse events of special interest associated with Pfizer's vaxgene. For Moderna's vaxgene, the increase in the risk of serious adverse events of special interest was 36% (57.3 per 10,000 vaccinated compared to 42.2 per 10,000 in the control group) (Fraiman et al., 2023). Within the category of adverse events of special interest of Brighton, the highest risk for both vaxgenes was 'coagulation disorders'.

Why were there marked differences between the FDA's analysis and interpretation (and that of other regulatory agencies worldwide) and Fraiman and colleagues' analysis? According to the authors of that study, it can be explained by the following reasons:

1) The FDA analysed the total number of participants who experienced a serious adverse event, while Fraiman and colleagues (2023) analysed the total number of serious adverse events (each event was counted, rather than counting only each person who experienced an event). The difference in their approach is significant: the FDA's approach does not accurately reflect the excess of multiple adverse events — almost twice as many people in the vaccine group had multiple adverse events compared to those in the control group.

2) The follow-up times and the technique for analysing non-fatal serious adverse events were different. The FDA reported that 0.6% (126 out of 21,621) of vaccinated participants had at least one serious adverse event compared to 0.5% (111 out of 21,631) of participants who received a placebo, leading them to say that there were no differences between the groups[130]. In contrast, Fraiman and colleagues' analysis (2023), which used the same FDA data, found

[130] Food and Drug Administration. Emergency Use Authorization for Pfizer-BioNTech COVID Vaccine Review Memo [Internet]. December 2020. Available at: https://www.fda.gov/media/144416/download

127 serious adverse events among 18,801 vaccinated volunteers and 93 serious adverse events among 18,785 volunteers who received a placebo. The discrepancy in the number of volunteers is because the FDA included 5,666 participants who received at least one dose, regardless of how long the follow-up lasted[131], while Fraiman and colleagues' study (2023) considered data from follow-ups of more than two months after the second dose. Therefore, the FDA's analysis included more than five thousand participants who had very little follow-up time, and most of whom had only received one dose.

I find it important to mention that on August 23, 2021, just nine months after Pfizer's COVID vaxgene was granted emergency authorization, the FDA granted it a license (approval) [132]. This led a group of doctors and scientists to request, under the legal framework of the Freedom of Information Act (FOIA), access to information about the data on which the approval of this vaxgene was based[133]. In response, the FDA asked a federal judge to grant them a 75-year grace period before providing the requested information. In other words, they requested that the information used for approval of the vaxgene wait be released until the year 2096. Therefore, a lawsuit was filed against the FDA in September 2021, demanding the release of the information before March 2022. The lawsuit proceeded[134], and in response, the FDA asked the court to allow the release of 50 pages per month (which would take exactly 75 years since the total information they reviewed for licensing consisted of almost half a million pages)[135]. Their request was denied, and on January 6, 2022, a federal court in Texas

[131] Food and Drug Administration. Pfizer-BioNTech COVID vaccine EUA review memorandum [Internet]. December 2020. Available at: https://www.fda.gov/media/144416/download

[132] US Food and Drug Administration. News release: FDA Approves First COVID Vaccine [Internet]. Available at: https://www.fda.gov/news-events/press-announcements/fda-approves-first-COVID-vaccine

[133] Public Health and Medical Professionals for Transparency. Document 091621 [Internet]. Available at: https://phmpt.org/pfizer-court-documents/

[134] Bloomberg Law "Why a Judge Ordered FDA to Release COVID Vaccine Data Pronto" [Internet] Available at: https://news.bloomberglaw.com/health-law-and-business/why-a-judge-ordered-fda-to-release-COVID-vaccine-data-pronto

[135] Freedom of Information Act. Case 4:21-cv-01058-P Document 22 Filed 12/06/21 [Document]- Available at: https://www.sirillp.com/wp-content/uploads/2021/12/FDA-Brief-and-Appendix-e3999de9aee38921cd4fbb035c33e304.pdf

ordered the accelerated release of documents, meaning they would have to release 55,000 pages per month[136], which they started in 2022.

A review of the released data showed inconsistencies between what was published as partial results of the phase 3 clinical trial of Pfizer's COVID vaxgene (Polack et al., 2022) and the original data (Michels et al., 2023). This could explain why, since the beginning of their administration, many more adverse events have been reported for COVID vaxgenes than for any other pharmacological product in history.

In the next chapter, the events recorded in adverse event monitoring systems that could be associated with COVID vaxgenes will be presented.

---

[136] Public Health and Medical Professionals for Transparency. Document ORDER_2022_01_06.pdf [Internet]. Available at: https://phmpt.org/pfizer-court-documents/

Chapter 3. Adverse event reporting in monitoring systems

Which was crazier, she wondered, seeing patterns when they weren't there, or ignoring patterns when they obviously were?

Lis Wiehl

The adverse event monitoring systems were created with the purpose of collecting data on the occurrence of specific events that occurred after receiving a vaccine or a drug, so that trends can be observed during the post-authorization period when they are already used in the general population. Their purpose is precisely to monitor and thus be able to detect when something out of the ordinary happens. In the past, adverse events detected during the post-authorization period in monitoring systems have led to the withdrawal of several vaccines from the market. Perhaps the most well-known case is the rotavirus vaccine, which had been administered to nearly a million children before it was recognized to be associated with an increased risk of intestinal intussusception[137], occurring in about 1 in every 10,000 vaccinated children (CDC, 2004). Other vaccines withdrawn from the market due to signals detected in monitoring systems include two influenza vaccines (Nasalflu and Pandemrix), the first associated with facial nerve paralysis (13 per 10,000 vaccinated) and the second with narcolepsy (13 per 100,000 vaccinated) (Hampton et al., 2021).

There are different epidemiological and pharmacological surveillance systems; some are national and others international. International systems rely on what each country reports. In that sense, they are indicators of 'good faith' about what is happening. If a country does not report or register what really occurs, those events will not be taken into account.

Some surveillance systems are passive, relying on people (depending on the surveillance system, they may be doctors, authorities, or the general public) to report events. This means that there are limitations in interpreting

[137] Occurs when part of the intestine slips within itself. It is a medical emergency that can be fatal if not detected and treated opportunely.

the data because there will almost always be underreporting (Sharma et al., 2021). It may also happen that reported events are not associated with what the person reporting believes, which could lead to overestimation; however, this is not frequent (Sandberg et al., 2022; Sharma et al., 2021).

By their very definition, data from monitoring systems do not constitute data that can be used for comparative epidemiological analysis or to demonstrate causality, as there is no denominator. In other words, there is no way to know, with the data from monitoring systems, how many adverse events occurred per 100,000 vaccinated individuals.

Internationally, the most recognized adverse event monitoring systems are:

- *Vigiaccess*[138]. Pharmacovigilance system for the early detection of adverse events possibly associated with drugs or vaccines. Created by the WHO in 1968.

- *Eudravigilance*[139]. Pharmacovigilance system for the early detection of adverse events possibly associated with drugs or vaccines. Created by the European Union in 2001.

By country, adverse event monitoring systems include:

- *VAERS*[140]. Pharmacovigilance system for the early detection of adverse events possibly associated with vaccines. Created in the United States by the Centres for Disease Control and Prevention (CDC) and the Food and Drug Administration (FDA) in 1990. It is a system that detects occasional vaccine harms to determine if the risk-benefit ratio is sufficiently high to justify continuing the use of a particular product and to identify preventable health problems in the population.

---

[138] World Health Organization. Vigiaccess [Internet]. Available at: https://www.vigiaccess.org/

[139] Eudravigilance. European Database of Suspected Adverse Drug Reaction Reports [Internet]. Available at: https://www.adrreports.eu/en/index.html

[140] US Department of Health and Human Services. Vaccine Adverse Event Reporting System [Internet]. Available at: https://vaers.hhs.gov/ and https://openvaers.com/

- FAERS[141]: Pharmacovigilance system for the early detection of adverse events possibly associated with drugs or vaccines in the United States. Created by the FDA in 1968. It is a system that detects occasional harms caused by drugs or vaccines to determine if the risk-benefit ratio is sufficiently high to justify continuing the use of a particular product and to identify preventable health problems.

- Yellowcard[142]: Pharmacovigilance system for the early detection of adverse events possibly associated with drugs or vaccines. Created by the UK Ministry of Health in 1964.

- Health Infobase[143]: Pharmacovigilance system for the early detection of adverse events possibly associated with drugs or vaccines in Canada.

- DAEN[144]: Adverse event reporting system for drugs and vaccines in Australia.

- PMDA[145]: Adverse reaction reporting system for drugs of the Pharmaceuticals and Medical Devices Agency of Japan. It is not accessible without being registered as a doctor in the system.

- SINAVE[146]: National Epidemiological Surveillance System of Mexico. Records are not accessible, and only monthly reports of adverse events associated with specific products are presented to the public.

---

[141] US Food and Drug Administration. FDA Adverse Event Reporting System (FAERS) Public Dashboard [Internet]. Available at: https://www.fda.gov/drugs/questions-and-answers-fdas-adverse-event-reporting-system-faers/fda-adverse-event-reporting-system-faers-public-dashboard

[142] Medicines and Healthcare Products Regulatory Agency. Coronavirus vaccine - summary of Yellow Card reporting [Internet]. Available at: https://www.gov.uk/government/publications/coronavirus-COVID-vaccine-adverse-reactions/coronavirus-vaccine-summary-of-yellow-card-reporting

[143] Reported side effects following COVID vaccination in Canada [Internet]. Available at: https://health-infobase.canada.ca/COVID/vaccine-safety/

[144] Therapeutics Goods Administration. Database of Adverse Event Notifications (DAEN) - medicines [Internet]. Available at: https://daen.tga.gov.au/medicines-search/

[145] Pharmaceuticals and Medical Devices Agency [Internet]. Available at: https://www.pmda.go.jp/english/safety/info-services/safety-information/0001.html

[146] Secretaría de Salud. Dirección General de Epidemiología (General Office of Epidemiology; Health Secretariat) [Internet; Spanish]. Available at: https://www.sinave.gob.mx

- SVI[147]: Integrated Surveillance System of the Chilean Public Health Institute. Not accessible to the general public, and only general monthly reports or reports on specific products are presented to the public.

- Medsafe[148]: Integrated Surveillance System of the Government of New Zealand. Not accessible, and only general bimonthly reports or reports on specific products are presented to the public.

Taking into account passive adverse event monitoring systems with accessible records, such as those in the United States (VAERS), the European Union (Eudravigilance), Canada (Health Infobase), Australia (DAEN), and the WHO (Vigiaccess), we can see an unprecedented number of adverse events possibly associated with COVID vaccination in the history of vaccinology. For example, as of September 22, 2023, VAERS had accumulated 22 times more reports of adverse events associated with COVID vaccines and vaxgenes in 33 months (1,595,001) than reported for all other vaccines in 592 months (931,993). This means that reports of adverse events associated with COVID vaccines and vaxgenes in the United States represent 63.12% of all accumulated adverse event reports since January 1, 1990 (2,526,994), occurring at a rate of 48,333 reports per month. In contrast, for all other vaccines combined, adverse event reports occur at a rate of 1,574 per month[149]. This implies that in the United States, there are 31 times more reports per month associated with COVID vaccines and vaxgenes than with all other paediatric and adult vaccines combined.

In Eudravigilance, as of October 9, 2023, 1,241,962 reports of adverse events possibly associated with Pfizer's vaxgene, 550,875 reports associated with AstraZeneca's vaxgene, 383,064 reports associated with Moderna's vaxgene, and 71,407 reports associated with Janssen's vaxgene have been accumulated[150]. This totals 2,247,308 reports associated with the

---

[147] Sistema de Vigilancia Integrada para la Comunicación de Eventos Adversos (System for the Integrated Monitoring of Adverse Event Communications) [Internet; Spanish]. Available at: https://svi.ispch.gob.cl/isp/index

[148] New Zealand Medicines and Medical Devices Safety Authority [Internet]. Available at: https://www.medsafe.govt.nz/COVID/vaccine-report-overview.asp

[149] US Department of Health and Human Services. Vaccine Adverse Event Reporting System [Internet]. Data updated to September 22 2023. Available at: https://openvaers.com/

[150] Eudravigilance. European Database of Suspected Adverse Drug Reaction Reports [Internet]. Data updated to October 9 2023. Available at: https://www.adrreports.eu/en/index.html

main COVID vaxgenes administered in the European Union, and according to their own reports, 45% of them have been serious[151].

On a more global scale, in Vigiaccess[152], the contrast between reports of adverse events associated with COVID vaccines and vaxgenes and reports associated with other vaccines is even more pronounced. The 5,192,490 reports associated with COVID vaccines and vaxgenes to date represent 80.74% of all adverse event reports associated with any vaccine between 1968 and 2023. Assuming a constant reporting rate, reports of adverse events associated with COVID vaccines and vaxgenes are accumulating at a rate of 157,348 per month, while reports associated with other vaccines have historically accumulated at a rate of 1,870 per month. In other words, there are 84 times more reports of adverse events associated with COVID vaccines and vaxgenes per month than with other vaccines.

Although it is not possible to use these reports as evidence of causality between the COVID vaxgenes and health disorders, adverse event monitoring systems are intended to detect patterns and trends that could be signals of safety problems with applied products. These can be investigated using the Bradford Hill criteria for causality (Hill 2015) to determine if they are indeed causal associations, as explained in Chapter 4.

You may consider the 5,192,490 reports of adverse events associated with COVID vaccines in the Vigiaccess global monitoring system as excessive. However, the situation is likely worse because, as mentioned earlier, monitoring systems suffer from underreporting issues (Sandberg et al., 2022; Sharma et al., 2021). A report by Harvard University researchers delivered to the US Department of Health and Human Services (DHHS) in 2011 found that less than 1% of adverse events are reported to the VAERS system[153]. While this underreporting factor is not universal, it likely varies

---

[151] The 1,645 ESAVI associated with the Novavax vaccine, 388 ESAVI associated with the Vidpretyn Beta vaccine, and 35 ESAVI associated with the Valneva vaccine reported until October 9, 2023 are excluded from the sum, since they are not vaxgenes.

[152] World Health Organization. Vigiaccess [Internet]. Data updated to October 10 2023. Available at: https://www.vigiaccess.org/

[153] Ross L. et al., 2011. Electronic Support for Public Health–Vaccine Adverse Event Reporting System (ESP:VAERS) [Document]. Available at: https://digital.ahrq.gov/sites/default/files/docs/publication/r18hs017045-lazarus-final-report-2011.pdf

depending on the type of adverse event, being more common for non-severe events than for severe ones.

To calculate the underreporting factor for adverse events, one must consider the *expected* number of adverse events, obtained by multiplying the total number of doses administered by the number of adverse events recorded in clinical trials. This number is then divided by the *observed* number of adverse events. According to the FDA's evaluation of preliminary results from the phase 3 clinical trial of Pfizer's vaxgene[154], 0.7% of those vaccinated experienced serious adverse events. Therefore, the underreporting factor for serious adverse events associated with this vaxgene in the United States was calculated as 31, using the number of reports and doses administered until August 2021 (Rose 2021). This implies that for every serious adverse event reported in VAERS associated with Pfizer's COVID vaxgenes, 31 unreported serious adverse events would be expected.

If we extrapolate this underreporting factor to the number of serious adverse events (only those resulting in deaths or hospitalizations) associated with COVID vaxgenes used in the United States and registered in the VAERS monitoring system from the start of vaccination until September 22, 2023[155], we would be talking about 6,550,564 serious adverse events possibly associated with COVID vaxgenes in the United States. This number was calculated as follows:

$$\{(36\ deaths\ + 210{,}138\ hospitalizations) \times 31\}$$

It would not be correct to use the same underreporting factor to calculate the expected number of adverse events globally, but you will understand

[154] Vaccines and Related Biological Products Advisory Committee Meeting December 10, 2020 [Internet] https://www.fda.gov/media/144245/download
[155] US Department of Health and Human Services. Vaccine Adverse Event Reporting System [Internet]. Data updated to September 22 2023 and not corrected with the underreporting factor. Available at: https://openvaers.com/covid-data

that it is undoubtedly more than the 5,192,490 reported by October 8, 2023, in Vigiaccess[156].

The adverse events listed in Vigiaccess as possibly caused by COVID vaccines and vaxgenes include the following:

- Pain and complications at the injection site (26%)
- Disorders of the nervous system (16%)
- Musculoskeletal and connective tissue disorders (10%)
- Gastrointestinal disorders (7%)
- Infections (5%)
- Respiratory and mediastinal disorders (4%)
- Cardiac disorders (3%)
- Vascular disorders (2%)
- Blood and lymphatic system disorders (2%)
- Reproductive and mammary system disorders (2%)
- Psychiatric disorders (2%)
- Auditory disorders (1%)
- Ocular disorders (1%)
- Immune system disorders (1%)
- Metabolic disorders (1%)
- Hepatobiliary disorders (<1%)
- Malignant, benign, and unspecified neoplasms (<1%)
- Renal and urinary disorders (<1%)

You might think that 1% is low, but when we're talking about over 5 million adverse events (without applying the correction factor for underreporting), even 1% becomes a number that cannot be ignored, as it would be more than 50,000 cases. Does it seem insignificant that there have been at least 100,000 cases of psychiatric disorders and 150,000 cases of cardiac issues associated with COVID vaccines? Moreover, these events have predominantly occurred in people aged 18 to 44, which is noteworthy because, generally, vaccines administered to the general population (from

[156] World Health Organization. Vigiaccess [Internet]. Data updated to October 8 2023. Available at: https://www.vigiaccess.org/

infants to the elderly), such as the influenza vaccine, do not show the highest number of adverse events in this age group (Fig. 12).

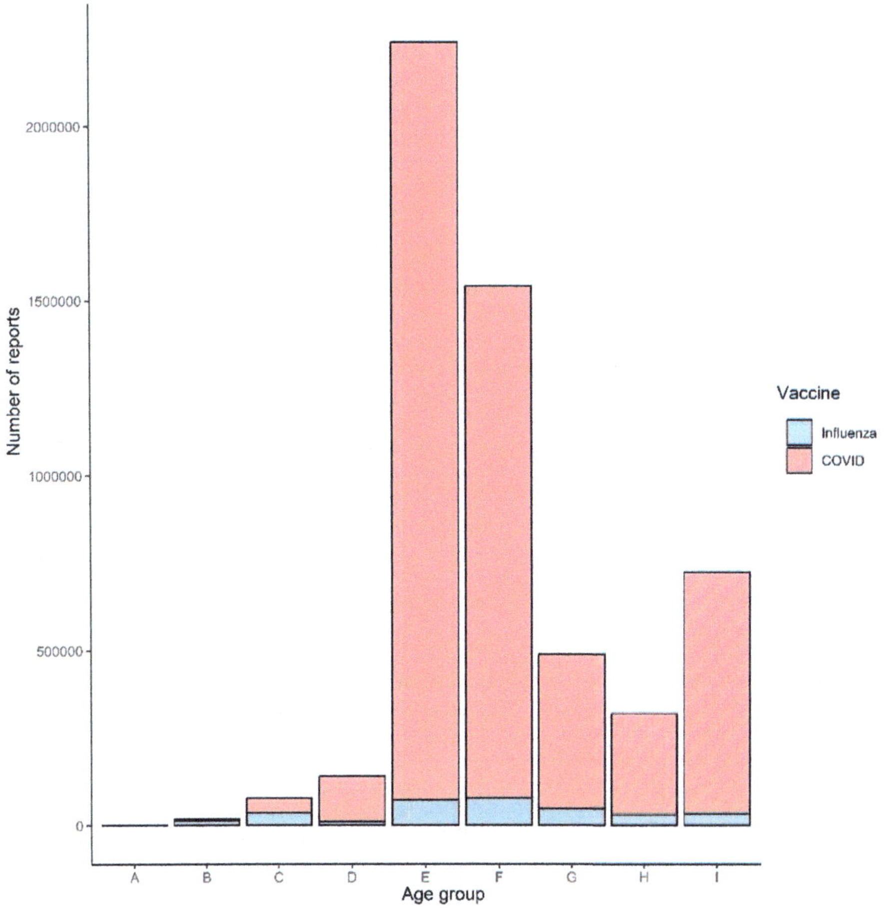

Figure 12. *Number of adverse event reports related to COVID vaccines and vaxgenes and related to flu vaccines according to age groups. Number of all reports for COVID products: 5,233,659 accumulated between December 2020 and November 2023; number of all reports for flu vaccines: 317,407 accumulated between December 1997 and October 2023. Age groups: A) 0-27 days, B) 1-23 months, C) 2-11 years, D) 12-17 years, E) 18-44 years, F) 45-64 years, G) 65-74 years, H) > 74 years, I) Age unknown. Source: Vigiaccess. Data updated to November 12 2023.*

Before continuing, it seems important to address a question frequently asked by people when they hear about adverse events: "*If they are so unsafe, why didn't anything happen to me (or my family or friends) after receiving the vaccine?*" It's a valid question and has two rational explanations:

1) We are biological organisms, not mathematical equations. This means that we vary in many aspects that influence our susceptibility (and therefore our risk).
2) Not all batches are associated with the same risk. This was known as early as October 2021, less than 12 months after the global vaccination campaign began (Bruce Yu et al., 2021).

More recently, from a statistical analysis of adverse event reports in Denmark, adverse events are not evenly distributed among vaxgene batches; there is a bias towards certain batches (Schmeling et al., 2023). Between December 27, 2020, and November 11, 2022, 701 million doses of Pfizer's vaxgene were administered in the European Union, associated with 971,021 suspected adverse event reports. Out of 7,835,280 doses from 52 lots administered to 3,748,215 people in Denmark, 43,496 adverse events were recorded in 13,635 people. This results in a rate of 3.19 ± 0.03 events per affected person. Adverse events were associated with doses from 1,531 (± 0.004) lots, and the rates of adverse events per 1,000 doses varied significantly between batches.

The results of the study by Schmeling and colleagues (2023) should not be underestimated, and certainly not ignored, as they imply that, at best, the heterogeneity in lots associated with adverse events could be due to variations in manufacturing and vial quality. If this were the case, it would pose a problem primarily for regulatory agencies, which should have ensured that the products their citizens were receiving had the same quality. At worst, the results could reflect intentional bias between lots, warranting an international judicial investigation. The authors noted that there should be uniformity in the manufacturing and quality of lots of COVID vaxgenes, but studies in this regard have not been conducted (Schmeling et al., 2023).

As mentioned before, we are not mathematical equations. Individual variability in various physiological and health characteristics undoubtedly influences susceptibility to adverse events. However, lot-to-lot variability also plays a significant role. Not all doses of each brand of COVID vaxgenes contain the same components, nor are they present at the same concentration.

Chapter 4. Causal inference

Everything happens for a reason! Mostly often because of the activities that precede it.

Peter Francis

Since ancient times, humanity has sought to explain events by attributing causality. The causalities attributed are not always accurate, and history is full of examples of false causality that has led to misguided decisions, especially in medicine. For instance, in Japan, there was a belief that a demon, a Hōsōshin, was the cause of the disease known as smallpox. This disease had been introduced to Japan in the year 734 (Suzuki, 2011), and given the beliefs of that time, it was easier to comprehend that people developed fever, vesicular lesions, and that a third of the affected individuals died in vengeance of a demon, rather than considering it could be due to a virus[157]. Therefore, under the belief and culture of that time, since the Hōsōshin of smallpox was afraid of red things, it is logical to understand that people displayed red dolls and wore red clothing. Others tried to appease the Hōsōshin through offerings of poems, dances, flowers, and incense. This belief persisted over time and space; from the 12th century in Europe, the idea of using or wearing red to ward off smallpox was imported and became known as the "red treatment". It was even common in royalty: King Charles V of France, who reigned in the mid-14th century, wore a red shirt, leggings, and mantle as protection against smallpox, and Queen Elizabeth I of England was wrapped in a red cloak when she fell ill with smallpox in the mid-16th century (Thèves et al., 2016). In West Africa, Sopona, the Yoruba god of smallpox, was represented dressed in red[158], and sacrifices with blood became common to appease the gods who sent smallpox as punishment, as occurred in China, parts of Africa, India, and Mesoamerica (Hartwig, 1984). All derived from the belief in causality between a god (or demon) and smallpox.

[157] By the way, 1,150 years had to pass to begin to understand that there were microorganisms smaller tan bacteria that could be associated with some diseases, and 50 years more to be able to see them with an electron microscope.

[158] CDC [Internet].; Accessed October 12, 2023. Available at: https://www.cdc.gov/museum/history/shapona.htm

Certainly, beliefs or the paradigm of the moment influence our understanding of events and how we can prevent or resolve them. Sometimes humanity 'hits the mark' with its assignment of causality, but other times it does not. Determining that an event is related to exposure to a specific factor or event (in other words, establishing a cause-and-effect relationship) is more complex than simply showing that the event occurred after exposure to the factor. To determine causality, causal inference is used (Rothman and Greenland, 2005).

To understand what causal inference is, it is first necessary to define what causality is. It is a concept that involves a lot of self-learning; even from an early age, we incorporate it into our perception of the world. For example, as children, if we spill a glass of milk and that earns us anger or punishment from our mother, we quickly establish causality between the action of spilling the milk and receiving punishment. It is understood, then, that our concept of causality, initially, is based on our own direct observations of effects that become apparent immediately. However, this first impression of causality is often not the complete story or is mistaken. Rothman and Greenland (2005) explain this well with a concrete example: the light switch. It is immediately apparent that if we flip the switch, the light turns on. However, the causal mechanism for the light to turn on goes far beyond flipping the switch. If, for some reason, there is no electricity in our house or the bulb is burnt out, then flipping the switch will not turn on the light. There are many factors that come into play between the switch and the incandescent light. Only if all the factors are present, the light turns on when the switch is activated. If one of them fails, the effect will not be seen.

It must be clear that, for epidemiology, causality is an interpretation based on the observation of two variables: an event and an exposure that vary together (covary) in time and space (Lucas and McMichael, 2005). This is because few diseases or conditions can be attributed to unequivocal causality, particularly for conditions with many risk factors. If we think about COVID, many will say 'the cause is infection with SARS-CoV-2', but if it were unequivocal causality, then everyone who became infected with SARS-CoV-2 would develop the disease known as COVID, and we know that is not the case. From the early weeks of the pandemic, it became clear that there were *risk factors* (such as age, inflammatory comorbidities, immunomodulation status, etc.). There were also people who could have some of the multiple and varied symptoms and signs of COVID without testing positive for SARS-CoV-2 in diagnostic tests. So, you can see that causality is a continuum, ranging from highly improbable to highly probable, and determining causality from a single study is not correct.

At this moment, we are facing a deluge of cases of deaths and health alterations in individuals vaccinated against COVID, many of whom had no medical history to explain their occurrence. That fact, it seems to me, cannot be debated or *verified* as false. Data is data, and these are official data. Reports of cases of cancer, cardiovascular and reproductive issues, autoimmune and autoinflammatory problems, as well as neurological and neuropsychological disorders in individuals who received COVID vaxgenes are accumulating (see Chapter 6). By saying 'more cases', I mean more cases than those observed annually in the five years before the start of vaccination. Of course, some people who consider COVID vaxgenes to be safe might argue that this increase has *nothing* to do with them and is due to there being more people now than before. Also, some argue that many people did not want to go to the doctor during 2020 due to fear of SARS-CoV-2, so there was an underestimation of cases that later 'added up' to 2021 and 2022, or that the increase is due to other factors such as climate change or stress. I'm not kidding; in reality, both have been used as explanations for the heart attacks and sudden deaths that are occurring at an unusually high rate in news reports and other media. Of course, it is a possibility that stress, or high summer (or low winter) temperatures play a role, but the hypothesis would need to be properly challenged before attributing causality, as is done now, without the minimum evidence required by causal inference.

To avoid falling into the same mistake that the media often makes, it is essential to learn to distinguish between causality and coincidence. There can be an apparent relationship between an event and a factor in a spurious, chance manner, or even if a relationship is statistically significant[159], it may

[159] This means that the statistical analysis identifies a relationship that, at least numerically, is not due to chance.

not have a shred of reality. Spurious correlations occur when two factors seem to be related but are not really. It can also be due to confounding factors, such as an unconsidered third variable that affects both study variables, and a small sample size. Therefore, studies with an appropriate experimental design that controls for all possible variables and sources of error are required (Gianicolo et al., 2020).

Tobías and colleagues (2019) demonstrated it elegantly in their article titled "*The FIFA World Cup and climate change: correlation is not causation*". At first glance, the title may seem like a joke, but it is not. In it, they show how a significant positive relationship can be demonstrated between the temperature anomaly and the number of penalties of countries in the World Cups, as well as an inverse, almost mirror-like relationship between the number of penalties and the minimum ice coverage in the Arctic (Tobías et al., 2019). Perhaps heat makes professional football players be prone to cheat?

I do not doubt for a moment that for those who promote a specific narrative, such correlations are like gold, but in reality, they are promoting fool's gold[160] and not real gold. In other words, the simplicity of a correlation does not allow us to see the complexity of a possible association (Tobías et al., 2019). Taking a correlation as evidence of causality without considering that it may be due to chance leads to erroneous interpretations. This is because a correlation simply describes the strength of a linear relationship between two variables. Can you imagine the number of variables that may seem to be related even if they are not really? For example, the number of pets per family and the number of dietary supplements consumed per family[161]. If we could obtain this data for one or more countries (or cities, it doesn't matter) and graph it, we would probably find a very good correlation. However, unless we consider that pets exert a physiological (or telepathic) pressure that compels us to buy dietary supplements, or that taking dietary supplements activates the expression of genes that make us more inclined to adopt pets, there is not much reason to think that there is a real association (i.e., not just a statistical association)

---

[160] Sulphuric mineral with the chemical formula FeS_2. It appears to be gold, but it is not.
[161] I mean vitamins and minerals.

between the two variables. In this hypothetical case, it is more plausible to interpret the observed relationship in the following way: both variables (i.e., the number of pets per family and the number of supplements bought per family) vary in the same way due to another related factor, which possibly would be the purchasing power of families.

One of the most common mistakes when trying to interpret correlations as if they were causations is ecological fallacies, i.e., what happens when conclusions about individual effects are drawn using grouped data (Piantadosi et al., 1988). For example, between countries, chocolate consumption *per capita* is positively correlated with the number of Nobel Prizes *per capita* (Prinz, 2020)[162]. This correlation may reflect causality. Perhaps eating chocolate, by stimulating serotonin production (Silva, 2010), creates a more relaxed and happier psychoneurological environment from which it is possible to be more creative and hardworking, increasing the chances of winning a Nobel Prize. However, we cannot assert that the correlation means that. This is because, with data grouped by countries, we cannot know if those who won the Nobel Prize are the ones who ate the most chocolate. And we would need to know this if we want to claim that the correlation implies causality. So, it's not that correlations observed from grouped data are not useful; in fact, they can be crucial for identifying problems and generating hypotheses (Pearce, 1999), but they are not unequivocal evidence of causality. Perhaps they are, but we won't know until we formulate hypotheses that can be challenged and conduct the corresponding studies.

Talking about the safety, or lack thereof, of COVID vaxgenes, in section 6.3, I will present how mortality due to dementia has behaved in Australia over time and, comparatively, during 2021 and 2020. This increase *could* be associated with vaxgenes. If we were to graph the number of vaccinated individuals in Australia in relation to the number of dementia-related deaths during 2021, it is highly likely that we would find a significant positive correlation in which, the more people vaccinated against COVID, the more cases of dementia-related deaths.

---

[162] Yes, someone took the time to study that topic.

If we stop there and take that result as unequivocal evidence that COVID vaxgenes cause death by dementia, we would be as irresponsible as the media when they say that the sudden deaths of young athletes are due to climate change. The relationship between cases of death by dementia and COVID vaccination coverage is a clear example of a correlation in grouped data. Do we know if those with dementia were vaccinated? In Australia, where vaccination was practically mandatory, it is highly likely, but with this data, we simply cannot know.

On the other hand, even if the cases of dementia deaths occurred only in vaccinated individuals, we still could not consider them *unequivocal* evidence of causality. To determine if it is possible and correct to deduce causality between an event (for example, deaths by dementia) and an exposure to something (for example, the COVID vaxgene), the observed relationship between the event and the cause must be evaluated against several criteria known as the Bradford Hill criteria (Hall, 2023; Fedak, 2015; Hill, 1965), which are:

1) Strength
2) Consistency
3) Specificity
4) Temporality
5) Biological gradient
6) Plausibility
7) Coherence
8) Experimentation
9) Analogy

Strength refers to the magnitude of the association. In Epidemiology, this is determined with measures like the odds ratio (OR) or relative risk (RR). The further away from 1, the stronger the association. Let's use an example of a clinical condition associated with COVID vaxgene in adverse event monitoring systems: the reactivation of herpesvirus (see section 6.6). One of the most significant findings is that individuals who received at least one COVID vaxgene have a higher risk of herpesvirus reactivation if they had a previous infection (Hertel et al., 2022), implying impairment in their immune system. The study was conducted with over a million people in two cohorts: the vaccinated and the non-vaccinated, and the incidence of herpesvirus reactivation was compared between the cohorts for 60 days after vaccination. They found that indeed, there were more cases of herpesvirus reactivation in the vaccinated cohort than in the non-vaccinated cohort, and the RR was 1.8 (with a 95% confidence interval of 1.680-1.932). In other words, the vaccinated have almost twice the risk of herpesvirus reactivation than those who were not vaccinated. If it were 1.2 instead of 1.8, the strength would be lower. If it were 10.8, the strength would be much greater. That is strength, and it holds for the relationship between COVID vaxgenes and herpesvirus reactivation.

Consistency refers to different studies finding similar results. Using the same example, there are, at the time of writing this chapter, 50 scientific articles published by different research groups and from different countries that found that individuals who received at least one dose of COVID vaxgene experienced herpesvirus reactivation. That is consistency, and it holds for the relationship between COVID vaxgenes and herpesvirus reactivation.

Specificity refers to the likelihood that the factor (in this case, the COVID vaxgene) is causal of the effect (in this example, herpesvirus reactivation) if it is only associated with that effect and not others. Before the more contentious readers exclaim, "*It doesn't hold because there is a wide variety of conditions reported as possibly associated with COVID vaccines!*", I invite you to pause for a second and think about the wide variety of adverse events known to be associated with smoking cigarettes. It not only affects the lungs; smoking has been associated with conditions in the cardiovascular system, skin, eyes, intestines, reproductive organs, etc. This criterion of causality is, in my opinion, one of the least relevant. As long as the biodistribution of the vaxgene and the described cellular interaction mechanisms allow us to understand why it could cause more than one effect, there is no reason to consider that the lack of specificity undermines the causal association between exposure and outcome.

Temporality refers to the factor (in this case, the COVID vaxgene) occurring before the effect (in this example, herpesvirus reactivation). If herpesvirus reactivates first and then the COVID vaxgene is received, it could not be a cause-and-effect relationship. That is temporality, and it holds for the relationship between COVID vaxgene and herpesvirus reactivation.

Biological gradient refers to the greater the exposure to the factor (in terms of frequency or amount), the greater the event (more severe or more likely to occur). In the case of herpesvirus reactivation, no study has been conducted yet to determine if the risk is higher with more doses of COVID vaxgene. It would be an interesting study, but it has not been done yet. What has been demonstrated is that the more COVID vaxgenes a person receives, the higher the risk of severe COVID illness (Shrestha et al., 2023). And that *is* a biological gradient.

Plausibility refers to knowing the biological mechanism through which the causal relationship between the factor and the event could be understood. It is evident that this criterion depends on the knowledge available on the topic. To determine if there is plausibility, it is useful to ask ourselves, '*Is it possible to imagine a mechanism that, if it had occurred, would produce the observed results?*' (Hoffler, 2005). When COVID vaccinations started, no studies had been conducted to identify the molecular and cellular interactions of the components of COVID vaxgenes in individuals receiving them. Now we have those studies, and we know, for example, that synthetic mRNA interacts with different molecules in the cell cytoplasm, activating various cellular processes and turning off others (see section 5.3), and that these changes translate into alterations in immune ability. We also have studies showing that COVID vaxgenes modify immune responses, increasing susceptibility to infections, including various herpesviruses (herpes zoster, herpes simplex, Epstein Barr virus), as well as other microorganisms, including SARS-CoV-2 (see section 6.6 and section 6.7). Therefore, we understand the mechanisms by which the relationship between exposure to something and the event could be explained. That is plausibility, and it holds for the relationship between COVID vaxgenes and herpesvirus reactivation.

Coherence is related to plausibility. The difference between the two criteria is that coherence refers to the relationship between exposure and outcome not conflicting with the available knowledge. This implies that it depends on the existing knowledge. Imagine Dr. Ignaz Semmelweis when he spoke about the causal relationship between doctors' lack of hygiene and puerperal fever (Kadar et al., 2018). Based on the knowledge available at that time, his proposal was not coherent because it conflicted with the premise that diseases could not be due to contagion but originated from foul odours. Therefore, we must be careful because knowledge changes. It is useful to ask the following to determine if there is coherence: '*If we assume that the established theory is correct, do the observed results fit into that theory?*' (Hoffler, 2005). The causal relationship between COVID vaxgenes and herpesvirus reactivation does not conflict with the available knowledge. We know the cause of reactivation well: it is due to immune suppression. The possible cause-and-effect relationship regarding the available knowledge about the possibility that multiple and repeated doses of vaxgenes lead to anergy or lymphocyte exhaustion (see section 6.6 and section 6.7) is also not incongruent, so there is no incoherence. Thus, with the available knowledge, a 'coherent whole' begins to be constructed. Through different pathways, we understand the observed relationship between exposure and outcome. That is coherence, and it holds for the relationship between COVID vaxgenes and herpesvirus reactivation.

Experimentation refers to having evidence from controlled experiments, in animals, or in humans (the latter is not always available for ethical reasons). When there is experimental evidence in animal models, it is essential to consider that sometimes differences in metabolism or physiology between species could mean that the cause-and-effect relationship in humans would be different from, for example, a mouse (see section 2.3). Experimental evidence of causality could come from studies showing that by eliminating the factor, the effect is reduced or eliminated. The lack of experimental evidence should not be a reason to dismiss possible causality during the causal inference process. In the example I am developing (COVID vaxgenes as a cause of herpesvirus reactivation), we lack controlled experimental evidence that has been published after peer review. However, based on the post-authorization report from Pfizer, which was released after a Federal court order in the United States[163], we can see that herpesvirus reactivation was detected in the vaccinated cohort during their phase 3 clinical trial and constituted a special adverse event of interest. That is experimentation, and it holds – even if partially – for the relationship between COVID vaxgenes and herpesvirus reactivation.

Analogy is considered the weakest criterion of causality. It refers to considering different analogies that help us understand the observed relationship. When proposing this criterion, Bradford Hill (1965) implied that when there is strong causal evidence for an exposure and an event, it can be accepted as evidence of causality that a similar factor could cause a similar event, even if the evidence is less strong. For example, based on their molecular structure and physicochemical properties, the hypothesis of the causal mechanism of carbon nanotube toxicity could be tested by analogy with what was already known about the toxicity mechanisms of asbestos fibres (Donaldson et al., 2010). Morphologically, carbon nanotubes were similar to asbestos fibres, so it could be expected that they could reach the lung if inhaled. Since asbestos fibres cause fibrosis and inflammation of the pleura and increase the risk of developing pleural mesothelioma[164] because cells divide more frequently to repair the damaged epithelium, a similar effect could be expected by analogy. This analogy was useful to later demonstrate that, indeed, exposure to carbon nanotubes causes events similar to those caused by exposure to asbestos fibres (Murphy et al., 2011). In the example I have been using so far, an analogy could be that, as it is known that herpesviruses can be reactivated when CD^{8+} T lymphocytes in immunoneural synapses are activated by the presence of antigens and an exacerbated inflammatory response (Freeman et al., 2007), COVID vaxgenes based on synthetic mRNA, which lead to the expression of the Spike protein for a long time and activate CD^{8+} T lymphocytes in addition to generating an exacerbated inflammatory response (see section 5.3), could generate a reactivation of herpesviruses.

---

[163] Bloomberg [Internet]. Accessed October 9 2023. Available at: https://news.bloomberglaw.com/health-law-and-business/why-a-judge-ordered-fda-to-release-COVID-vaccine-data-pronto

[164] Cancer that starts in the layer of cells that line the lungs, known as pleura.

This would need to be addressed experimentally, of course, but the lack of an analogy is not evidence that there is no causality, but, at least from the perspective of some epidemiologists, it is a sign of a lack of creativity on the part of the scientist (Hoffler, 2005). Other epidemiologists consider that the opposite effect may occur: that there is an excess of 'inventive imagination' in scientists looking for analogies everywhere[165]. Therefore, the value of the analogy is not to confirm causality but to allow the generation and testing of mechanistic hypotheses about causality (Fedak, 2015).

I have used a concrete example (herpesvirus reactivation) to show how, through the process of causal inference, evidence of causality can be determined. It is clear that all or most of Bradford Hill's criteria (Hill, 1965) are met to establish the causal relationship between COVID vaxgenes and herpesvirus reactivation. With time and effort, the same could be done to determine whether there is causality between COVID vaxgenes and the many types of adverse events that are being recorded.

Obviously, Bradford Hill's criteria are not rules but standards. Only one of the criteria is a *sine qua non*[166] condition for establishing causality (I refer to temporality). The other criteria are guidelines that support, if met, the causal relationship between exposure and effect. Without a doubt, in the case of COVID vaxgenes, the relationship between the vaccines and adverse events goes beyond a possibility or a spurious relationship, and almost all the criteria for causality are met.

In the next chapter, I will explain the biological mechanisms through which the adverse events associated with COVID vaxgenes can be understood. This includes the scientific basis for the *biological plausibility* of these adverse events.

---

[165] Encyclopaedia of Biostatistics, Online © 2005 John Wiley & Sons, Ltd. [Internet] Doi: 10.1002/0470011815.b2a03072.

[166] Latin expression that means "without which it does not" and it is used to refer to an indispensable condition for something to occur.

Chapter 5. Physiopathology of adverse events associated with COVID vaxgenes

Nothing in life should be feared, just understood.

Marie Curie

As I explained in the previous chapter, to determine causal relationships between COVID vaxgenes and the wide range of reported adverse events it is not enough to say '*there are many reports on the adverse event monitoring pages*' as evidence that vaxgenes are the culprits. We need to demonstrate biological plausibility, in addition to other criteria (Shimonovich et al., 2021; Kundi, 2007), which I explained in Chapter 4. In this chapter I will present the mechanisms by which COVID vaxgenes can cause various adverse events. Although this does not unequivocally establish that there is a cause and effect relationship, it is a first and important step to be able to elucidate whether what is reported on the adverse event monitoring pages (see Chapter 3) is indicative of causality.

5.1 Allergies and hypersensitivity to the components of vaxgenes

Shortly after the start of mass vaccination against COVID, allergies and hypersensitivity reactions[167] began to be reported (Cabanillas and Novak, 2021). For decades, it has been known that vaccines can trigger these reactions in susceptible individuals. This is because traditional vaccines in the vaccination schedule contain components such as egg-derived albumin, gelatine, and milk proteins, to which some people[168] are allergic (McNeil et al., 2016). However, these components are not present in the COVID vaxgenes, leading many doctors to assert that they would not cause hypersensitivity reactions, let alone cases of anaphylaxis[169]. It was also

[167] A hypersensitivity reaction occurs after having been exposed to a chemical or biological agent that activates a danger signal in the organism and, consequently, leads to an excessive immune response that causes tissue damage. An allergy is a type of hypersensitivity caused by the effects of excessive production of E type immunoglobulin (IgE).
[168] It remains unknown how many people are allergic to albumin worldwide, although a recent study showed that 0.5 to 2.5% of children examined have this allergy (Rona et al., 2007).
[169] Acute allergic reaction that if not treated opportunely, can be lethal.

argued that although foreign RNA can cause allergic reactions (Casavant and Youmans, 1975; Weis et al., 2017), synthetic mRNA COVID vaxgenes supposedly have a lower risk of allergic reactions because all uridines in the sequence were replaced by N1-methylpseudouridine (see section 1.1), which should prevent cytotoxic responses (Parr et al., 2020). However, it should be noted that the presence of degraded RNA, truncated RNA, double-stranded RNA, protein residues, and bacterial DNA (Krutzke et al., 2022; Tinari 2021; Thacker 2021; Greinacher et al., 2021), resulting from the manufacturing process (Baiersdörfer et al., 2019; Karikó et al., 2011), detected in vaxgene vials (see section 1.4), could generate acute or delayed hypersensitivity responses (Barrios et al., 2022).

It is true that health authorities in many countries issued recommendations that individuals allergic to any of the components of vaxgenes should not be vaccinated. However, few people knew the components of the vials when agreeing to be vaccinated, in part because the informed consent forms (in those countries that implemented them) did not explicitly list the components[170], nor did they indicate the possibility of an acute or delayed hypersensitivity reaction (Little et al., 2021; Mazraani and Barbari, 2021). On the other hand, it is highly likely that most of the population is unaware of whether they are allergic to the components of COVID vaxgenes.

Among the components of COVID vaxgenes reported by pharmaceutical companies (see section 1.1), the lipids they contain could be the cause of hypersensitivities. Unfortunately, some of these components lack studies to determine their potential as allergens[171] (Cabanillas and Novak, 2021). Both Pfizer and Moderna vaxgenes contain cholesterol and DSPC, in addition to ionizable aminolipids that help compact synthetic mRNA and are essential for it to enter the cellular cytoplasm (Schoenmaker et al., 2021). It is highly unlikely that vaxgene recipients are allergic to

[170] Public Health England. COVID vaccination: consent form and letter for adults [Internet]. Available at: https://www.gov.uk/government/publications/COVID-vaccination-consent-form-and-letter-for-adults, Department of Health and Aged Care. Formulario de Consentimiento para la Vacunación COVID. [Internet]. Available at: https://www.health.gov.au/resources/publications/COVID-vaccination-consent-form-for-COVID-vaccination?language=es

[171] Chemical or biological substance that leads to an allergic reaction.

cholesterol, as it is an essential component of cell membranes and a precursor to other cellular components. However, DSPC could play a role in allergies. This is because it is a substrate for phospholipase A2, a molecule with a pro-inflammatory effect by mediating the release of eicosanoids (Hatziantoniou et al., 2021), as well as activating the complement pathway and lysosome[172] action, which can cause anaphylaxis, particularly in asthmatic patients (Pniewska and Pawliczak, 2013).

In addition to DSPC, vaxgenes contain ionizable aminolipids (ALC-0315 in the case of Pfizer, while in the case of Moderna, it is likely[173] to be heptadecane-9-8-2-hydroxyethyl-6-oxo-6-undecyloxy-hexyl-amino-octanoate; Moghimi, 2021). They also contain PEGylated lipids that serve to stabilize LNPs through esterification[174] (Schoenmaker et al., 2021). In the case of Pfizer's vaxgene, this component is ALC-0159, while Moderna's vaxgene uses another lipid coupled with PEG (1,2-dimyristoyl-rac-glycero-3-methoxyPEG2000), according to the data provided by the pharmaceutical company to regulatory agencies (see section 1.2).

PEG is precisely one of the components that can explain most cases of anaphylaxis in vaccinated individuals (de Vries, 2020) since these reactions are known to occur in individuals who received PEGylated drugs (Kozma et al., 2020). A decade ago, 22-25% of the healthy population had anti-PEG antibodies, compared to 0.2% in the last decade of the 20th century (Garay et al., 2012), implying that the risk of hypersensitivity to PEG in the population could be more common than previously thought (Stone et al., 2019). The increase in antibody prevalence may reflect the extensive use of PEG in various drugs, cosmetics, and processed foods in recent decades, exposing a substantial portion of the population to the chemical. A recent study found that the prevalence of anti-PEG antibodies in the blood of

[172] Eicosanoids are lipid molecules, originated by the oxidation of fatty acids, which have activities related to inflammation. The complement cascade is a series of sequential steps that increase activity og antibodies and immune cells to eliminate microorganisms and damaged cells, as well as to promote inflammation. Lysosomes are cell organelles that have enzymes that degrade proteins, nucleic acids, carbohydrates and lipids.

[173] Specific information was not available.

[174] It relates to the process of combining an organic acid with an alcohol, to form ester and water.

people who had never received PEGylated drugs ranged from <1% to 72%, depending on the population studied (Hong et al., 2020).

Vaxgenes based on adenoviral vectors contain polysorbate 80, a non-ionic detergent included as an excipient because it solubilizes proteins and helps them cross cell membranes (Cortés et al., 2020). Polysorbates are chemicals composed of a sorbitan molecule linked to four PEG chains; one of the chains is attached to a fatty acid, and this attachment determines the number by which polysorbate is identified (Nappi et al., 2023). Specifically, polysorbate 80 inhibits reflux pumps in the blood-brain barrier and contributes to solubility, allowing its passage into the brain after intravenous administration, making it useful for various pharmacological applications (Rocha et al., 2013). This trait helps understand why, after intramuscular administration, recombinant AdV in vectorized vaxgenes can reach the nervous system.

Polysorbate 80 can cause anaphylactic reactions (Banerji et al., 2020), a risk which has even led to its removal or replacement in many formulations (Bollenback et al., 2022; Schwartzberg and Navari, 2018). For this reason, it is not possible to rule out that some of the immediate anaphylactic reactions and delayed hypersensitivities are due to this chemical compound (Moghimi et al., 2020) present in AstraZeneca, Janssen, Sputnik, and CanSino vaxgenes.

It is worth noting that at the end of 2021, the pharmaceutical company Moderna issued safety recommendations regarding its synthetic mRNA COVID vaxgene[175]. In its statement, the company indicates that the "*Moderna COVID vaccine should not be administered to individuals with a history of severe reactions (anaphylaxis) to any component of the vaccine*". It also emphasizes the need for immediate access to appropriate medical treatment for acute anaphylactic reactions following the administration of its vaxgene. This caution was issued in 2020 when

[175] Moderna. U.S. CDC Advisory Committee on Immunization Practices Recommends Booster Vaccination with Moderna's COVID-19 Vaccine [Internet]. Available at: https://news.modernatx.com/news/news-details/2021/U.S.-CDC-Advisory-Committee-on-Immunization-Practices-Recommends-Booster-Vaccination-with-Modernas-COVID-19-Vaccine/default.aspx.

anaphylactic reactions to vaccination began to occur. However, to my knowledge, no health agency or epidemiological control institution has implemented a program to detect antibodies or risk markers for hypersensitivity reactions to the components of vaxgenes, despite the known risk (Moghimi et al., 2020; Stone et al., 2019). This risk could be exacerbated with repeated exposure to PEG with each additional dose received, as observed in certain types of cutaneous (Puangpet et al., 2013), food (Fukutomi, 2019), and respiratory hypersensitivity (Kulhankova et al., 2009; Larsen et al., 2007).

Typically, if a person is allergic to the lipid components found in vaxgenes, the hypersensitivity reaction tends to occur within minutes of receiving the injection (Picard et al., 2023; Wang C. W. et al., 2023; Park et al., 2022; Laisuan, 2021). In the United States' adverse event monitoring system, VAERS, at the time of writing this chapter, there are 10,664 reports of anaphylaxis and 46,500 reports of severe allergies occurring immediately after the administration of the COVID vaxgene. Of the anaphylaxis reports, 10,168 (95%) are associated with vaxgenes based on synthetic mRNA (Pfizer and Moderna), and the same applies to severe allergy reports (43,577, corresponding to 94%)[176].

I already explained (see Chapter 3) that it is not possible to calculate the incidence of adverse events or compare the rates of adverse events between vaxgenes and vaccines based on the data recorded in monitoring systems. However, the tens of thousands of cases recorded following the authorization of vaxgenes deserve attention. A literature review shows that, despite an initial CDC study (Shimabukuro, 2021) finding a frequency of hypersensitivity cases of 0.09% in those who received an COVID vaxgene (i.e., just under 1 per 1,000 vaccinated individuals), subsequent studies have found a higher frequency of cases. For example, one study estimated the occurrence rate of severe hypersensitivity reactions or immediate anaphylaxis in response to COVID vaxgenes to be three times higher (Beatty et al., 2021). However, even considering the lower incidence of 7.91 cases of anaphylaxis per million doses of COVID vaxgenes estimated in

---

[176] US Department of Health and Human Services. Vaccine Adverse Event Reporting System [Internet]. Data is updated to October 22 2023 and have not been corrected using the underreporting factor . Available at: https://www.openvaers.com/vaersapp/reports.php

early 2021 (Greenhawt et al., 2021), if we consider that as of now, 13,510,000,000 doses have been administered[177], most of them being vaxgenes, we could be talking about more than 100,000 immediate anaphylactic reactions globally among vaccinated individuals.

As mentioned before, most hypersensitivity reactions are immediate; however, some people may develop delayed hypersensitivity (Barrios et al., 2022), and others are at risk of developing late sensitization due to repeated exposure to allergens, which would occur with multiple doses of the vaccine. These cases have already been reported (e.g., Loli-Ausejo et al., 2023; Pignatti et al., 2023; Beyaz et al., 2022; Blumenthal et al., 2022; Dash et al., 2022; Fasano et al., 2022; Larson et al., 2022; Maoz-Segal et al., 2022; McMahon et al., 2022; Mohta and Sharma, 2022; Pitlick et al., 2022; Stoyanov et al., 2022; Wang et al., 2022; Kempt et al., 2021; Johnston et al., 2021; Lindgren et al., 2021; Robb and Robb, 2021; Sprute et al., 2021). In some cases, clinical signs appeared up to six months after vaccine administration (Papadimitriou et al., 2022).

To get an idea of what these delayed reactions can cause, I have included a photograph of maculopapular lesions due to a delayed hypersensitivity reaction to the third dose of AstraZeneca's vaxgene (Fig. 13).

[177] Our World In Data [Internet]. Data updated to October 8 2023. Available at: https://ourworldindata.org/explorers/coronavirus-data-explorer

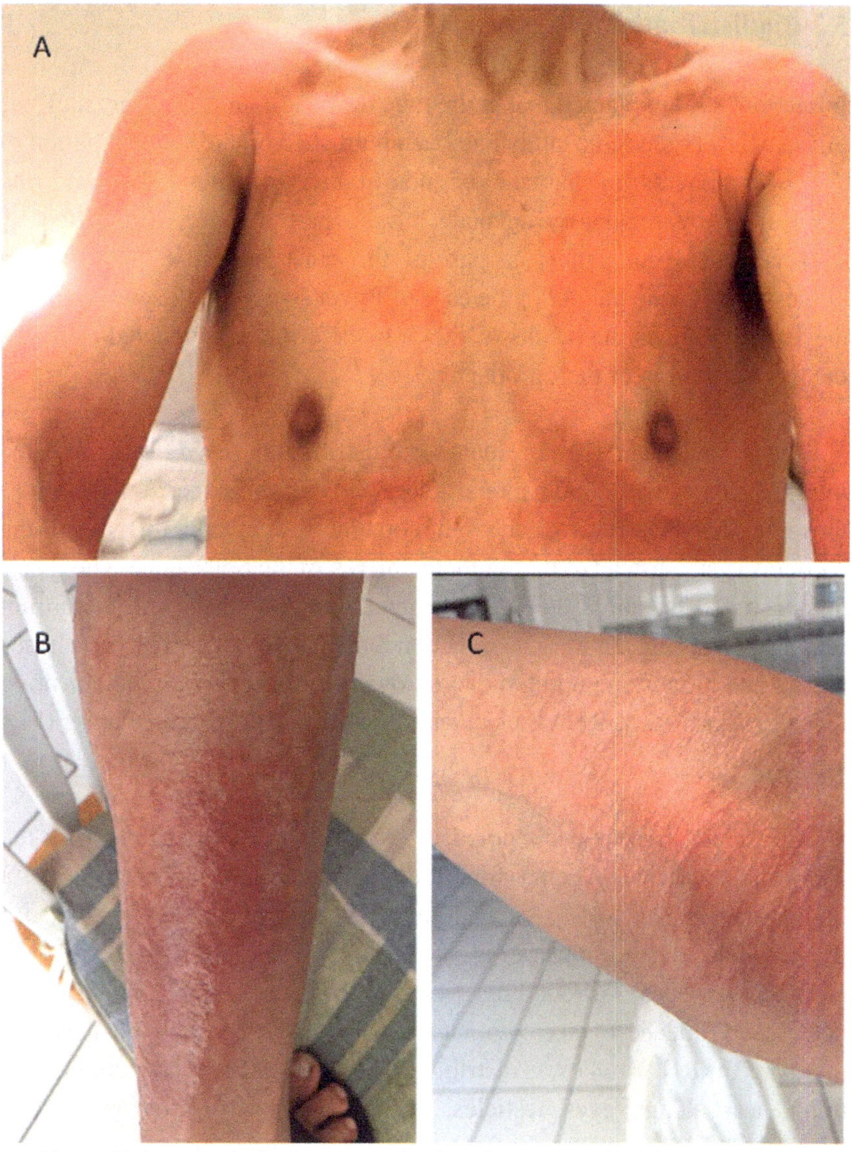

Figure 13. *Maculopapular lesions on the skin of a 68-year-old male patient, with no concomitant diseases or history of dermatological medical conditions. Lesion appeared one week after receiving the third dose of AstraZeneca's vaxgene. A) Injuries to the chest and abdomen. B) Back of the right leg. C) Internal arm fold. Credit: Dr. Adriana Quezada. Used with permission.*

5.2 Biodistribution of vaxgenes

In section 2.3, I explained that at the time of authorizing the emergency use of COVID vaxgenes, no study had been published on the biodistribution of their components in humans or non-human primates. However, the evaluations by regulatory agencies of the partial reports submitted by pharmaceutical companies as part of the emergency use authorization process were made public. In the case of Pfizer's vaccine, the evaluation by the EMA[178] shows the results of the only experiment conducted to assess the biodistribution of their product.

The experiment to evaluate biodistribution used rats injected intramuscularly with lipid nanoparticles (NPL) of the same composition as those in the COVID vaxgene but containing synthetic mRNA of the luciferase gene instead of the synthetic mRNA of the Spike gene. The report demonstrated that lipid nanoparticles containing synthetic mRNA do not remain at the site of muscle injection but quickly distribute to various tissues and organs, including the liver, ovaries, lungs, and brain, indicating that NPL-synthetic mRNA molecules can cross the blood-brain barrier (Fig. 14).

The same observation is noted in the intermediate assessment by the European Medicines Agency for Moderna, which also did not conduct a biodistribution study of its vaxgene in primates. Instead, they evaluated it by intramuscular administration of LNP (differing from those in their COVID vaxgenes) surrounding synthetic mRNA "1647" containing the complete sequence of six cytomegalovirus genes. They found that, "*as expected*", mRNA-1647 was distributed throughout the body, including the brain, heart, lungs, eyes, testicles, liver, spleen, and nearby and distant lymph nodes. The synthetic mRNA "*did not persist* [in rats] *for more than*

[178] European Medicines Agency. Committee for Medicinal Products for Human Use (CHMP) Assessment Report Comirnaty. EMA/707383/2020 Corr.1*1 [Document]. Available at: https://www.ema.europa.eu/en/documents/assessment-report/comirnaty-epar-public-assessment-report_en.pdf

1 to 3 days in tissues other than the injection site, lymph nodes, and spleen"[179].

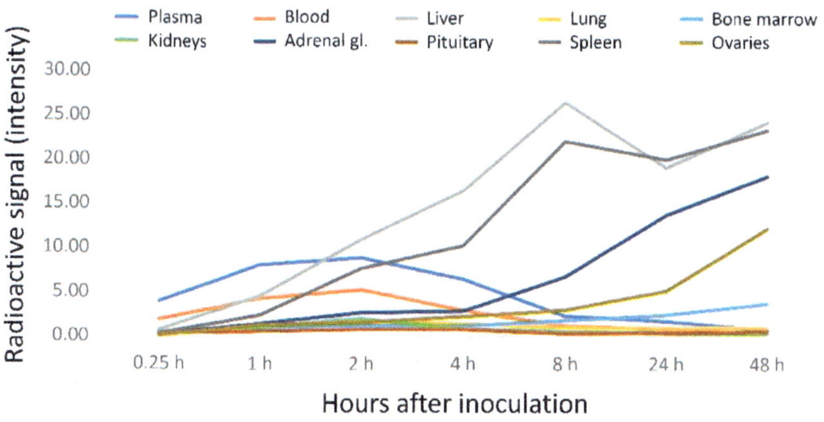

***Figure 14**. Biodistribution of lipid nanoparticles and synthetic mRNA after intramuscular inoculation in mice. Prepared based on the intermediate evaluation of the technical report EMA/707383/2020 on Pfizer's COVID vaxgene by the European Medicines Agency*[180].

In both cases, it is evident that synthetic mRNA and the lipid nanoparticles (NPL) enveloping it do not remain at the injection site or in proximal lymph nodes but distribute to all organs, including the central nervous system. It's worth noting that, for both vaxgenes (Pfizer and Moderna), the biodistribution studies conducted and presented to regulatory agencies contradict the regulatory guidelines for RNA therapeutics (Vervaeke et al., 2022).

---

[179] European Medicines Agency. Committee for Medicinal Products for Human Use (CHMP). Assessement Report Moderna EMA/15689/2021 Corr.1*1 [Internet] Available at: https://www.ema.europa.eu/en/documents/assessment-report/spikevax-previously-covid-19-vaccine-moderna-epar-public-assessment-report_en.pdf

[180] European Medicines Agency. Committee for Medicinal Products for Human Use (CHMP) Assessment Report Comirnaty. EMA/707383/2020 Corr.1*1 [Internet]. Available at: https://www.ema.europa.eu/en/documents/assessment-report/comirnaty-epar-public-assessment-report_en.pdf

What is interesting is that, to date, no independent scientific articles (aside from the reports from the pharmaceutical companies) have been published studying the biodistribution and pharmacokinetics of these products in non-human primates. This is highly relevant since both pharmaceutical companies only assessed the behaviour of the NPL complex with synthetic mRNA in rats, despite marked metabolic differences compared to humans (Fig. 15). Regulatory pharmacological guidelines caution against using such dissimilar species to evaluate the biodistribution and pharmacokinetics of a drug or therapeutic product intended for human use (Martignoni et al., 2006; Vervaeke et al., 2022).

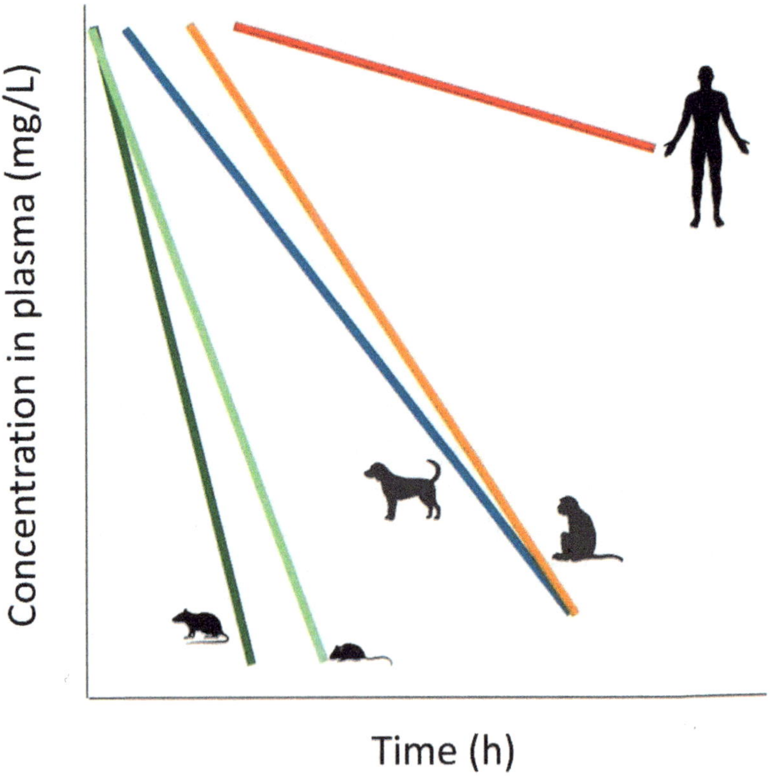

Figure 15. *Plasma concentration of valproic acid after administration in different species. Figure based on Nau (1986).*

Regardless of these two experiments, biodistribution results could be inferred from a scientific article published in 2017, showing similar outcomes to those reported by Pfizer and Moderna. The study, conducted in rats to explore the immunogenicity of synthetic mRNA vaxgenes against influenza viruses, found that NPL and the synthetic mRNA they contain distribute rapidly throughout the animals' bodies, even crossing the blood-brain barrier (Bahl et al., 2017).

In line with the interim assessments of regulatory agencies regarding the synthetic mRNA vaxgenes from Pfizer, which observed a systemic distribution of lipid nanoparticles (NPL), it has been found that synthetic mRNA can be present in the breast milk of vaccinated women (Hanna et al., 2022). This presence persists even 45 hours after vaccination, albeit in small quantities and with reduced viability (Hanna et al., 2023). The significance of this transfer to infants remains unknown as of the writing of this chapter (Banoun, 2023).

As for vaxgenes based on adenoviral vectors, the EMA's interim assessment of AstraZeneca's report[181] indicated that the biodistribution study (study 514559) was still ongoing. Instead, they presented results from *another* study conducted with a different adenoviral vector (ChAd63, as opposed to ChAdOx1, the adenoviral vector used in their COVID vaxgene). Quoting AstraZeneca's report, "*ChAd63 is closely related to ChAdOx1, and it is believed that the two viruses have the same infectivity and tissue tropism*" (page 47 of the report). The biodistribution analysis of the ChAd63 vector, administered to mice by intradermal injection rather than intramuscular, showed that no viral particles of that adenovirus were found anywhere other than the injection site. However, they noted that "*the methods used for the determinations are not clearly defined and/or validated*".

Unfortunately, when the pharmaceutical company completed the biodistribution study 514559 with the ChAdOx1 vector administered to

[181] European Medicines Agency. Committee for Medicinal Products for Human Use (CHMP). Assessment Report AstraZeneca EMA/94907/2021 [Internet]. Available at: https://www.ema.europa.eu/en/documents/assessment-report/vaxzevria-previously-COVID-vaccine-astrazeneca-epar-public-assessment-report_en.pdf

mice intramuscularly (published by the UK Medicines Regulatory Agency in January 2022, two years after its emergency authorization), it was evident that the vaxgene was distributed through the blood to various tissues, including the sciatic nerve, bone marrow, liver, spleen, and mammary glands[182]. The results of AstraZeneca's vaxgene biodistribution trial were not unexpected, as a study published in 2008 had shown that when recombinant adenovirus vectors were injected into rabbits intramuscularly, the virions were detectable in various organs, indicating that the entry of adenoviruses is not limited to muscle cells at the injection site but involves systemic distribution (Sheets et al., 2008). This risk had been highlighted in a letter to the editor of the British Medical Journal in July 2021[183].

The results of AstraZeneca's biodistribution study 514559, finally published in January 2022 (almost a year after its emergency authorization), showed that the recombinant adenoviruses (AdV) of their COVID vaxgene can indeed be found up to 29 days after a single-dose inoculation in various tissues of vaccinated mice. These tissues include bone marrow, spleen, inguinal lymph nodes, sciatic nerve, and the injection site. At nine days post-injection, the adenovirus was also found in the liver (Stebbings et al., 2022), suggesting a broad biodistribution of adenoviral vectors. Despite these results, the study's authors concluded that the distribution is not broad and that the vectorized vaxgene is safe. These conclusions are flawed because they ignore the observed systemic distribution and metabolic differences between rodents and humans (see Figure 15). Therefore, we could reasonably assume that the persistence of adenoviral vectors in humans who received this type of vaxgene will be prolonged.

Regarding Janssen's COVID vaxgene, the report submitted to the European Medicines Agency (EMA)[184] indicated that "*no biodistribution*

[182] Medicines and Healthcare Products Regulator Agency. Public Assessment Report National procedure Vaxzevria PLGB 17901/0355 [Internet]. Available at: https://assets.publishing.service.gov.uk/government/uploads/system/uploads/attachment_data/file/1148800/CMA_UKPAR_COVID_19_Vaccine_AstraZeneca_PAR_PAR_update_Annex_1.pdf

[183] Merchant H. Rapid Response to COVID: Regulators warn that rare Guillain-Barré cases may link to J&J and AstraZeneca vaccines "Autoimmune damage to the nerves following Covid vaccines: EMA issued warning to patients and healthcare professionals". The British Medical Journal [Internet]. Available at: https://www.bmj.com/content/374/bmj.n1786/rr-0

[184] European Medicines Agency. Committee for Medicinal Products for Human Use (CHMP). Assessment Report Janssen EMA/158424/2021. [Internet]. Available at:

studies were conducted with the specific COV2.S construct[185] *as discussed and agreed upon during the scientific recommendations of the applicant* [regulatory agency]" (page 50). Biodistribution studies in rats, conducted with another vector construct, showed that the recombinant Ad26 virus was detectable at the intramuscular injection site, lymph nodes, and spleen. Based on the EMA's assessment, it is not possible to determine if they sought the presence of the Ad26 virus in all organs or only in these. What they did mention is that the recombinant Ad26 DNA was detectable in the lymph node of one animal up to 180 days after the administration of the vaxgene.

It's worth noting that beyond the EMA's interim report, information on the biodistribution of COVID vectorized vaxgenes has not been publicly disclosed. However, studies conducted with Ebola vaxgene candidates based on adenoviral vectors showed that, while not common, the recombinant viral vector can be found in other tissues (Planty et al., 2020). Please be aware that, at the time of writing this chapter, there is no published scientific information on the biodistribution of Sputnik, Sputnik Light, and CanSino vectorized vaxgenes.

The systemic biodistribution of lipid nanoparticles (LNP), synthetic mRNA (Pfizer and Moderna) and adenoviral vectors (AstraZeneca, Janssen, CanSino, Sputnik, and Sputnik Light) could be even greater if the vaxgene penetrates the blood vessels that supply the deltoid muscle. This could lead to the rapid dissemination of the fluid and its components to distant tissues (Merchant, 2022; Rahamimov et al., 2021). Given the large number of volunteers needed for the administration of vaccines and vaxgenes to billions of people in a short period and the WHO's recommendation not to aspirate before pushing the syringe plunger (Merchant, 2022), the possibility that vaxgenes were inadvertently injected into the capillary blood vessels of the arm of some people should not be ignored.

---

https://www.ema.europa.eu/en/documents/assessment-report/COVID-vaccine-janssen-epar-public-assessment-report_en.pdf

[185] In this context, the word 'construct' refers to the recombinant AdV.

5.3 Pathophysiology of synthetic mRNA

A literature review on the PubMed platform reveals that, at the time of writing this chapter, 1,514 case reports associated with adverse events following the administration of COVID vaxgenes have been published[186]. Among these, 778 case reports specifically correspond to adverse events associated with the receipt of synthetic mRNA-based vaxgenes (Pfizer and Moderna)[187]. The published clinical cases reflect similar types of events as those reported by the WHO's adverse event monitoring system, in addition to the list of adverse events of special interest from the Brighteon Collaboration (see section 2.15).

As the mass administration of vaxgenes began, evidence and hypotheses started to emerge regarding the mechanisms through which synthetic mRNA can initiate molecular cascades impacting various organs and tissues[188], leading to various pathologies, including sudden deaths due to thrombosis. Medical professionals are being alerted to the need to be aware of this risk in vaccinated patients (Roncati et al., 2022).

It is understandable that, given the diversity of systemic effects reported by individuals who received COVID vaxgenes, questions arise about how such a wide range of adverse events could be explained. However, this question begins to be answered by examining the reports that pharmaceutical companies submitted to regulatory agencies as part of the authorization process for their product. The components of COVID vaxgenes are distributed to various organs and tissues after intramuscular administration. Upon entering the cells of these organs and tissues, the components of the vials can trigger various molecular and cellular cascades, with a consequential clinical impact.

---

[186] National Library of Medicine. PubMed [Internet]. Available at: https://pubmed.ncbi.nlm.nih.gov/ [Search done August 21 2023 using the search terms: (COVID AND vaccine AND adverse) AND (case report) NOT review]

[187] National Library of Medicine. PubMed [Internet]. Available at: https://pubmed.ncbi.nlm.nih.gov/ [Search done August 21 2023 with the search terms: (COVID AND vaccine AND adverse) AND (mRNA OR Pfizer OR Moderna) AND (case report) NOT review]

[188] Remember what I explained in Section 5.3; the components of the vaxgenes are distributed to various tissues and organs after intramuscular administration.

Based on their pathophysiology, adverse events associated with the administration of synthetic mRNA vaxgenes that have been reported to monitoring systems and published as clinical cases can be grouped into five categories: 1) autoinflammatory, 2) immunosuppressive, 3) autoimmune, 4) prothrombotic, and 5) degenerative. These categories are not mutually exclusive; in fact, they often occur simultaneously, and their impact on overall health can be exacerbated.

The presence of synthetic mRNA can dysregulate the functioning of the immune system, with a specific impact on the expression of type I interferon[189], interfering with the production of microRNAs (Stati et al., 2023). This can lead to suppression of innate and adaptive responses (Seneff et al., 2022). MicroRNAs are small non-coding RNAs[190] that regulate mRNA transcription by silencing or degrading them. MicroRNAs play a crucial role in regulating various biological processes, including cell differentiation (allowing a stem cell to become a specific cell type during embryogenesis[191]), cell proliferation, apoptosis[192], embryonic development, tissue growth, and function at a paracrine[193] level. Dysregulated expression of microRNAs can be significant in the development of various diseases, such as cancer, autoimmune diseases, type 2 diabetes, and amyotrophic lateral sclerosis (ALS) (Shi et al., 2021; Bravo-Vázquez et al., 2021; Liu J. et al., 2022).

Synthetic mRNA COVID vaxgenes can dysregulate the expression of microRNAs (Stati et al., 2023). Recent findings concur in that they have detected exosomes containing microRNAs associated with severe inflammatory responses in some individuals who received this type of vaxgene (Miyashita et al., 2022). Specifically, the expression of a microRNA (miR-92a-2-5p) was found to be low in individuals who received at least one dose of synthetic mRNA vaxgene and who experienced adverse effects. It's worth noting that the downregulation of miR-92a-2-5p

[189] Molecules (generically known as cytokines) that play an important role in inducing inflammation, regulating immune responses, directing responses by lymphocytes, causing programmed cell death (apoptosis) and preventing tumour formation.
[190] They do not contain information that ribosomes will use to make any protein, as does mRNA.
[191] Stages during which an embryo is formed.
[192] Programmed cell death.
[193] That it induces changes in the cells that are near.

is associated with cell proliferation issues that may lead to cancer (Zhuang et al., 2022). Additionally, low expression of miR-92a-2-5p is associated with other diseases (Mogilyansky and Rigoutsos, 2013), including diabetic cardiomyopathy (Li et al., 2019).

In the case of synthetic mRNA vaxgenes, it's essential to consider that once the synthetic mRNA enters a cell, it can activate various intracellular cascades (Trougakos et al., 2022b). One of these cascades leads to sustained production of type I interferon and the transcription of foreign pattern recognition receptors (such as MDA5[194], RLRs[195], and MAVS[196]), putting the cell in a pro-inflammatory "antiviral" state. Another intracellular process activated by synthetic mRNA is the activation of long interspersed nuclear elements type 1 (LINE-1)[197], which can retrotranscribe the sequence of synthetic mRNA and introduce it into the nucleus (Aldén et al., 2022; Domazet-Lošo, 2022).

The activation of LINE-1 is not trivial, so I'll dedicate a few paragraphs to explain. LINE-1 is, in fact, a retrotransposon. This means it's a "mobile" DNA sequence that, when transcribed (copied as an mRNA sequence), exits to the cytoplasm, is read by ribosomes, and two of its genes are translated into proteins (ORF1 and ORF2). These proteins associate with the LINE-1 RNA sequence, forming a ribonucleoprotein complex (RNP) in the cytoplasm. The RNP returns to the nucleus, where the LINE-1 ORF2 protein carries out the retrotranscription[198] of the RNA sequence and introduces it into other locations of the genome (Wells and Feschotte, 2020). This process generates more copies of LINE-1 in the genome (Boissinnot and Sookdel, 2016). I've summarized the entire process graphically to make it easier to understand (Fig. 16).

[194] Protein 5 associated with melanoma differentiation.
[195] Retinoic acid-inducible gene-like receptors.
[196] Antiviral mitochondrial signalling factor.
[197] I will explain this in the next page.
[198] Conversion of an RNA sequence into DNA using an enzyme called retrotranscriptase or reverse transcription.

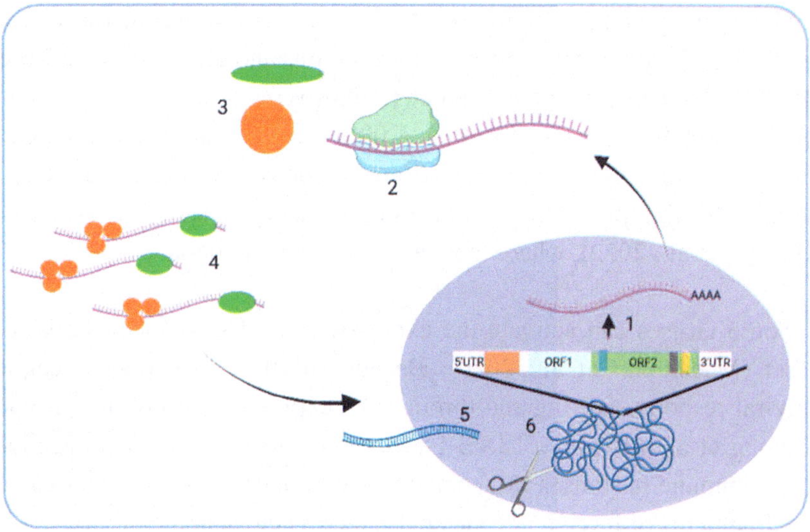

Figure 16. *Steps of LINE-1 activation. 1. Transcription of LINE-1 generates an mRNA. 2. This leaves the nucleus and is read by the ribosomes. 3. Two proteins (ORF-1 and ORF-2) are produced from the information from the ORF1 and ORF2 genes. 4. These proteins associate with the LINE-1 mRNA, or with mRNA sequences that are in the cytoplasm at that time and the ribonucleoprotein complex (RNP) is formed that is transported to the nucleus. 5. The ORF2 protein acts as a reverse transcriptase and generates a double strand of DNA from the mRNA sequence. 6. The double strand of DNA from the genome is cut and the new copy of LINE-1, already transcribed as DNA, is inserted into a random chromosome. Figure created in BioRender.*

In the human genome, there are over 500,000 copies of LINE-1 (Sánchez-Luque et al., 2019), although only about 150 are complete and capable of self-copying and transposing to other genetic regions when activated (Brouha et al., 2003). These new insertions accumulate in germline cells (ovules and sperm) and stem cells (Mastora et al., 2021). Of course, LINE-1 expression is carefully regulated. Its expression is high during certain phases of embryonic development within the maternal placenta (Percharde et al., 2018) and is indispensable for early development after implantation (Kohlrausch et al., 2022). This is because, during the early stages of embryogenesis, LINE-1 expression is key to generating functional diversity in the developing embryo (Faulkner and García-Pérez, 2017).

Generally, functional copies of LINE-1 are silenced in somatic cells and germline cells, although some cells, like neurons and glial cells, can express LINE-1, albeit in a regulated manner (Bedrosian et al., 2018), aiding in neuron formation (Ormundo et al., 2020). LINE-1 is also expressed in mature T lymphocytes, where it is crucial for controlling the activity of these cells and preventing them from entering a state of exhaustion (Marasca et al., 2022), where they are no longer functional.

Some viruses can activate the expression of LINE-1 in the cells they infect (Macchietto et al., 2020). Because of this activation, a cellular antiviral response is triggered through the expression of interferon type I (Chuong et al., 2016), so LINE-1 can be considered part of intracellular innate immune responses (Macchietto et al., 2020). Its activation explains how fragments of foreign nucleic acids (such as the genome of viruses) can be inserted into the cells' genome, as RNP complexes can form between LINE-1 ORF1 and ORF2 proteins and foreign RNA sequences found in the cytoplasm. This has been known for decades, as fragments of the genomes of viruses like Ebola, Marburg, and lymphocytic choriomeningitis virus have been found within the genome of infected cells (Belyi et al., 2010; Geukin et al., 2009), and even SARS-CoV-2 (Zhang et al., 2021). I clarify that it's not the entire genome of the virus that is inserted into the cell's genome, only fragments of that foreign genome. The problem with activating LINE-1 expression in cells where it's normally silenced is that it can lead to pathological processes such as autoimmune diseases, cancer, cellular senescence (Gázquez-Gutiérrez et al., 2021; Grandi and Tramontano, 2018), and even neuropsychiatric diseases if high levels of LINE-1 are expressed in neurons (Terry et al., 2020).

Now, beyond understanding what LINE-1 is and does, it is crucial to comprehend that the synthetic mRNA in COVID vaxgenes can activate LINE-1 expression (Aldén et al., 2022). This was observed in a study conducted with cultures of cancerous liver cells transfected with the COVID Pfizer vaxgene. Shortly after transfection, LINE-1 was found to be activated. Furthermore, the complete sequence of the synthetic mRNA for the Spike protein contained in the vaxgene was present in the cell nucleus, transcribed as DNA (Aldén et al., 2022). This can only be understood as a consequence of LINE-1, which was activated by the presence of this foreign genetic material.

Certainly, being an *in vitro* study done on cultured cancer cells (where LINE-1 expression tends to be more active than in healthy cells; McKerrow et al., 2022), it is not accurate to generalize these results or interpret them as unequivocal evidence that the same will happen in the cells of vaccinated individuals with these vaxgenes. However, since this study showed that LINE-1 expression in cancerous liver cells that only received saline solution (i.e., the control experimental group) was significantly lower, the result should not be ignored. There is no logical argument to assume that this phenomenon could not occur *in vivo* in healthy cells. What Aldén and colleagues' (2022) study implies is that the synthetic mRNA from vaxgenes can activate LINE-1 in the cells it enters, and retrotranscription of the synthetic mRNA sequence can occur. If nuclear integration of the retrotranscribed sequence occurs, there is a possibility of chromosomal instability[199] and insertional mutagenesis[200], whose consequences may include the silencing of tumour suppressor gene[201] expression or the activation of proto-oncogenes[202], increasing the risk of cancer (Langer et al., 2013).

The second consequence of LINE-1 activation by the synthetic mRNA in the vaccine is the initiation of a pro-inflammatory signal (Tiwari et al., 2020) through pattern recognition receptors mentioned earlier, such as MDA-5 and RIG-I (Brisse and Ly, 2019). This would exacerbate the pro-inflammatory state, that was initiated by the persistent presence of synthetic mRNA in the cytoplasm, as explained earlier. If this pro-inflammatory antiviral state is sustained, it can lead to various pathological autoinflammatory and autoimmune conditions (Funabiki et al., 2014).

---

[199] It occurs when there is an abnormally high rate of chromosome missegregation during mitosis due to defective cell cycle quality control mechanisms. It can cause the number of copies of chromosomes to be greater than the 46 that human somatic cells should have..

[200] Generation of mutations in the DNA of a cell due to the addition of one or more nucleotides in the sequence.

[201] They are genes that, when expressed, inhibit the proliferation of cells and the development of cancerous tumours

[202] Group of genes that allow cell division. They can cause cancer when mutated or when turned on out of time.

Considering that the modifications made to the synthetic mRNA sequence in Pfizer's and Moderna's vaxgenes precisely allow it to persist for a long time within the cytoplasm, a scenario in which there is chronic activation of antiviral and pro-inflammatory innate immune responses and persistent LINE-1 activation is plausible. This, in turn, would further promote antiviral and pro-inflammatory innate immune responses—a true vicious circle due to the persistence of this synthetic foreign genetic material from the vaxgenes (Acevedo-Whitehouse and Bruno, 2023).

The third consequence of LINE-1 activation by the synthetic mRNA in the vaxgene is that it can cause breaks in DNA strands (Gasior et al., 2006). This occurs precisely because when LINE-1 is expressed and inserts more copies of its sequence or other retrotranscribed mRNA into the genome, it needs to cut the DNA strands to "paste" the new copies (see Fig. 16). DNA breaks caused by LINE-1 action may be associated with a higher risk of cancer (McKerrow et al., 2022), especially when they impact the p53 tumour suppressor gene, whose expression is essential to prevent a transformed cell from proliferating (Kyriakopoulos et al., 2022). In other words, abnormal LINE-1 activation leads to chromosomal instability, which has been described for breast cancer, ovarian cancer, colon cancer, liver cancer, and endometrial cancer. Furthermore, LINE-1 activation also negatively impacts the ability to repair DNA damage (McKerrow et al., 2022; Situ et al., 2019), posing an additional risk for cancer development.

An additional mechanism through which synthetic mRNA could increase the risk of cancer relates to the codon optimization of the RNA sequence used (see section 1.2). As explained earlier, there is a higher GC (guanine and cytosine) content in the synthetic mRNA sequences of Pfizer and Moderna vaxgenes than in the mRNA sequence of the SARS-CoV-2 Spike gene (Seneff et al., 2022). This high GC content means that more secondary structures, including something known as G-quadruplexes (G4 structures), can form in the synthetic mRNA molecule during translation. The abundance of G4 structures could increase the chances of binding to microRNA sequences and RNA-binding proteins, disrupting the regulation of gene expression (Valdes Angues and Perea Bustos, 2023) and negatively affecting microRNA expression, which can impact cancer progression and other degenerative diseases (Seneff et al., 2022).

Finally, it has been reported that the synthetic mRNA in COVID vaxgenes (such as Pfizer and Moderna) can destroy the structure of ribosomal RNA (Tanaka et al., 2022). This was observed in a study that analysed ribosomal alterations in people who had been vaccinated with Pfizer's COVID vaxgene. The study included healthy volunteers and cancer patients, whether they were receiving adjuvant oncology therapy with the *Trametes robinophila* fungus, known as Huaier therapy[203]. The study found that the quality of RNA extracted from blood samples of volunteers shortly after receiving the first dose of Pfizer's vaxgene was abnormally low. Additionally, the structure of ribosomal RNA was drastically altered, affecting its translation capacity. These changes became more prominent with additional vaccine doses. Signs of accelerated cellular senescence[204] were also detected (Tanaka et al., 2022).

The relevance of the Tanaka et al. (2022) study is significant: causal associations have already been described between mutations affecting ribosomal biogenesis and an increased risk of developing cancer or rapid cancer progression (Pelletier et al., 2018). Despite being a preliminary study conducted with a small number of samples, it is important to consider because it demonstrates biological plausibility for the association between synthetic mRNA vaxgenes and the occurrence of neurodegeneration and cancer (see section 6.9). It is concerning that the study by Tanaka and colleagues (2022) found that the destruction of ribosomal RNA structures was different from that caused by immunotherapy used in some cancer cases, and that it continued to progress even six months after the first dose. Frankly, I cannot imagine any oncologist who can read that study and not at least consider that synthetic mRNA vaxgenes may pose a risk to their patients.

A graphic summary of the different intracellular processes that can be impacted by the presence of synthetic mRNA when it enters cells can be seen in Figure 17.

---

[203] Therapy with *Trametes robinohila* has an anticancer effect because it decreases cell proliferation (Narayanan et al., 2023).

[204] Cellular senescence is the aging process of cells. If accelerated, it contributes to neurodegenerative pathologies (Martínez-Cue and Ruedas, 2020) and cancer (Schmitt et al., 2022).

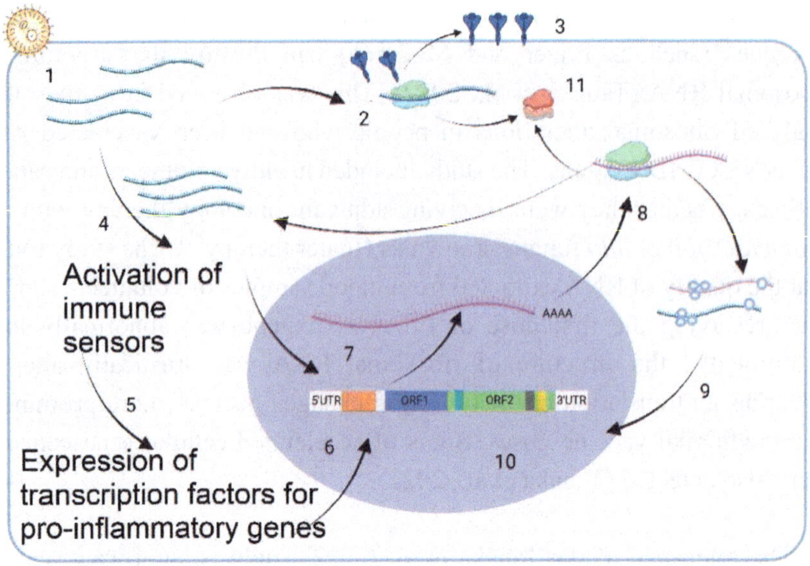

***Figure 17**. Intracellular processes triggered by the presence of synthetic mRNA of Pfizer's and Moderna's COVID vaxgenes. 1) The synthetic mRNA is released to the cytoplasm after the lipid nanoparticles are fused with the cell membrane. 2) A part of the synthetic mRNA is translated by ribosomes to express the Spike protein. 3) The Spike protein is expressed in the cell membrane. 4) The synthetic mRNA is accumulated in the cytoplasm for weeks or months and by persisting it activates immune sensors. 5) Immune sensors activate transcription factors leading to a pro-inflammatory and antiviral state in the cell. 6) The expression of LINE-1 is activated. 7) The presence of foreign RNA in the cytoplasm also activates the expression of LINE-1. This leads to its transcription and translation by ribosomes. 8) Ribonucleoprotein complexes (RNP) are formed with the LINE-1 sequences and with sequences from the synthetic mRNA of the vaccine. 9) RNPs enter the nucleus, break the DNA strands and integrate into the genome. 10) Genomic instability can occur. 11) The ribosomal structure is destroyed. Figure created in BioRender based on Acevedo-Whitehouse and Bruno, 2023.*

5.4 Pathophysiology of the adenoviral vector

As I explained in Chapter 1, vectors used for COVID AstraZeneca vaxgenes, Janssen, Sputnik, Sputnik light and CanSino are human or chimpanzee adenovirus (AdV). In all these vaxgenes, the AdV used are replication-deficient, which is achieved through the elimination of the viral E1 gene (Fallaux et al., 1998). Many times, the viral E3 gene of the AdV is also eliminated to have more space (up to 8,000 base pairs) to insert in the desired genetic sequence the AdV genome. In the case of COVID vectorized vaxgenes, that sequence is the S gene, which contains the instructions for cells to produce the SARS-CoV-2 Spike protein. Once this gene is inserted into the genome of the replication-deficient AdV, it is now considered a recombinant AdV.

To make this type of vaxgenes, it is necessary to culture the recombinant AdVs, and this is done in cells that are compatible with the AdVs. Human embryonic renal cells HEK293 or human embryonic retinal cells PER.C6 are usually used (Suleman et al., 2022). These cells have been genetically modified to express the viral E1 gene that was removed from recombinant AdVs. If they did not, the AdVs could not replicate as they are replication deficient. The culture process of recombinant AdVs should prevent the risk of the generation of competent AdV (Kovesdi and Hedley, 2010) and ensure that they are not present in the vaccine[205].

To be able to produce these vaxgenes at a large-scale, required to produce billions of COVID vaxgenes, culture of human cells and recombinant AdV is performed in bioreactors with optimal growth conditions (Lesch et al., 2015). Then the cells are lysed and the AdVs are purified to obtain a suspension of AdV virions without cellular remains (Suleman et al., 2022). If purification was not adequately done, the vaxgenes could contain protein debris and human cellular DNA (hcDNA) from the cell culture. If hcDNA is present in the vials, there is an implicit risk that the cells in which the vaxgene enters become malignant and

---

[205] European Medicines Agency. Guideline on Scientific Requirements for the Environmental Risk Assessment of Gene Therapy Medicinal Products. EMEA/CHMP/GTWP/125491/2006 [Document]. Available at: https://www.ema.europa.eu/en/documents/scientific-guideline/guideline-scientific-requirements-environmental-risk-assessment-gene-therapy-medicinal-products_en.pdf

cancerous tumours be formed (Dumont et al., 2016; Yang, 2013). This is because the hcDNA can enter the nucleus of the cells and become integrated, affecting the expression of tumour suppressor genes, which are responsible of controlling the cell cycle, and can also activate proto oncogenes (Sheng-Fowler et al., 2009). Both events could increase the risk of cancer. This is why even the WHO and FDA recommend that vectorized vaxgenes should not exceed 10 ng of hcDNA per dose and that the size of residual hcDNA fragments be less than 200 base pairs (Yang et al., 2013).

Up to now, only one published study has reported not finding hcDNA in vials of COVID vectorized vaxgenes (Krutzke et al., 2022). However, it's not only hcDNA that can be problematic in vectorized vaxgenes. To date, two studies have examined the components of vials of these products. The first reported the presence of around 1,000 cellular and viral proteins in the vials, at a concentration of 70-80 μg of protein per mL, of which up to 50 μg corresponded to proteins derived from HEK293 cells (Greinacher et al., 2021). The second study analysed four batches of vectorized vaxgenes (from AstraZeneca) and found evidence of more than 1,200 cellular proteins (Krutzke et al., 2022). What can be inferred from both studies is that the purification process of these vectorized vaxgenes was not adequate. Additionally, it's worth noting that in the EMA report on AstraZeneca (EMA/94907/2021), they indicated that no data on the amount of human DNA and cellular remnants present in their vaxgenes were provided[206], and they committed to delivering this data by March 2021 when these vaxgenes had already been administered to millions of people worldwide. However, as of the writing of this book, there is no available evidence that AstraZeneca has provided this data to the EMA.

In the case of the vectorized vaxgene from Janssen, the EMA report (EMEA/H/C/005737/II/0071/G) [207] indicated that the vaxgene "*contains only trace levels of human cellular proteins and human DNA. Levels of*

[206] European Medicines Agency. Committee for Medicinal Products for Human Use (CHMP). Assessment Report AstraZeneca EMA/94907/2021. [Document]. Downloadable at: https://www.ema.europa.eu/en/documents/assessment-report/vaxzevria-previously-COVID-vaccine-astrazeneca-epar_public-assessment-report_en.pdf

[207] European Union Risk Management Plan. JCOVDEN (VAC31518 [Ad26.COV2.S] [Document]. Downloadable at: https://www.ema.europa.eu/en/documents/rmp-summary/COVID-vaccine-janssen-epar-risk-management-plan_en.pdf

human cellular proteins were significantly below the residual levels of human cellular proteins reported in other commercial vaccines produced in human cells". For the other three COVID adenoviral vector-based vaxgenes (CanSino, Sputnik, and Sputnik Light), this information is not available. I will explain the possible biological consequences of the contaminating proteins found in AstraZeneca's COVID vaxgenes a little later (section 5.7).

The potential harmful effects of adenoviral vectors are varied and depend on the AdV used. A review summarized the risks that could be considered for vectorized COVID vaxgenes (Baldo et al., 2021), and these include:

- Intrinsic harmful properties (causing damage, being toxic, causing allergies, and promoting tumour formation).

- Reconversion abilities of AdV through recombination, rearrangement, or complementation mechanisms between the replication-deficient AdV used as a vector and circulating AdV in the population, which could produce an unknown variant.
- Abilities for dissemination or elimination after administration, release to others through faeces or mucous membranes (known as shedding), biodistribution, and possible vertical transmission.

On the other hand, the risks related to the S gene sequence of SARS-CoV-2 that are inserted into the adenoviral vector of the vaxgenes are:

- Intrinsic harmful properties (causing damage, being toxic, causing allergies, and promoting tumour formation).

- Impact on host range, tropism, biodistribution, and elimination to others (Wang et al., 2003), especially when changes in the AdV surface occur due to genetic modifications.

- Impact of the insert on replication efficiency.

- Probability of recombination due to homology with circulating seasonal coronaviruses (Walls et al., 2020).

One of the risks of vectorized vaxgenes is the development of a condition known as thrombotic thrombocytopenia. The consequences of this process will be explained in more detail in section 6.2, but it's relevant to explain here that the phenomenon has already been described for vectorized vaxgenes after experimental challenges with cells and laboratory animals (Greinacher et al., 2021). In a pro-inflammatory environment, due to the electronegative surface charge of the hexon proteins of recombinant AdVs (Marietta et al., 2022), they can induce conformational changes in the PF4 molecule[208], leading to the formation of anti-PF4 antibodies, which can cause thrombotic thrombocytopenia (Marietta et al., 2022). The EDTA present in the vials (see section 1.1) also promotes capillary extravasation at the inoculation site (Gao et al., 2000), worsening inflammation. Extravasation allows viral and human proteins present in the vaxgene to enter the blood, as observed for other vaxgenes based on the same adenoviral vector used in AstraZeneca's product (Greinacher et al., 2021).

Immediately after the injection of the vectorized vaxgene, its components, which include around 50 billion AdV virions (Marietta et al., 2022), in addition to EDTA and more than 1,000 cellular and viral proteins (Greinacher et al., 2021), interact with platelets. Due to their negative electric charges, AdV hexon proteins can bind to platelets, replacing heparin and causing platelet activation, with the consequent release of PF4. The interaction of AdV proteins with PF4 causes conformational changes in this molecule and induces the generation of anti-PF4 antibodies that will bind to PF4 (Toh et al., 2022). This leads to the formation of aggregates of platelet-bound PF4 molecules, which together can reach over 120 nm in diameter (Greinacher et al., 2021). In other words, a large blood clot.

Along with the aggregates formed between PF4 and vaxgene components, viral proteins (Sallard et al., 2022), and human proteins derived from cell cultures are recognized by natural antibodies (Pfueller et

---

[208] Remember that PF4 is the acronym for plasminogen activating factor 4, as I mentioned in Chapter 2.

al., 1990), generating immune complexes, which, in turn, activate the complement system via the antibody crystallizable fraction receptor (Fcγ) [209], causing further tissue damage (Khandelwal et al., 2018), and activating monocytes and neutrophils, thus exacerbating an inflammatory cascade (Marietta et al., 2022). This, in turn, stimulates B lymphocytes to produce more antibodies against PF4.

The scenario I describe is similar to a well-recognized pathology. I am referring to heparin-induced immune thrombocytopenia (HIT, Greinacher et al., 2017). The cascade of events is sustained, activating more platelets that release more PF4 and communicate molecularly with neutrophils[210], generating a process called NETosis. NETosis occurs when the DNA of dying neutrophils is released into the extracellular space, where it binds to circulating PF4 and generates more complexes that recruit more anti-PF4 antibodies, culminating in massive activation of different immune cells and endothelial cells (Arepally and Oadmanabhan, 2021).

A natural way to regulate the process and avoid this cascade of events is the action of extracellular DNA-degrading enzymes since they eliminate NETs. This point is important because it has been observed that patients who developed vaxgene-induced thrombotic thrombocytopenia after receiving a dose of AstraZeneca's product had low activity of these enzymes (Greinacher et al., 2021). In this sense, it appears that the vectorized vaxgene can cause a cascade of events that culminate in a "molecular storm" within the blood vessels.

The result of the cascade of these pathological processes is clinically observed as a picture of thrombotic thrombocytopenia with a high risk of blood clot formation, which have been detected even in atypical sites, such as cerebral venous sinuses, splenic veins, and arteries (Marietta et al., 2022). In section 6.2, I will describe some of these clinical cases.

---

[209] The crystallizable fraction of antibodies is the 'tail' part of an antibody that interacts with the Fc receptors of various immune cells. It is the region of antibodies that activates the complement system and other immune processes.

[210] Cells of the immune system that are the first to arrive when there is a sign of damage, or a molecule associated with a microorganism considered pathogenic. They are the most abundant immune cells in the blood.

It's possible that the risk of platelet activation is higher for AstraZeneca's COVID vaxgene than for those of Janssen, Sputnik, and CanSino, because the adenoviral vector used in AstraZeneca (ChAdOx1) has a higher negative charge on the surface of its hexon proteins than AdV26 (used in Sputnik) and Ad5 (used in Janssen, CanSino, and Sputnik) (Marietta et al., 2022). If so, it could explain why the incidence of thrombotic thrombocytopenia post-vaccination seems to be higher in people who received doses of AstraZeneca than in those who received any of the other vectorized vaxgenes (Ledford, 2021).

It's worth noting that the prothrombotic events I have described so far occur independently of the Spike protein; they are due to the components of the vectorized vaxgene *before* it begins to operate within cells to generate the target protein (which is Spike protein in the case of COVID vaxgenes). It's not that the Spike protein cannot cause prothrombotic events (of course, it can! and I will explain it in the next section), but on their own, the components of the vials of vaxgenes based on adenoviral vectors can have pathophysiological effects, just like what I have described for synthetic mRNA. It's crucial to understand this fact because it implies that, beyond COVID, if vaxgenes with this same genetic technology are produced for other infectious or non-infectious conditions, they would have an intrinsic risk of harm that should not be ignored.

5.5 Pathophysiology of SARS-CoV-2 Spike protein

Vaxgenes based on synthetic mRNA or adenoviral vectors contain instructions to produce the complete Spike protein of SARS-CoV-2. This glycosylated protein[211], with a weight of 180 to 200 kDa[212] and a sequence of 1,273 amino acids, is present in all betacoronaviruses and is clustered on the virus surface in sets of three copies (Fig. 18).

[211] Process by which a protein is linked to a carbohydrate (typically a sugar molecule).

[212] A Dalton (Da) is the unit of atomic mass of a protein. One kilodalton (kDa) is 1,000 Da. The Spike protein, with a mass of 180 to 200 kDa has a molecular weight of 180,000 to 200,000 grams per mole.

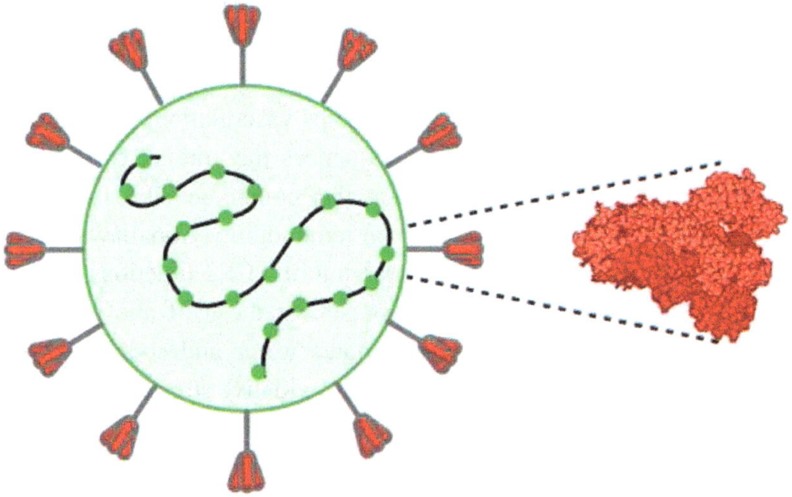

Figure 18. *SARS-CoV-2 Spike protein. The figure shows the basic structure of a SARS-CoV-2 virion with the Spike proteins protruding from its membrane. The dotted line shows the conformation of Spike trimers in their prefusion state.*

Each Spike copy is composed of two subunits: the S1 subunit and the S2 subunit, and in extracellular SARS-CoV-2 virions, these subunits are in a 'stable form', also known as the prefusion conformation. When the Spike protein interacts with its cellular receptor (angiotensin-converting enzyme 2, or ACE2), changes in the Spike structure occur, exposing the anchoring site of the S2 subunit. At this anchoring site is a part of the protein called the fusion peptide, which allows the SARS-CoV-2 virus membrane to fuse with the cell membrane to enter the cytoplasm and initiate its replication (Huang Y. et al., 2020).

The Spike protein is one of the most relevant virulence factors of SARS-CoV-2, implicated in some of the symptoms that constitute the clinical picture of severe COVID (Parry et al., 2023; Saadi et al., 2021; Theoharides and Conti, 2021). This is because when Spike binds to the ACE2 of vascular endothelial cells, it dysregulates the renin-angiotensin-aldosterone (RAA) axis (Trougakos et al., 2022a; Lei et al., 2021).

Before proceeding, it is relevant to explain a bit about ACE2 and its role in maintaining the homeostasis of the RAA axis. ACE2 is a zinc-dependent metalloproteinase that cleaves angiotensin II, generating angiotensin I (Imai et al., 2007). By doing so, it promotes vasodilation, regulates blood sodium concentration (natriuresis), influences the amount of fluid in the blood (diuresis), and facilitates actions that counteract fibrosis, oxidative stress, inflammation, and cardiovascular remodelling (Gopallawa and Uhal, 2014). In other words, adequate expression of ACE2 functions as a tissue protector. These functions are antagonistic to those of another enzyme, ACE, which is vasoconstrictive, promotes water and sodium retention, induces inflammatory responses, promotes oxidative stress, and contributes to cardiovascular remodelling (Patel et al., 2016). In balance, together, ACE and ACE2 regulate the RAA axis and modulate blood pressure and many other physiological functions (Zhang H. et al., 2020).

It is known that the Spike protein can dysregulate the RAA axis by decreasing the expression of ACE2. This occurs through the activation of intracellular signals by Spike when it is present in high quantities within the cytoplasm (Gao et al., 2022). By decreasing the expression of ACE2, it increases the concentration of angiotensin II in the blood, leading to an increase in blood pressure, osmotic balance disturbances, endothelial damage, and inflammation, which were described as clinical signs in patients with severe COVID (Zhang H. et al., 2020). Additionally, the S1 subunit of Spike, when present in moderate to high amounts within the cell, can alter the function of the blood-brain barrier, as demonstrated *in vitro* (Buzhdygan et al., 2020). This explains why some patients with severe COVID presented inflammation of the central nervous system (Lee et al., 2021; Rhea et al., 2021).

Regardless of the cascade effect produced by the Spike protein when inside the cell, there is another issue, and that is molecular mimicry. By this, I refer to the similarity of some domains of the Spike protein to human proteins found in the endothelial cell membrane. The resemblance between fragments of a foreign protein and human proteins is a problem because it increases the risk of triggering immune responses against our own proteins, leading to the subsequent destruction of the endothelium (Marino

Gammazza et al., 2020; Paladino et al., 2020), which would be an autoimmune response.

The similarity between the Spike protein and various human proteins has been investigated since 2020 (Adiguzel et al., 2021; Beaudoin, et al., 2021; Obando-Pereda 2021; Vojdani et al., 2021; Kanduc and Shoenfeld, 2020). It has been found that the Spike protein of SARS-CoV-2 has many regions whose amino acid sequence is identical to that of various human proteins (Kakoulidis et al., 2023; Kanduc 2023; Cuspoca et al., 2022; Khavinson et al., 2021). The regions with similarity include heptamers[213] and octamers[214] (Fig. 19).

Another study found that a part of the Spike protein with the sequence TQLPP[215] is identical to a part of thrombopoietin, a molecule essential for platelet production. The similarity is not only in terms of sequence but also in terms of structure and antibody-binding properties (Nuñez-Castilla et al., 2022). The antigenic similarity is very relevant because if an immune response against thrombopoietin is triggered due to exposure to the TQLPP of the Spike protein produced by the cells of those who receive the vaxgene, it could lead to thrombocytopenia. On the other hand, they also found that another part, ELDKY[216] of the Spike protein is very similar to several human proteins, including some related to platelet activation (human PRKG1 protein) and muscle contraction and relaxation (human tropomyosin protein). Triggering autoimmune reactions against these proteins could lead to heart disease and coagulation disorders (Nuñez-Castilla et al., 2022).

---

[213] Protein fragment composed of seven amino acids.
[214] Protein fragment composed of eight amino acids.
[215] Threonine-Glutamine-Leucine-Proline-Proline.
[216] Glutamic acid-Leucine-Asparagine-Lysine-Tyrosine.

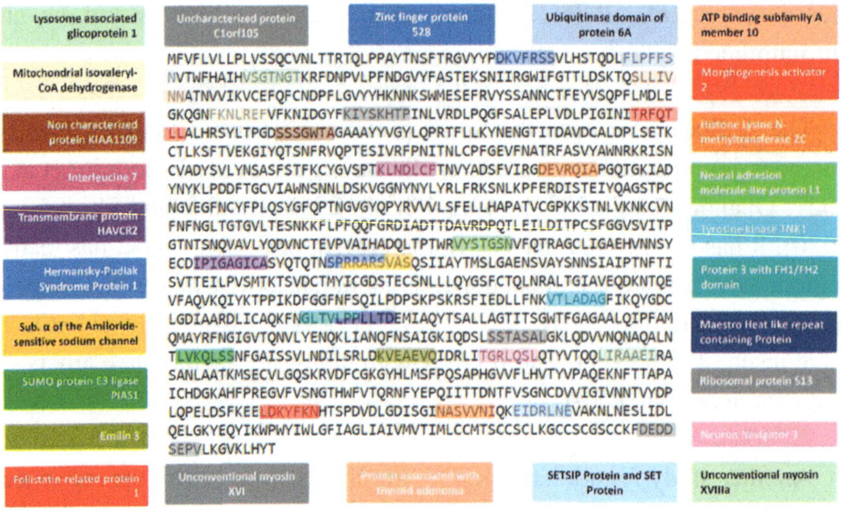

Figure 19. *Complete sequence of the amino acids that form the SARS-CoV-2 Spike protein (https://www.uniprot.org/uniprotkb/P0DTC2/entry). The boxes show the identities of human proteins that are homologous to the coloured sections in the Spike sequence, according to Khavinson and collaborators (2021).*

Other human proteins that show similarity to the Spike protein of SARS-CoV-2 are found in the nervous system (Cuspoca et al., 2022). Specifically, there are 39 proteins related to the functioning and homeostasis of axons and myelin, including phosphacan, the major proteoglycan of the extracellular matrix of the central nervous system that mediates communication between neurons and support cells of the nervous system[217] (Garwood et al., 2023), attractin, which is an important protein for the binding between neurons that is crucial for countering neurodegeneration (Paz et al., 2007), and teneurin 4, which regulates the differentiation of oligodendrocytes[218] and myelination of small axons (Suzuki et al., 2012). This led the authors of the study to call for a reconsideration of using the Spike protein as the target for COVID vaxgenes (Cuspoca et al., 2022). Unfortunately, despite the risk posed by such similarity for the development of neurodegenerative conditions due to autoimmunity, all countries

[217] These are cells that help neurons, either by providing them with nutrients, isolating them, or defending them. They are collectively known as glial cells.
[218] Cells that produce myelin for neurons in the central nervous system.

proceeded with the use of the Spike protein as the target for the vaxgenes and protein-based vaccines.

Let's recall that synthetic mRNA remains viable in the cell cytoplasm for a longer time than cellular mRNA (Fertig et al., 2022). Its presence has even been detected in the germinal centres of lymph nodes for up to 30 days (Krausson et al., 2023) or 60 days after vaccination (Röltgen et al., 2022). Therefore, it is not surprising that the self-production of the Spike protein by the cells of those who received a COVID vaxgene is greater than what occurs with most infections (Appelbaum et al., 2022). Its production is also much more prolonged than assumed at the time of emergency authorization for these products (Brogna et al., 2023; Krauson et al., 2023; Mörz et al., 2023; Samaniego-Castruita et al., 2023; Baumeier et al., 2022; Fertig et al., 2022; Magen et al., 2022; Röltgen et al., 2022). Additionally, as indicated in section 5.2, Spike protein production can occur in virtually all organs and tissues of the vaccinated individual's body.

This is because that protein is the most important virulence factor[219] of SARS-CoV-2 (Parry et al., 2023; Saadi et al., 2021). Physiological effects of Spike are not only on the RAA axis, as explained before, and can include the following effects:

1) Formation of blood clots through direct contact with cellular proteins (Trougakos et al., 2022a).

2) Marked pro-inflammatory effect by binding to Toll-like receptors 2 and 4 (TLR2 and TLR4)[220], activating the expression of the NF-κB transcription factor[221] (Kircheis et al., 2022; Khan et al., 2021),

---

[219] A virulence factor is that which most explains the effects it causes..

[220] Toll-like receptors 2 and 4 are proteins that are expressed in the cell membrane and play an important role in regulating the inflammatory process. Its activation leads to exacerbated local and systemic inflammation..

[221] The transcription factor NF-κB has the function of allowing the expression of genes that participate in innate and adaptive immune responses. Its activation induces, among other things, sustained inflammation.

affecting macrophage[222] function (Zhao et al., 2021), and damaging vascular endothelium (Robles et al., 2022).

3) Alteration of the transmembrane glycoprotein CD147[223], impacting red blood cells (erythrocytes) and heart pericytes[224], leading to haemolytic anaemia, blood hyperviscosity, and myocarditis (Al-Kuraishy et al., 2022; Avolio et al., 2021; Wang et al., 2020).

4) Binding to the oestrogen receptor (ER alpha) (Solis et al., 2022), potentially causing menstrual disturbances (Laganá et al., 2022).

5) Interaction with the tumour suppressor genes P53 and BRCA (Seneff et al., 2023; Singh and Singh, 2020) which increases the risk of cancer development.

6) Inhibition of the function of nicotinic acetylcholine receptors (α7nAChR) in the cholinergic nervous system[225] (O'Brien et al., 2023) due to similarity of Spike to neurotoxic proteins with affinity to α7nAChR receptors (Changeux et al., 2020). This can lead to disruptions in neuromuscular junctions and regulation of inflammation (Farsalinos et al., 2020).

There is an additional trait of SARS-CoV-2 Spike protein that warrants attention. I am referring to its prion and amyloid traits (Bhardwaj et al., 2023; Burnap et al., 2023; Cao et al., 2023; Chesney et al., 2023; Mir et al., 2023; Aksenova et al., 2022; Azzaz et al., 2022; Ma et al., 2022; Nyström and Hammarström, 2022; Seth and Sakar, 2022; Actis et al., 2021; Hsu et al., 2021; Liu S. et al., 2021). Amyloid proteins are characterized by the formation of aggregates, which are fibril structures associated with various degenerative and inflammatory diseases. To date, there are 36 proteins with

---

[222] Immune cells that specialize in the detection, phagocytosis, and destruction of bacteria and other microorganisms. After phagocytosing, they present the T lymphocytes with the fragments of the bacteria and other microorganisms they 'ate', which activates inflammation and ultimately leads to the generation of antibodies and cytotoxic responses.

[223] The CD147 protein is on the membrane of many cells, where it helps regulate cell division, programmed cell death (apoptosis), as well as tumour cell migration and metastasis.

[224] Pericytes are cells found on the inner wall of capillaries.

[225] The cholinergic nervous system includes neurons in the basal forebrain, cerebral cortex, and hippocampus. Cognition depends on the functioning of this cholinergic system.

an amyloid behaviour (Picken, 2020), although those that are more frequently associated with neurodegeneration are amyloid beta protein (β-amyloid), Tau and α-synuclein, which are associated with Alzheimer's disease, Parkinson's disease, and Lou Gehrig's disease or amyotrophic lateral sclerosis (Sengupta and Kayed, 2022), antibody light chains, which are associated with AL amyloidosis (Falk et al., 2016), transthyretin, which is associated with ATTR amyloidosis (Muchtar et al., 2021) and serum protein A, which is associated with AA amyloidosis (Deshayes et al., 2016). AL, ATTR and AA can affect the liver, kidneys, heart and intestine. In all cases, the functioning of that organ or system is altered.

Prions are a special type of amyloid protein, found mainly in the nervous system. They are characterized by misfolding and by inducing other proteins to misfold. There are various prion diseases that affect mammals, and in humans, the most common is Creutzfeldt-Jakob disease, that can be hereditary, due to somatic mutations, due to iatrogenesis (medical error) or by eating contaminated products (Uttley et al., 2020; Sigurdson et al., 2019). Invariably, these are diseases with progressive nervous deterioration that leads to death within a short time after diagnosis (Sikorska et al., 2012).

Given that a domain (that is, a section) of the SARS-CoV-2 Spike protein shares characteristics with prions, it is reasonable to consider the possibility that sustained exposure to Spike could lead to neurodegeneration due to misfolding of proteins in the central nervous system (Seneff et al., 2023; Tetz and Tetz, 2022). This could contribute to explaining the unusually high number of neurological events reported in individuals who have received the vaxgene, as indicated by international adverse event monitoring platforms (see section 6.3).

The risk of prion-like diseases resulting from cerebral exposure to the Spike protein was raised in early 2021. It was discovered that the Spike protein of SARS-CoV-2 contained a prion-like domain, absent in the Spike protein of SARS virus (the coronavirus that appeared in 2002; Stadler et al., 2003). The presence of this prion-like domain in the Spike protein of SARS-CoV-2 was suggested to contribute to some of the neurological signs and symptoms observed in individuals infected with SARS-CoV-2 (Tetz and

Tetz, 2022), a suggestion later corroborated by an independent publication (Seneff et al., 2023).

The implication of the Spike protein containing prion-like domains is significant, as all but two of the emergency-use authorized COVID immunization products are based on the Spike protein. This includes vaxgenes, which instruct our cells to produce the protein (such as Pfizer, Moderna, AstraZeneca, Janssen, Sputnik, and CanSino vaccines) or vaccines that are based on pre-made Spike protein (such as Novavax and Soberana vaccines). Therefore, almost all COVID vaccines and vaxgenes carry the risk of prion-like diseases developing in the vaccinees. The risk is even higher for COVID vaxgenes, as the self-production of Spike in vaccinated individuals lasts at least six months (Brogna et al., 2023).

Additionally, the Spike protein has been found to modify the production and release of exosomes from the cell (Mishra and Banerjea, 2021). Exosomes are membrane-bound vesicles containing cellular products, including microRNAs[226]. These microRNAs travel to different organs and tissues, including the brain and spinal cord, initiating severe pro-inflammatory immune responses (Mishra and Banerjea, 2021). This occurs because when exosomes enter nervous system cells, they suppress the expression of a gene known as ubiquitin peptidase 33, disrupting the levels of another gene, interferon regulatory factor 9, crucial for inflammation and antiviral responses. This, in turn, activates a cascade of events orchestrated by the transcription factor NF-κB (Kircheis et al., 2022; Khan et al., 2021).

5.6 Pathophysiology of undeclared contaminating nucleic acids

Evidence is mounting that COVID vaxgenes, particularly those using synthetic mRNA, contain degraded RNA and double-stranded RNA (Tinari, 2021; Thacker, 2021), as well as fragments of DNA, including DNA plasmids (McKernan et al., 2023), possibly due to methodological errors or quality issues during the manufacturing process (Baiersdörfer et al., 2019; Karikó et al., 2011), as mentioned in section 1.4.

---

[226] Specifically, they contain microRNAs miR-148a and miR-590.

The news that degraded RNA had been found in Pfizer vaxgenes in quantities greater than those reported for batches used in clinical trials raised concerns because even slight degradation of synthetic mRNA molecules in the vaxgene can halt or slow down the efficiency of protein translation (in this case, the Spike protein of SARS-CoV-2), reducing its expected effectiveness (Crommelin et al., 2021). Considering what I've explained in section 5.5, it is reasonable to suggest that a decrease in the efficiency of translating the Spike protein in the cells of vaccinated individuals might not be a bad idea. Still, as this book does not focus on the effectiveness or lack thereof of COVID vaxgenes, I won't delve further into the consequences of degraded RNA in synthetic mRNA vaxgenes (Tinari, 2021).

However, what is relevant to this book is the presence of double-stranded RNA in mRNA vaxgenes, which unequivocally reflects issues in the manufacturing of synthetic mRNA vaxgenes and, consequently, deficiencies in the quality control process. This is because one of the most common contaminants when generating synthetic mRNA and not adequately purifying the synthetic mRNA molecules is precisely double-stranded RNA (Baiersdörfer et al., 2019; Karikó et al., 2011). The presence of double-stranded RNA in vials is concerning because, if it enters cells, it can trigger cellular and molecular reactions leading to severe inflammatory states (Shao et al., 2018). This effect has been well-known for a long time; it is, in fact, part of the vertebrate innate immune responses and is highly effective against viral infections (Kawai and Akira, 2008; Samuel 2001), if it is modulated correctly. Once double-stranded RNA is detected by pattern recognition receptors, it initiates a cascade of molecular events that activate the expression of type I interferon (Thoresen et al., 2021), which, in turn, activates various immune cells that collectively generate inflammation (Kang and Tang, 2012). The inflammatory response generated against double-stranded RNA is so potent that synthetic analogues, such as polyinosinic-polycytidylic acid (Poly I:C), have been used as adjuvants in some vaccines (Hafner et al., 2013). The problem with the potent inflammatory response induced by double-stranded RNA is that if it persists in cells or is administered exogenously, it can cause sustained pro-inflammatory reactions and even lead to autoinflammatory and autoimmune conditions, such as lupus erythematosus, as experimentally demonstrated in a study with mice receiving the synthetic double-stranded RNA analogue (Steinberg et al., 1969). Unfortunately, this adverse effect has not prevented its continued use, and there is ongoing preclinical research on a sublingual vaccine against SARS-CoV-2 containing Poly I:C (Yamamoto et al., 2023).

We must remember that synthetic mRNA vaxgenes contain lipid nanoparticles (NPL) that, due to their electrical and biochemical properties, surround nucleic acids. Therefore, not only synthetic mRNA but also double-stranded RNA would be surrounded by these nanoparticles, easily entering the vaccinated individual's cells and initiating pro-inflammatory molecular cascades. This means that the presence of double-stranded RNA in the vials would be an additional mechanistic explanation, not exclusive, possibly acting synergistically with other mechanisms described earlier (see section 5.3 and section 5.5) that explain the reported autoinflammatory and autoimmune disorders as adverse events (see section 6.5). Furthermore, since the presence of double-stranded RNA in Pfizer's and Moderna's vaxgenes reflects quality control issues during manufacturing, it could also explain variations in the numbers of adverse events disproportionately associated with some batches of vaxgenes and not others, as explained in Chapter 3.

In addition to double-stranded RNA, the presence of plasmid DNA used in the production of synthetic mRNA vaxgenes is highly relevant (McKernan et al., 2023). Based on different genetic and molecular techniques, copies of the plasmid used in Pfizer's and Moderna's vaxgenes could be identified. It was observed that the plasmid found in Pfizer's vials contains a 72 bp sequence corresponding to the enhancer of the SV40 virus genome (Lednicky and Butel, 2001), a primate polyomavirus[227] associated with an increased risk of developing various types of cancer (such as primary brain tumour, lymphoma, bone cancer, and malignant mesothelioma) in laboratory animals and humans (Vilchez and Butel, 2004). The 72 bp fragment of the SV40 promoter found in the vials belongs to non-coding regulatory regions of the SV40 genome, covering the virus's

[227] Despite the name, polyomaviruses have nothing to do with the polio virus. That is an enterovirus and has a small, RNA genome, while polyomaviruses are DNA. You can read more at ViralZone Expasy [Internet]. Available at: https://viralzone.expasy.org/148?outline=all_by_species

replication initiation site, as well as the virus promoter and enhancer. This enhancer, 72 bp in size, is known as the "minimal transcriptional enhancer" (MTE) of the virus (Firak and Sybramanian, 1986).

It is crucial to note that the tumorigenic properties of SV40 are primarily attributed to one of its genes, from which a protein known as the 'large T antigen' (T-ag) is expressed, essential for the virus to complete its replication cycle. The T-ag protein of SV40 alters cell cycle control and inhibits the tumour suppressor proteins of the cell (Sullivan and Pipas, 2002; Sáenz-Robles et al., 2001). These actions of T-ag help explain the tumorigenic properties of SV40 (Vilchez and Butel, 2004). I mention this because it was not the T-ag gene that McKernan and colleagues found but the MTE. However, the presence of MTE in the vials is also concerning because its sequence has a nuclear localization signal that allows it to traverse the nuclear membrane, even in cells not in mitosis (Prasad and Rao, 2005; Dean et al., 1999). This characteristic is precisely why this region of the SV40 genome is included in plasmids constructed for use in gene therapy (Vacik et al., 1999), as it helps foreign DNA enter the cell nucleus (Prasad and Rao, 2005). Another reason for using the MTE of SV40 is that it promotes the expression of the desired gene for a more extended period (Wang et al., 2016). The elements contained in the plasmid used by Pfizer in its vaxgenes would indeed be used for gene therapy due to their efficient expression in mammals (Makrides, 2003).

There are various safety issues associated with the plasmid DNA found in synthetic mRNA vaxgenes:

1) By persisting for an extended period in the cytoplasm due to its stability, foreign DNA could cause anaphylactic reactions (Kurth, 1995), as well as lead to the generation of anti-nuclear antibodies against double-stranded DNA (Pisetsky et al., 2022; Donnelly, 1997). This may contribute to the development of systemic lupus erythematosus (Pisetsky, 2016).
2) Foreign DNA can enter the nucleus, where it interacts with the DNA of the chromosomes of the cells it entered and can integrate into their genome (Bai et al., 2017). While the risk might be low (Ledwith et al., 2000), regulatory agencies acknowledge that the

risk exists (Klinman et al., 2010). It was indeed one of the arguments used to 'validate' the use of synthetic mRNA to manufacture vaxgenes. I quote Pardi and colleagues (2018, page 1571) verbatim: "*Compared with other nucleic acid-based systems, mRNA combines several other positive attributes, including the lack of integration into the host genome...*" and another quote from Pardi (2018), who wrote the review most used to argue that synthetic mRNA vaxgenes are safe: "*In vaccinated individuals, the theoretical risks of infection or vector integration into the host cell's DNA are not a concern for mRNA. For these reasons, mRNA vaccines have been considered a relatively safe vaccine format*" (Pardi et al., 2018b, page 274).

The key issue to consider is that the genomic integration of a plasmid is not a *theoretical* risk. The mechanism of action of DNA-based gene therapy is, precisely, its insertion into the genome, although attempts are made for it to integrate in an orderly manner at a specific site, either eliminating the defective gene or inactivating its expression (Kaufmann et al., 2013). However, sometimes it integrates elsewhere, causing a genetic debacle that can be catastrophic. In the words of Sadelain (2004, page 569), "*Insertional mutagenesis is an inevitable consequence of the transposition of genetic material. Whether involving an integrative virus, a transposable element, a replication-deficient vector, or plasmid DNA, ectopic chromosomal integration is a mutagenic event that can alter chromatin or genetic structure, thereby affecting gene transcription, its regulation, and/or coding sequences*". '*Well, OK; but, in practical terms*' - some might think – '*Where is the evidence of genetic integrations of plasmid DNA used in gene therapy?*' Well, for starters, the FDA itself is aware of this evidence. In June 2022, the FDA held a meeting on "*the risk of insertional oncogenesis with Eli-cel, Lovo-cel, and Beti-cel*", which, despite their somewhat playful names worthy of a comic, are gene therapy drugs with very serious and formal names (elivaldogene autotemcel, lovotibeglogene autotemcel, and betibeglogene autotemcel). These medications were recently approved by the FDA to treat cerebral adrenoleukodystrophy, sickle cell anaemia, and transfusion-dependent β-thalassemia, respectively[228]. The FDA's Advisory Committee on Gene, Cell, and Tissue Therapies reported a 98% rate of DNA integration of the Eli-cel product into the Ectopic Viral Integration Site 1 gene (EVI1, also known as MECOM), located on human chromosome 3q26.2 (Liu and Tirado, 2019), which could explain at least three cases of myelodysplastic syndrome in the 67 volunteers who received it. It was not the only gene in which this unwanted insertion occurred, although it was the most common. You can see more details by consulting the Advisory Committee's report[229].

If genetic integration of the plasmid DNA found in the vials of Pfizer's vaxgene occurs, it could lead to *i*) a silent insertion (one that causes no changes) if it inserts into a non-coding region (Kurth, 1995), *ii*) limited or absent effects if silenced by cellular elements causing its methylation or cleavage, *iii*) cell death if it inserts into essential genes, *iv*) insertional mutagenesis, i.e., the activation of proto-oncogenes or inactivation of tumour suppressor genes that can lead to cancer (Langer et al., 2013; Medjitna et al., 2006), and *v*) chromosomal instability caused by DNA breaks and genetic rearrangements (Dunbar and Larochelle, 2010).

It is known that plasmid DNA can enter the nucleus, although only 1% to 10% of plasmids transfected into the cytoplasm achieve this (James and Giorgio, 2000). In the case of Pfizer vaxgene, the finding by McKernan and colleagues (2023) was replicated by Speicher and colleagues (2023) using a broader sample of vials and different batches. This implies that those who receive these vaxgenes are at risk of genomic integration, as the plasmid contains the SV40 promoter, including an enhancer fragment with nuclear localization signals that increase the entry of the plasmid into the nucleus (Dean et al., 1999), thereby opening the possibility of integration into the cellular genome, either randomly or by homologous recombination. This latter possibility is plausible due to the similarity between some sequence

[228] National Organization for Rare Disorders. Sickle Cell Disease [Internet]. Available at: https://rarediseases.org/rare-diseases/sickle-cell-disease/

[229] Cellular, Tissue, and Gene Therapies Advisory Committee (CTGTAC) Meeting FDA, June 6, 2022 [Internet]. Available at: https://www.fda.gov/media/159130/download

fragments of the Spike gene and human genes (see section 5.5), which increases the chances of recombination when the plasmid enters the cells.

In section 5.3, I presented evidence that synthetic mRNA can activate the expression of LINE-1, allowing the retrotranscription of synthetic mRNA into DNA and entry into the nucleus (Aldén et al., 2023), with the potential for integration and causing insertional mutagenesis, chromosomal instability, and DNA damage. The plasmid found in Pfizer and Moderna vaxgenes could generate the same effect even without the need to have first activated LINE-1. These are not mutually exclusive mechanisms; rather, they are two different mechanisms that can cause similar consequences, thereby increasing the risk of the previously described health alterations.

Finally, considering that the fate of plasmid DNA in the cell when injected into animals is unknown (Medjitna et al., 2006), and due to the widespread biodistribution of NPLs in the vaccinated individual's body (see section 2.3), the consequences of plasmid presence in synthetic mRNA vaxgenes could occur in any organ. It is essential to consider that, given the biodistribution of NPLs, if the plasmids from these vaxgenes were to enter the gametes (ovules and sperm) of a vaccinated person, they could cause changes in these cells with the potential to be inherited by their offspring (Glenting and Wessels, 2005), as acknowledged by the EMA[230],, and as has been experimentally demonstrated in rats (Gallot et al., 2002).

5.7 Pathophysiology of contaminating cellular proteins

In section 1.4 I explained that one of the various contaminants that has been detected in vials of the COVID vaxgene from AstraZeneca are cellular and viral proteins (Krutzke et al., 2022). '*Wait a second!*'– some might argue – '*is it not normal that there are viral proteins if these vaxgenes are based on a virus?*'. Very astute, but the thing is that what has been detected are unbound, free viral proteins, that are not a part of the adenoviral vectors that make up the vaxgene. With a proteomic analysis of the vials, one would

---

[230] European Medicines Agency: Report from the *ad hoc* meeting of CPMP Gene Therapy Expert Group. 2003, 23–24 January 2003. EMEA-5382-03-Final [Document]. Available at: https://www.ema.europa.eu/en/documents/committee-report/committee-medicinal-products-human-use-chmp-february-2003-plenary-meeting-monthly-report_en.pdf

expect to find the four external proteins of the adenovirus (hexon, penton, protein III1 and fibre protein; see Kulanayake and Tikoo, 2021). The problem is that the analysed vials have a different protein pattern to what is expected (Fig. 20), including adenoviral non-structural proteins, such as DNA binding proteins (DBP), an unidentified 52/55 kDA protein and an unidentified 10 kDA protein. Up until this moment, the only thing that could be inferred about the finding would be that the vaxgenes were not well purified. Adenoviral DBP proteins are antigenic to humans (meaning that we generate immune responses against them) (Guo et al., 2013). The consequence of generating immune responses against these proteins would be that the effectiveness of the following doses of these vaxgenes would probably be lower. However, the presence of human cellular proteins is much more worrying. This is because they can lead to autoimmune responses (see section 6.5).

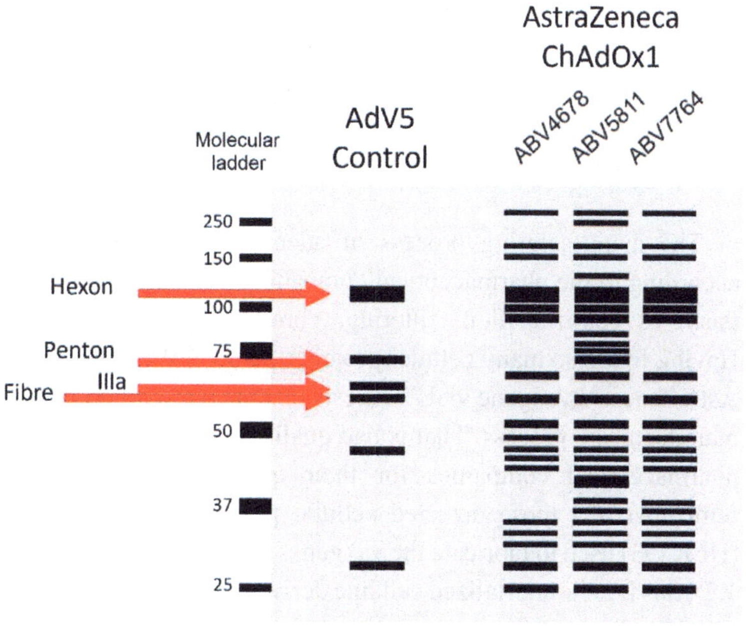

Figure 20. *Proteins found in AstraZeneca's vaxgene vials. On the far left you can see the banding pattern expected if the vials contained only adenovirus (AdV) virions (AdV5 Control), and the banding pattern of the three lanes corresponds to proteins detected in three vials from different lots. Figure based on Krutzke et al., 2022.*

It would be wholly understandable for you to think that, as these are cellular proteins, and we have immune tolerance towards our own proteins and antigens (except for some in the crystalline, sperm and myelin as they are 'sequestered antigens' that were never presented to our lymphocytes; Forrester et al., 2018), the fact that they were detected in AstraZeneca's vaxgene vials should not cause any concern. However, immune tolerance is specific to each tissue (Matsumoto et al., 2020) and depends on our proteins being intact. When they are, in general, even if they are injected, we would not expect an immune response against them. I mean that, if we try to 'immunize' an individual with its own proteins (autologous proteins), we should not normally get an immune response against them (Unanue et al., 2016). However, if the protein is denatured or altered, then it is likely that an immune response against it occurs, which can lead to an autoimmune disease. This is known since at least 70 years ago, when rabbits were injected with denatured autologous thyroglobulin and an autoimmune thyroiditis ensued (Weigle, 1965). Similar results were found when injecting encephalitogenic protein to rabbits (Swanborg and Radzialowski, 1970). Exposure to autologous proteins that are altered or denatured are one way in which an autoimmune reaction can occur (Yin et al., 2013).

The manufacturing process of adenovirus-based vaxgenes includes, according to the pharmaceutical companies, physical purification methods (such as centrifugation, filtering, chromatography and ultrafiltration). Having found so many cellular proteins, some of the in high abundance, in AstraZeneca's vaxgene vials suggests that the purification failed during the manufacturing process. That is bad quality control! But beyond failing the pharmaceutical companies for their quality control issues, we must remember that those detected cellular proteins come from the cell line (HEK293) used to fabricate the vaxgenes. As I explained earlier (see section 1.2), this is an immortalized cell line derived from human embryonic kidney cells. The issue is that being immortalized cells, there are differences with normal cells. For instance, there are unique amino acid variations in some of their proteins that can affect their folding (Choong and Sung, 2022). In other words, alter them. As I mentioned above, it is not a good idea to be exposed to altered self-proteins because this can lead to autoimmunity (Zhang et al., 2019; Atassi and Casali, 2008).

On the other hand, proteins can become altered if heated or cooled relative to ambient temperature (Pastore et al., 2007). These changes affect the secondary and tertiary structure of the proteins, which means they denature. This is why vaccines, antibodies, enzymes and any drug based on proteins must be stored and distributed without breaking the cold chain (Chen et al., 2017). Exposure to denatured proteins is one of the mechanisms that increases the risk of losing T-regulatory (T-reg) lymphocytes' tolerance to these proteins (Goswami et al., 2022). A clear example of this is an experiment carried out on mice that showed that those that were immunized with autologous denatured insulin generated immune responses against it (Thomas et al., 1989).

To date, there does not appear to be any published study about the rates at which the human cellular proteins detected in AstraZeneca's vaxgene vials denature (Krutzke et al., 2022). Despite the WHO having recommended that AstraZeneca include in the public documentation of its vaxgene that it must be kept between 2°C and 8°C for a maximum of six hours, the pharmaceutical company preferred to include a statement that there was no problem with maintaining their product at 30°C for six hours at a time when mass vaccinating. If we consider that many non-industrialized countries are located at mid latitudes with high environmental temperatures and that it is difficult to maintain the cold chain during vaccination campaigns, it is not unreasonable to consider that there is a high probability that in many countries those vials were kept at more than 30°C for more than six hours. If so, this could cause a certain amount of protein degradation within the vials[231].

Among the human cellular proteins that have been detected in AstraZeneca's vaxgene using mass spectrometry (Krutzke et al., 2022), one is of particular interest if we wish to understand one aspect of their plausible pathophysiology. I mean the autoantigenic nuclear sperm protein (NASP, for its acronym in English) can be found in the supplementary material file[232] of the study by Krutzke and colleagues (2022). The NASP protein

---

[231] Abcam Inc. [Internet]. Available at: https://www.abcam.com/help/protein-stability-tips-and-tricks

[232] The file contains a list of proteins detected by mass spectrometry in vials from three batches of AstraZeneca's vaxgene. Supplementary material from Krutzke et al., 2022. Elife [Internet]. Available

(with identifications P49321, Q5T624, E9PI86, H0YF33, H0YDS9, and E9PPQ8) was detected in the analysed vials from batches AVB4787, ABV5811, and AVB7764, ranking fifteenth in abundance among the 1238 detected human cellular proteins. It is a protein that transports histone proteins[233] into the nucleus to stabilize chromosomes (Richardson et al., 2006). There are two isoforms of the NASP protein, encoded by the NASP gene[234]. The somatic isoform (NASPs), consisting of 421 amino acids, is expressed in all dividing cells (mitotic cells, such as lymphocytes and epithelial cells), and the testicular isoform (NASPt), consisting of 773 amino acids, is expressed by testicular cells and embryonic tissue (Richardson et al., 2000). In the testicles, the NASP protein is expressed in different locations of germ cells during spermatogenesis: in the cytoplasm of spermatocytes, in the nucleus of sperm cells, and in the periacrosomal[235] region of mature spermatozoa (Fig. 21). The function of the NASP protein is essential for the normal development during embryo formation (Fin et al., 2012).

Given the data presented in the supplementary material in Krutzke and colleagues' study (2022), that reports a 788 amin acid sequence, it stands to reason that the isoform detected in the vials is the testicular isoform. The little problem that NASPt was detected in the vials analysed is that if autoantibodies against this protein are generated, it can lead to male infertility (Chereshnev et al., 2021; Lu et al., 2008). For you to get an idea of the relevance of this possibility, more than three decades ago, induction of autoimmunity via inoculation of NASPt in 'infertility vaccines' was considered as a viable option. This is because the blood-testis barrier makes the testicles be an 'immune privileged' tissue (Fijak and Meinhardt, 2006). This is precisely what makes many of the proteins expressed late in spermatogenesis be 'sequestered antigens'. Furthermore, many of the auto

at: https://cdn.elifesciences.org/articles/78513/elife-78513-fig2-data1-v2.xlsx. Downloaded October 15, 2023.

[233] Histone proteins bind to DNA, and they help chromosomes have an adequate structure. They also help regulate gene expression..

[234] Uniprot. NASP protein. [Internet]. Available at: https://www.uniprot.org/uniprotkb/Q99MD9/entry

[235] The acrosome is a structure that covers the frontal part of the head of a sperm cell. It contains hydrolitic and protein-degrading enzymes that the sperm cell uses to penetrate the ovule.

antibodies against NASPt are generated after a testicular infection or trauma, or after vasectomy (Batova et al., 2000).

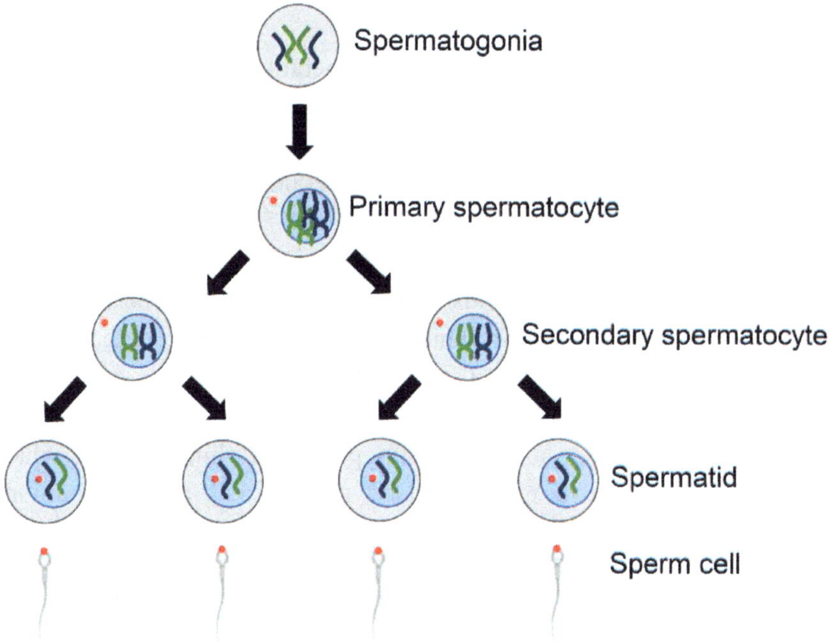

Figure 21. *Stages of spermatogenesis. Red dot shows the place where NASPt is expressed.*

The impact of immunization with NASPt on fertility was investigated experimentally on mice. One group of female mice was injected with a fragment of autologous NASPt, and another with a fragment of synthetic human NASPt. Both groups of mice generated high levels of anti-NASPt antibodies. Female mice that had been vaccinated against NASPt had lower fertility when mating fertile male mice. This was because anti-NASPt antibodies prevented the union between the sperm and the ovule, as well as the fusion of the gametes (Wang et al., 2009). This coincides with what had been described earlier for women with anti-NASP antibodies, as they had significantly lower implantation and pregnancy rates (Kikuchi et al., 2003). Additionally, in men, the presence of anti-NASPt antibodies is associated, together with antibodies against other testicular proteins, to infertility due to autoimmunity (Chereshnev et al., 2021). Given all that I have explained, it is not unreasonable to postulate the possibility that the presence of NASPt, both native as degraded, could increase the risk of infertility in those who received this vaxgene.

It is worth mentioning that the risk of generating anti-NASP antibodies is not exclusively related to fertility; they can also increase the risk of developing autoimmune diseases due to anti-nuclear antibodies, such as systemic lupus erythematosus (Batova et al., 2000).

To end this chapter, I want to specify that it is possible that the detected proteins are present in a few vials of this vaxgene, and that perhaps it is a small fraction of vaccinees in which these effects occur, if they do so. However, we cannot ignore it as a possible mechanism of damage, especially considering some of the adverse events and abnormalities reported in monitoring systems and in published clinical cases, which encompass reproductive problems (see section 6.4) and autoimmune problems (see section 6.5), among others.

5.8 Repeated mono antigenic stimulation

All blood cells are produced in the bone marrow of long bones, including lymphocytes, of which there are two main lineages: B lymphocytes and T lymphocytes. When these are produced they are 'naive' cells that migrate to peripheral lymph nodes throughout the body. They are naive because they have yet to contact a specific foreign antigen or an altered self-antigen[236]. Once they do so, they are activated and differentiate into effector cells, roughly seven to 10 days after the start of the acute infection or after vaccination (Henning et al., 2018). To differentiate, lymphocytes need to integrate multiple molecular signals that are communicated by other immune cells. These signals lead activated lymphocytes to become mitotic (that is, to start dividing), thus generating thousands of identical copies, or clones. Most of these clones will be effector cells that will participate in the

---

[236] Remember that antigens are small fragments of proteins, lipids or carbohydrates that cells show (present) to other cells. This process is essential to trigger adaptive immune responses, which involve the production of antibodies and the activation of T lymphocytes.

immune response against a specific antigen, and part of the clones will become memory cells that will remain in the bone marrow of the long bones (Henning et al., 2018). Those lymphocytes that become memory cells acquire the ability to renew and to re-enter mitosis without the need for antigenic stimulation (Kurachi, 2019). This is a normal process pertaining to all vertebrates that, like us, have true jaws (Flajnik, 2014; Kasahara and Sutoh, 2014).

B lymphocytes are the only cells that, when activated, synthesize antibodies[237] against specific antigens. To do this, they need to establish a molecular "dialogue" with a subpopulation of T lymphocytes, known as T helper cells (or, more formally, as $CD4^+$ T lymphocytes). The other important subpopulation is that of the cytotoxic T lymphocytes ($CD8^+$ T lymphocytes) that are essential to detect antigens that are presented to them by different cells throughout the body[238]. If they recognize these antigens as foreign or self but altered, they will destroy these cells. This is an important way to control and resolve viral infections, intracellular bacterial infections and to destroy cancer cells (Reina-Campos et al., 2021).

When chronic infections cause repeated and constant antigenic stimulation or when cancer leads to constant expression of altered antigens, the normal response program of memory $CD8^+$ T lymphocytes changes (McLane et al., 2019; Hashimoto et al., 2018). As a consequence of this change, they progressively lose their ability to function, alter their metabolism, and decrease their ability to clonally expand their population (Gallimore et al., 1998). Eventually, they start expressing receptors that inhibit their action and become unable to migrate to tissues in response to signals (Hsiung et al., 2023). The set of these events is known as lymphocyte exhaustion (Verdon et al., 2020).

There is experimental evidence that repeated exposure of $CD8^+$ T lymphocytes to the same antigen precisely leads to this state of exhaustion

---

[237] Secreted proteins that bind to antigens on the surface of viruses or bacteria and thus activate different immune responses that end up resolving a disease process associated with these microorganisms.
[238] That is, they display them through proteins known as the MHC (Major Histocompatibility Complex) that they have in their membrane. MHC proteins associate with antigens that are inside the cell.

and lymphocyte senescence (Li and Chen, 2019; Ventura et al., 2017; Ferris et al., 2014), and this can also happen with B lymphocytes (Illingworth et al., 2013). We could then think that antigenic stimulations caused by the vaxgenes have the same risk as antigenic stimulations caused by exposure to specific microorganisms. However, unlike what happens during an infection by a virus or bacteria, where the adaptive immune system is exposed to many diverse antigens of the microorganism (Pandey et al., 2022; Grifoni et al., 2021), vaxgenes induce the production of a single protein, and this is expressed for months, as mentioned in section 5.5 (Brogna et al., 2023; Krauson et al., 2023; Mörz et al., 2023; Samaniego-Castruita et al., 2023; Baumeier et al., 2022; Fertig et al., 2022; Magen et al., 2022; Röltgen et al., 2022). That means the foreign antigen will intensely and persistently activate specific lymphocyte activities against it (Seneff et al., 2022; Townsend et al., 2022). The result is chronic mono antigenic stimulation, which can lead to lymphocyte exhaustion. There is even experimental evidence from studies with mice that repeated stimulation with a traditional attenuated or inactivated vaccine can alter the balance between protective immune responses and induce lymphocyte exhaustion (Johnson et al., 2011). In this case, it's not a single antigen, but several, but repeated stimulation with these same antigens in a short time simulates a scenario that would not occur naturally.

Another mechanism by which vaxgenes can impact immune function is the induction of a class switch in immunoglobulins (Irrgang et al., 2023). The class switch is a process that occurs within B lymphocytes and is key for the maturation of the antibody-based immune response (Senger et al., 2015). What happens is that when B lymphocytes are activated (i.e., they 'realize' that there are antigens they react to), these cells can change the expression of the immunoglobulin class (also known as isotype). This means changing from producing IgM (immunoglobulin M) to IgG, IgE, IgA, or IgD.

To facilitate the class switch of immunoglobulin, a DNA recombination event occurs within the nucleus of lymphocytes. This event is unique—it happens nowhere else in the body except in lymphocytes! Recombination refers to a change in the genetic segments carrying information for the constant region of the heavy chain (Xu et al., 2012). So, it's the genes of the heavy chain that determine which class of immunoglobulin will result.

Immunoglobulin IgG can exist in four different subclasses: IgG1, IgG2, IgG3, IgG4. Among these, IgG1 is generated in response to the presence of soluble and membrane antigens, making it the most common subclass produced in response to a viral infection. In contrast, IgG4 is produced when there has been repeated or prolonged exposure to the same antigen. This typically doesn't occur (we usually resolve infections quickly, and it's not common to be infected with the same pathogen many times once we have developed immunity), with exceptions such as gastrointestinal parasite infections. In these cases, due to their recurrence and our less efficient immune response (we resemble those worms too closely, making it challenging for our immune system to differentiate between them and us), we often reach immune tolerance and stop mounting a strong response against them. The shift of an activated lymphocyte from producing IgG1 to IgG4 is mediated by a cytokine (interleukin 10 or IL10). The presence of IgG4 signals immune tolerance.

An experimental study detected and quantified the IgG subclasses in individuals who had received three doses of the COVID vaxgene (Irrgang et al., 2023). The findings were significant and worrying: 10 days after the second dose of Pfizer's synthetic mRNA vaxgene, the IgG4 levels increased and remained high, rising even further after the third dose. IgG4 is an antibody of tolerance, not for antigen elimination. Moreover, the accumulation of IgG4 can lead to a pathological condition characterized by fibrosis in various tissues, which may result in organ failure and death (Dassanayaka et al., 2023; Spandorfer et al., 2023).

The results from Irrgang and colleagues' study provide clear evidence that the vaxgene alters the immune response of those vaccinated, shifting it towards tolerance. In other words, there is no longer a reaction when exposed to SARS-CoV-2. Additionally, IgG4 increased in abundance in the blood with each administered dose, further enhancing tolerance. The authors of the study reported that the class switch to IgG4 takes a few months to occur after lymphocyte maturation. Interestingly, the phenomenon of immunoglobulin class switching did not occur in people who received AstraZeneca's vaxgene, suggesting that it is something triggered by synthetic mRNA and not solely due to the constant presence of the Spike protein in the body (Irrgang et al., 2023).

Unfortunately, to date, the possibility of lymphocyte depletion due to repeated doses leading to a mono antigenic stimulus has not been studied for COVID vaxgenes. The lack of evidence that repeated doses of vaxgenes do not increase the risk of lymphocyte depletion led the European Medicines Agency to express its doubts about the justification for administering a fourth booster dose[239]. Similar to many other risks associated with the vaxgenes, this pronouncement was ignored. According to official WHO data as of September 16, 2023, 64.85% of the world's population (equivalent to 5,170,000,000 people) had received the complete vaccination scheme[240]. Additionally, since mid-2021, some countries began offering booster doses, and by December 31, 2021, over 500 million booster doses had been administered to various countries (of high and upper-middle socioeconomic status), representing up to 15% of the daily doses given to their populations (Bert et al., 2022). This occurred despite a lack of evidence that receiving additional doses was safe or even necessary (Kunal et al., 2021). As of September 16, 2021, according to WHO data, 35% of the global adult population had received at least one additional booster dose[241]. In April 2023, the FDA authorized a second booster for Pfizer's second vaxgene (the bivalent one), implying that in the United States, some people have received the two doses of the original vaccination schedule, plus the booster (third dose), plus the bivalent vaxgene (fourth dose), plus the bivalent booster (fifth dose), all in just under 2.5 years. Since most vaccinations have been carried out using vaxgenes and most countries' authorized boosters were synthetic mRNA vaxgenes, it can be estimated that nearly a billion humans have been repeatedly exposed to the same

---

239 Reuters. "EU drug regulator expresses doubt on need for fourth booster dose". 11/01/2022 [Internet https://www.reuters.com/business/healthcare-pharmaceuticals/eu-drug-regulator-says-more-data-needed-impact-omicron-vaccines-2022-01-11/; https://www.larepublica.co/globoeconomia/la-ue-advierte-que-los-refuerzos-repetidos-podrian-debilitar-el-sistema-inmunologico-3285008

240 Our World in Data. [Internet]. Data updated to September 16 2023. Available at: https://ourworldindata.org/explorers/coronavirus-data-explorer

240 Our World in Data. [Internet]. Data updated to September 16 2023. Available at: https://ourworldindata.org/explorers/coronavirus-data-explorer

241 Our World in Data. [Internet]. Data updated to September 16 2023. Available at: https://ourworldindata.org/explorers/coronavirus-data-explorer

antigen (Spike protein) in a short period. Considering the lack of profound understanding of the impact of vaxgenes on the regulation of immune function and the absence of a single study on the medium-term and long-term effects of receiving multiple doses in a short time, it becomes necessary to question the possibility that lymphocyte depletion could occur in some individuals.

Potential lymphocyte depletion in people who received doses of Pfizer's or Moderna's vaxgenes would be a complex and multilateral process. This is because not only do they sustainably produce the Spike protein, but the synthetic mRNA of the vaxgene itself impacts several cascades within the cell, leading to a greater risk of developing autoinflammatory states, with constant activation of innate immune responses (Acevedo-Whitehouse and Bruno, 2023; Seneff et al., 2022). There is also a possibility of decreasing adaptive immune responses (Seneff et al., 2022; Volloch and Volloch, 2021), as I explained in section 5.2. If this occurs, in the long run, the immune responses of people who have received these doses would be affected in different ways.

The consequence of a state of lymphocyte exhaustion due to mono antigenic hyperstimulation would be an increase in the risk of various pathological processes occurring, including a greater predisposition to infections and a greater probability of developing cancer. It should be noted that, to date, there has not been a single experimental or observational study that evaluates the possibility of lymphocyte depletion and immune dysregulation with repeated doses of vaxgenes.

5.9 '*Shedding*' or vaxgene elimination with the possibility of transmission to others

One of the most frequent questions asked by people who have understood the relevance of all the pathophysiology mechanisms of vaxgenes is: '*Can vaxgenes be transmitted from a vaccinated person to an unvaccinated person?*'. A valid answer is '*it is not known*', because this possibility has not really been studied (see section 2.3). However, it seems to me that the question requires a more in-depth analysis before discarding the issue due to lack of information.

Firstly, it is necessary to define what vaccine elimination (a phenomenon known as 'shedding') refers to. In section 1.3 I explained the differences between a vaccine and a vaxgene. Let us remember that attenuated vaccines contain microorganisms that are viable but have been forced to replicate in difficult conditions, so they should not cause disease but rather stimulate a protective immune response. Attenuated vaccines are used with the intention that the copies of the virus or bacteria they contain reproduce (or replicate[242], in the case of viruses), but without causing the disease. However, since they are viable, their offspring can be transmitted to others if they are eliminated from the body of the vaccinated, and there is the possibility that during this reproduction or replication, the vaccine microorganisms have reacquired their traits of virulence[243]. This is well known for some attenuated vaccines, such as the Sabin oral poliomyelitis ('polio') vaccine (Okayasu et al., 2011).

Children vaccinated with the Sabin oral vaccine will be infected with the attenuated virus for weeks (up to seven weeks; Chorin et al., 2023). This means that the attenuated virions of the polio-associated virus replicate in the intestinal cells of the vaccinated child and will be eliminated in their faeces for some time (Altamirano et al., 2018; Martinez et al., 2004). Consequently, other children who did not have immunity acquired by natural infection or by vaccination and that are exposed to the vaccine virions contained in the faeces of vaccinated children (through contaminated water or food, for example), can become infected with the vaccine virus and acquire immunity against it. That is, attenuated vaccines are transmitted to others because the microorganisms within them remain viable. However, by continuing to replicate, attenuated virions of the polio-

[242] The difference between reproducing and replicating goes beyond semantics. All organisms, from bacteria to whales, reproduce. This means creating a new individual from another. This can be achieved by sexual or asexual reproduction. If sexual, two individuals participate to create one or more progeny. If asexual, a single individual creates progeny. However, replication is different. It is done by non-cellular organisms; namely, viruses. During replication, the virus that entered a cell disassembles until only its instructions (genetic material) is left, and this is used as the blueprint so that the cell in which it entered makes more copies of the virus. Thus, with replication, new individuals are not created from another one; rather, the cell they are in makes them from the original genetic material of the virus.

[243] Virulence is the degree of damage that is observed in a host. It can be a trait of the microorganism that infected the host, or it can be due to the response of the host (i.e. virulence can be due to an exaggerated immune response against a microorganism).

associated virus can 'revert to pathogenicity'. This occurs when they acquire one or more mutations during their replication process and become like the wild type virus again. In that case, instead of the virions that appear in the faeces of vaccinated children potentially immunizing other exposed children without causing problems, they can cause the disease that was sought to be prevented (Burns et al., 2004). This has already happened and has caused outbreaks of vaccine polio in about 40 countries, most in Africa and Asia (Alipon et al., 2022; Alleman et al., 2021; Tseha 2021), but also in England, the United States and Israel (John and Dharmapalan, 2022).

Although it is the best known case, the attenuated vaccine against the virus associated with poliomyelitis is not the only one in which the elimination of vaccine virions occurs. It has also been reported for attenuated vaccines against rubella (Detels et al., 1971), against rotavirus gastroenteritis (Hsieh et al., 2014) and against influenza (Jackson et al., 2020), among others.

In contrast to attenuated vaccines, the elimination of vaccine virions does not occur in inactivated vaccines, since the bacteria or viruses they contain are not viable, if the inactivation process has been carried out correctly (Green and Humadi 2017).

Now, what do we know about the elimination of active compounds found in the vaxgenes from a vaccinated person to others? Remember that as we established in section 1.3, vaxgenes *are* gene therapy. According to the FDA[244], the elimination of gene therapy products is defined as: "*The removal of bacterial or viral gene therapy products from the patient by any or all of the following routes: excreta (faeces), secretions (urine, saliva, nasopharyngeal fluids, etc.), or through the skin (pustules, lesions, wounds)*". The FDA emphasizes in the same document the importance of studying the elimination of gene therapy-based products: "*Elimination studies should be conducted for each virus- or bacteria-based gene therapy or oncolytic product to provide information on the possibility of*

[244] US Food and Drug Administration "Design and Analysis of Shedding Studies for Virus or Bacteria-Based Gene Therapy and Oncolytic Products" [Internet]. Available at: https://www.fda.gov/regulatory-information/search-fda-guidance-documents/design-and-analysis-shedding-studies-virus-or-bacteria-based-gene-therapy-and-oncolytic-products

transmission to untreated individuals since historical data alone may not predict the elimination profile." (Page 3).

In the case of vaxgenes based on adenoviral vectors, i.e., recombinant adenoviruses (AdV), if these vectors are truly replication-deficient (see section 1.3), the risk of transmission to others through their elimination is reduced. Note that I wrote '*the risk is reduced*'; I did not write '*there is no risk*'. This is because two scenarios can explain the potential elimination and transmission of adenoviral vectors from a vaccinated person to an unvaccinated person, even if the AdV are replication-deficient:

1) That the genetic modification of recombinant AdV to make them replication-deficient was not adequately done. There is evidence that at least one brand of this type of COVID vaxgene had non-replication-deficient AdV in the vials (Moutinho and Wadman, 2021); see section 1.1.

2) That the AdV from the vaxgene recombine with wild-type AdV (Shenck-Braat et al., 2007). There are more than 100 species of AdV in humans (Omidi et al., 2022), and they circulate widely in the population. Furthermore, the phenomenon of recombination easily occurs, even between human adenoviruses and animal adenoviruses when they coinfect a cell (Lockett and Both, 2002). This homologous recombination[245] would restore the replicative capacity of the vaxgene AdV (i.e., it would become competent for replication again).

In both scenarios described above, individuals who received one or more doses of this type of vaxgene could indeed eliminate recombinant AdV and thereby 'vaccinate' others.

It is also essential to consider that AdV uses the Coxsackievirus and Adenovirus receptor (CAR), as well as some glycoproteins (GD1a) and desmoglein 2, among others (Stasiak and Stehle, 2020). These are very common cellular receptors (Vogels et al., 2003), making it easy for AdV to

[245] Homologous recombination is a mechanism by which two DNA molecules that are compatible are swapped. Viruses can use this mechanism when they coinfect the same cell.

infect various cell types, whether the cells are dividing or not (Lai et al., 2002). This is precisely why they have been considered useful for use as gene therapy vectors (Havenga et al., 2002).

Adenoviruses generally transmit in a faecal-oral manner, and virions of AdV can be eliminated in the faeces for a long time (Vogels et al., 2003). So, considering that after intramuscular administration of the vectorized vaxgene, virions are distributed to various organs (see section 5.2), it is not unreasonable to suggest the possibility that those who received vaxgenes based on recombinant AdV could transmit these virions to others as they eliminate them for weeks in secretions and excretions[246].

At the time of writing this book, I am not aware of any studies that have determined whether AdV from COVID vectorized vaxgenes are detectable in the saliva, urine, faeces, semen, or breast milk of vaccinated individuals. However, there are studies conducted on other gene therapy products that use recombinant AdV as replication-deficient vectors. Out of 50 publications investigating the elimination phenomenon, in 42% (21 studies), no vector elimination was observed when the drug was administered intra-arterially, intramuscularly, intranasally, or by inhalation, nor by intrapleural, intravitreal, intratumoural, and intramyocardial routes (reviewed by Shenck-Braat et al., 2007). In contrast, in 58% (29 studies), the presence of vector DNA or infectious virions was reported in various excretions, depending on the route of administration and the post-inoculation time at which the measurement was taken. Saliva and nasopharyngeal fluids from patients who had received gene therapy intranasally or by inhalation frequently eliminated virions or vector DNA (reviewed by Shenck-Braat et al., 2007), up to 90 days after a single application of the product (Griscelli et al., 2003). Other administration routes did not seem to have a high risk of shedding of the gene therapy drug.

In the case of vectorized vaxgenes, according to information published by the FDA on January 8, 2020, AdV virions can be shed in faeces for up

---

[246] Secretion is the release of substances, both useful and harmful, from cells and the body. Breast milk would be the product of a secretion; There are also secreted elements in saliva. Excretion is the process of removing waste or waste from the body. Urine, faeces and sweat are examples of excretions.

to 28 days[247]. Furthermore, in 2007, a critical review was published on the possibility of vector virion shedding (Shenck-Braat et al., 2007). I include the exact quote from this review due to its importance: "*A major environmental safety concern for the use of a viral vector for gene therapy is the potential for vector spillage into the environment via patient excretions. This phenomenon is called shedding. Depending on national regulations on the use of genetically modified organisms, shedding is a significant issue in the regulatory application process for a gene therapy clinical protocol. If gene therapy is considered a deliberate release of a genetically modified organism into the environment, the clinical investigator must conduct an environmental risk analysis on the likelihood of shedding and its potential consequences*". How is it possible that these studies have not been conducted? Could it be that evidence emerged between the publication of this review and the emergency authorization of COVID vectorized vaxgenes, indicating that virion elimination was not a problem?

Based on what we know thanks to studies that were performed on other gene therapy drugs that are based on recombinant AdV (not vaxgenes), it is possible for these virions to be eliminated and the risk seems to be taken seriously by the regulators that authorized or approved the drugs based on this technology. Let's see some examples of non-immunizing gene therapy in which recombinant virions or their DNA have been found to be eliminated for a long time:

1) Nadofaragene firadenovec-vncg (brand name: Adstiladrin; used to treat refractory bladder cancer). According to the FDA, which approved the gene therapy in January 2023, it is a replication-deficient recombinant Adenovirus (AdV) containing the human interferon-alfa 2b gene (IFNα2b). In the product information document[248], it is mentioned in section 5.2 that there is a risk of disseminated adenovirus infection, especially in immunocompromised individuals (including those undergoing

[247] Centres for Disease Control and Prevention. Vaccine Information Statement (VISs). Adenovirus VIS [Internet]. Available at: https://www.cdc.gov/vaccines/hcp/vis/vis-statements/adenovirus.html
[248] Food and Drugs Administration. Highlights of prescribing information. Adstiladrin. [Internet]. Available at: https://www.fda.gov/media/164029/download?attachment

immunosuppressive therapy). This risk is attributed to "*the possibility of low levels of replication-competent adenovirus*". Individuals with immune system deficiencies "*should not come into contact with Adstiladrin*". The document also indicates that after the administration of Adstiladrin, human IFNα2b protein is detectable in urine, and AdV DNA is found in blood and various tissues (liver, kidneys, and gonads). Preclinical trial animals had AdV vector DNA in the bladder on days 8 and 98 (seven days after the first and second doses, respectively), and one animal had AdV vector DNA in the kidney even on day 148 after exposure. Studies of biodistribution and elimination of Adstiladrin were also conducted in humans, revealing that most patients had AdV DNA in urine 12 days after the administration of Adstiladrin. Finally, the product document states that patients and their caregivers should be informed that transient and low-level elimination of Adstiladrin (i.e., recombinant AdVs) in urine may occur, and they "*should disinfect urine with chlorine in the toilet for 30 minutes before flushing*".

2) Voretigene neparvovec (brand name: Luxturna; used to treat vision loss due to inherited retinal dystrophy). This gene therapy drug, approved by the FDA in June 2022, does not use an AdV but a recombinant adeno-associated virus (AAV[249]). According to the FDA, each dose contains 150 billion virions and is administered intraocularly. The product information document[250] states, "*Transient and low-level vector shedding may occur in the patient's tears. Patients and caregivers should be advised to handle dressing material, tears, and nasal secretions properly, which may include storing waste material in sealed bags before discarding them in the trash. These precautions should be followed for 14 days after the*

---

[249] AAV adeno-associated viruses are satellite viruses with a genome that is made up of a single strand of DNA of 4.7 kb. They are unable to replicate unless a 'helper' virus, such as adenovirus or herpesvirus, is present. AAVs are used for gene therapy because they generate a poor immune response, integrate into the genome and do not cause systemic damage (Fragkos et al., 2008). Comparatively with AdVs, AAVs are chosen when we want to have a low level of genetic expression for a longer time, and when the therapeutic gene is small, because they have less space in their genome. They can be inserted into the genome of cells in a targeted manner (Lai et al., 2002).

[250] European Medicines Agency. Luxturna Product Information [Document]. Available at: https://www.ema.europa.eu/en/documents/product-information/luxturna-epar-product-information_en.pdf

administration of voretigene neparvovec. It is recommended that patients and caregivers use gloves to handle dressings and trash, especially under conditions of pregnancy, lactation, or caregiver immunodeficiency. Patients treated with Luxturna should not donate blood, organs, tissues, or cells for transplantation".

3) Onasemnogene abeparvovec-xioi (brand name: Zolgensma; used to treat spinal muscular atrophy caused by a mutation in the survival motor neuron 1 gene, SMN1). The drug was FDA-approved in October 2023. According to information about this drug[251], recombinant AAV virions are eliminated in faeces, urine, and saliva between two weeks and two months. The FDA recommends that, given the "*temporary elimination of the ZOLGENSMA vector primarily occurs through bodily excretions*", caregivers of patients should "*properly handle the patient's faeces*", "*procedures including sealing disposable diapers in plastic bags before throwing them away are recommended*", instructions on "*proper hand hygiene when in contact with patient bodily waste*" should be given to caregivers and family members, and "*these precautions should be maintained for one month after* [administering] *the ZOLGENSMA infusion*".

4) Valoctocogene roxaparvovec-rvox (brand name: Roctavian; used to treat severe congenital haemophilia A[252]). This drug, FDA-approved in June 2023 for use in the United States, is essential to mention. According to information presented by the regulatory agency about this drug[253], recombinant AAV virions from this drug are eliminated in saliva, semen, faeces, and urine for an extended period. Although the maximum concentration of vector DNA in blood was observed up to nine days post-injection, elimination continues steadily in excretions and secretions. According to the product information, "*In patients from two clinical trials, vector-encapsulated DNA (potentially transmissible) was detectable in plasma up to 10 weeks*

---

[251] Food and Drugs Administration. Highlights of prescribing information. Zolgensma. [Internet]. Available at: https://www.fda.gov/media/126109/download?attachment

[252] Haemophilia is a genetic condition that prevents coagulation from occurring properly.

[253] Food and Drugs Administration. Highlights of prescribing information. Roctavian. [Internet]. Available at: https://www.fda.gov/media/169937/download?attachment

after ROCTAVIAN administration". The FDA document also indicates that all patients stopped having vector DNA in semen at 36 weeks, and the maximum time for vector DNA to no longer be detectable in semen was 12 weeks. It is alarming that the maximum time to stop having detectable DNA (of the vector) was eight weeks in urine, 52 weeks in saliva, and 131 weeks in faeces. Yes, you read that correctly: 131 weeks.

5) Delandistrogene moxeparvovec-rokl (brand name: Elevidys; used to treat cases of Duchenne muscular dystrophy (DMD) with a confirmed mutation in the DMD gene). This drug, FDA-approved in June 2023, uses a recombinant AAV as a gene vector. According to the FDA, vector DNA can be found in serum, excreta, saliva, faeces, and urine[254]. Although the maximum average concentration is reached at 5 hours in serum, 7 hours in saliva, 6 hours in urine, and 14 days in faeces, the average time for the vector DNA to no longer be detectable is 63 days in serum, 50 days in saliva, 123 days in urine, and 162 days in faeces. The FDA recommends that caregivers and patients "*be careful to wash their hands when in contact with patient bodily waste, and that materials contaminated with bodily waste be placed in sealed bags before disposal for one month after receiving the Elevidys intravenous infusion*".

6) Etranacogene dezaparvovec-drlb (brand name: Hemgenyx; used to treat cases of congenital haemophilia B due to factor IX deficiency). This drug, FDA-approved in November 2022, uses a recombinant AAV as a gene vector. According to the FDA[255], the vector elimination study showed that vector DNA was detectable in blood, saliva, nasal secretions, semen, urine, and faeces. The maximum observed time for the vector DNA to no longer be found was 22 weeks in urine, 26 weeks in saliva and nasal secretions, 40 weeks in faeces, 52 weeks in semen, and 159 weeks in blood (three years). In the clinical efficacy study, at 24 months after receiving Hemgenyx,

---

[254] Food and Drugs Administration. Highlights of prescribing information. Elevidys. [Internet]. Available at: https://www.fda.gov/media/169679/download?attachment

[255] Food and Drugs Administration. Highlights of prescribing information. Hemgenyx. [Internet]. Available at: https://www.fda.gov/media/163467/download?attachment

56% (30 out of 54) of subjects stopped eliminating vector DNA in the blood, and 69% (37 out of 54) stopped eliminating vector DNA in semen. The FDA thus indicates that "*vector distribution in the blood and vector elimination in semen and other excretions and secretions may occur post-infusion. It is unknown how long this will continue. Patients should not donate blood, organs, tissues, or cells for transplants*".

In other words, the FDA has taken seriously the risk of elimination-transmission of recombinant AdV virions and recombinant AAV virions, which form the basis of gene therapy drugs that they have approved for use. It's great that they acknowledge the importance of this risk. However, I find it challenging to understand how the world's most important regulatory agency could recognize the significance of this risk in drugs intended for treating rare conditions[256], while seemingly having no concern about the same risk when authorizing AdV vectorized vaxgenes against COVID to be used in the global population, including children, and in both healthy and sick individuals. Could it be that they didn't care because they lacked data on potential elimination and the possibility of transmission to others? Something like '*if I don't see it, it doesn't exist*'? Furthermore, not only will there be few potential users of these gene therapy products because, as mentioned earlier, they are for rare conditions, but even fewer people will use them since they cost between $850,000 and $3.2 million per treatment[257]. In comparison, COVID AdV vectorized vaxgenes have been administered (with the cost subsidized by each country) to billions of people. In the European Union alone, nearly 100 million doses of this type of vaxgene have been administered at the time of writing this book; in

[256] Rare diseases are those that occur in fewer than 1 in 2,000 people. Source: Eurordis [Internet]. Available at: https://www.eurordis.org/information-support/what-is-a-rare-disease. To put it into numbers, Duchene muscular dystrophy affects 2.9 out of every 100,000 boys (Crisafulli et al., 2020), spinal muscular atrophy is even less common: it affects one in every 10,000 children born alive (Lally et al., 2017), hereditary retinal dystrophy affects one in every 1,380 children (Ben-Yosef, 2022).
[257] Forbes. "Non-Profit Says $850,000 Gene Therapy Is At Least Twice As Expensive As It Should Be" [Internet]. Available at: https://www.forbes.com/sites/matthewherper/2018/01/12/non-profit-says-850000-gene-therapy-is-at-least-twice-as-expensive-as-it-should-be/?sh=4d8d2574b979; The New York Times. "A dilemma for governments: How to pay for million dollar therapies" [Internet]. Available at: https://www.nytimes.com/2023/01/24/health/gene-therapies-cost-zolgensma.html#; ABC News "$2.9 million gene therapy for severe haemophilia is approved by FDA" [Internet]. Available at: https://abcnews.go.com/Health/wireStory/gene-therapy-severe-hemophilia-approved-fda-100508758#; Sarepta prices Duchenne gene therapy at $3.2M [Internet]. Available at; https://www.biopharmadive.com/news/sarepta-duchenne-elevidys-price-million-gene-therapy/653720/

Canada, just over three million; in the United States, nearly 19 million. Latin American countries opted for this type of vaxgene more than others: in Argentina, more than 43 million doses were purchased; in Peru, more than 8 million doses; in Ecuador, 5.5 million doses; in Chile, 1,236,465 doses; in Mexico, almost 105 million doses. That's a lot of doses! According to the latest update from WHO, UNICEF, and the World Bank, 2,073,005,334 doses of AstraZeneca, Janssen, Sputnik, and CanSino COVID vaxgenes have been sent to more than 100 countries worldwide[258]. If we consider that an average of two doses has been administered per person, we would be talking about more than a billion people who have received two doses of these products. How can regulatory agencies not be at least a little concerned about the risk of elimination-transmission of recombinant AdV virions when they would be administered to more than an eighth of the world's population?

It is true that the intramuscular administration route has comparatively less risk of viral elimination than other administration routes for adenoviral vectors, such as inhaled, intranasal, intravenous, and intraperitoneal routes (Tiesjema et al., 2010). However, remember that if precautions are not taken to prevent the vaccine from reaching a blood vessel during its application (see section 5.2), the contents of an intramuscular injection can reach the bloodstream (Merchant, 2022). When gene therapy based on recombinant AdV is administered through the bloodstream, between 10,000,000,000 and 1,000,000,000,000 viral particles have been detected in urine, rectal swabs, and oral swabs, and up to 10,000,000,000 viral particles in semen (reviewed in Tiesjema et al., 2010). Therefore, if the AstraZeneca, Janssen, Sputnik, or CanSino COVID vaxgenes were to enter a blood vessel when injected into the deltoid muscle of the arm, it would be plausible for the vaccinated individual to eliminate recombinant AdV in faeces, urine, saliva, semen, and breast milk.

Of course, it is unlikely that *all* individuals who received a AdV vectorized vaxgene would eliminate recombinant AdV to others (Lichtenstein and Wold, 2004), but we cannot rule out that it is a possible

---

[258] IMF-WHO COVID Vaccine Supply Tracker, UNICEF COVID Vaccine Market Dashboard, and IMF staff calculations. Data updated to January 2022 [Internet]. Available at: https://www.imf.org/en/Topics/imf-and-covid19/IMF-WHO-COVID-Vaccine-Tracker

scenario. Although specific studies will be necessary to determine if elimination occurs, how frequently transmission is happening in the population, and what it represents for public health, it is not unreasonable to consider it as a risk for this type of vaxgene.

In the case of vaxgenes based on synthetic mRNA, as explained in section 1.1, these do not contain any virus. Therefore, it would not be possible for viral elimination to occur. One might think this settles the discussion. However, before saying '*then there can be no shedding and transmission of synthetic mRNA vaxgenes*', we need to remember that these products contain genetic material wrapped in lipid nanoparticles (LNP), and these particles are distributed to virtually all organs in the body (see section 5.2). If shedding were to occur in those who received a synthetic mRNA vaxgene (Pfizer, Pfizer bivalent, Moderna, or Moderna bivalent), it would involve the active compound, i.e., the modified synthetic mRNA wrapped in LNP.

Let's examine the available evidence regarding the *possibility* of transmission of LNP and synthetic mRNA compounds:

1) In the report of the partial results of Pfizer's clinical trials evaluated by regulatory agencies, it was indicated that 50% of ALC-0159 and approximately 1% of ALC-0315 are excreted in the faeces for 14 days after intramuscular administration of a dose (in experiments conducted with rats)[259].

2) In the report of the partial results of Pfizer's clinical trials evaluated by regulatory agencies, it is indicated that the presence of the vaxgene could be detected in the salivary glands, bladder, skin, and uterus (see section 5.2), which could imply elimination through urine, sweating, and genital secretions.

---

[259] Centres for Disease Control. CDC 2021-0034-1148. Pfizer COVID vaccine. [Document]. Available at: https://downloads.regulations.gov/CDC-2021-0034-1148/attachment_1.pdf

3) In the protocol of its phase 3 clinical trial[260], Pfizer excluded individuals who were exposed to its vaxgene through skin contact or inhalation of vaccinated individuals. Specifically, investigators were required to report 'environmental exposures'. For Pfizer, environmental exposures included the following cases: "*Male participants who are receiving the study intervention* [i.e., the vaxgene] *or have discontinued study participation and have exposed a female partner before or around the time of conception; female family member or healthcare provider who reports being pregnant after exposure to the study intervention through inhalation or skin contact; male family member or healthcare provider who has been exposed to the study intervention through inhalation or skin contact and subsequently exposes his female partner before or around the time of conception; women who are breastfeeding while being exposed to the study intervention* [...] *through inhalation or dermal contact*". These indications cannot be interpreted as evidence that synthetic mRNA from the vaxgene is excreted through exhalation, sweat, and semen, and has the potential to be transmitted to others, but it is noteworthy that they explicitly made these indications to the investigators in the clinical trial protocol. What can be interpreted from the clinical trial protocol is that any close contact, from sexual contact to skin contact and exhalation, with someone who received the synthetic mRNA vaxgene has the potential for transmission of this active compound (Banoun, 2022).

4) A study showed that in 13 lactating women who had received two doses of the synthetic mRNA vaxgenes, low amounts of partially degraded synthetic mRNA could be detected up to 45 hours after vaccination. It was found in extracellular vesicles in breast milk. However, it is worth mentioning that when HT-29 cells were exposed to these vesicles, the expression of the Spike protein was not induced (Hanna et al., 2023).

[260] SARS-CoV-2 mRNA Vaccine (BNT162, PF-07302048). 2.6.4 Summary statement of the pharmacokinetic study [Document]. Available at: https://ia902305.us.archive.org/28/items/pfizer-confidential-translated/pfizer-confidential-translated.pdf

At the time of writing this book, we lack available information on shedding studies for any synthetic mRNA drug (intended for gene therapy or immunization) that would allow us to assess that risk. This is even though the first gene therapy products based on synthetic mRNA were tested on cells (in *in vitro* experiments) in 1996 (Boczkowski et al., 1996). To date, there are more than 30 registered clinical trials evaluating gene therapies based on nanolipids and liposomes[261] containing synthetic mRNA (reviewed in Lorentzen et al., 2022), with at least three of them administered intramuscularly, similar to synthetic mRNA vaxgenes. However, none of these trials are evaluating the possibility of the elimination of synthetic mRNA in excretions and secretions, and I could not find a single preclinical study that assessed this risk in animal models. This is despite the identified risk and the recommendation that these studies be conducted (Vervaeke et al., 2022). Undoubtedly, we are walking blindly on the gene therapy highway, which is problematic when considering that synthetic mRNA technology is proposed to be the "unlimited future" of medicine (Damase et al., 2021).

Finally, there is the possibility that the Spike protein, generated by cells that received the synthetic mRNA vaxgene or the AdV from vectorized vaxgenes, can be transmitted to others through excretions or secretions to unvaccinated individuals or other vaccinated individuals. Remember that there is already evidence that the vaxgene-induced Spike protein is produced for months in some people who received these products (see section 5.5). If a vaccinated person produces high amounts of the Spike protein for an extended period, it will mean that individuals in contact with their excretions and secretions *may* experience some of the adverse events related to the Spike protein's pathophysiology, whether vaccinated or not (Parry et al., 2023).

Up to the time of writing this book, and to the best of my knowledge, no study had been published on potential shedding of the AdV vectorized vaxgene, synthetic mRNA vaxgene, or of shedding of self-produced Spike protein from a vaccinated person to an unvaccinated person. What we have are testimonials, both from the general public and from doctors, reporting

---

[261] A liposome is a series of cationic lipids that associate with RNA due to their electrical polarity.

cases of unvaccinated individuals experiencing various effects, such as general discomfort, headache, fatigue, fever, nausea, diarrhoea, skin rashes, epistaxis (nosebleeds), and uterine bleeding after cohabiting with individuals who had recently received one or more doses of COVID vaxgenes.

It is difficult to understand how the risk of vaccine shedding vaxgenes, which would be used in billions of people, was not taken seriously, not only as an 'option' but in many countries as a mandate. In February 2022, COVID vaccination was mandatory in Austria, Costa Rica, Ecuador, Italy, Greece, Malaysia, Micronesia, Indonesia, Tajikistan, Turkmenistan, and the Vatican[262], and it was mandatory for doctors and other healthcare professionals in most countries, while in other countries such as Australia, New Zealand, and most countries in Europe, North America, Asia, and Latin America, COVID vaccination was required to work, attend university, use sports facilities, enter cinemas, restaurants, museums, and travel, which meant a kind of *de facto* requirement for those who wanted to carry out their activities and keep their jobs (Mtimkulu-Eyde et al., 2022).

We have covered a lot of material in this chapter, and I know that there are many complex concepts for the non-specialized public, but it is essential that the different mechanisms through which damage can occur at the cellular level, with an impact on tissues, organs, and the complete system. Only in this way can the following chapter, in which I describe the main adverse events that have been associated with COVID vaxgenes, be understandable.

To make what has been learned in this chapter easier, I have included a summary of the damage mechanisms known to date for each of the components of vaxgenes, and you can see it on the next page (Table 3).

---

[262] Statista [Internet]. Available at: https://www.statista.com/chart/25326/obligatory-vaccination-against-COVID/

Table 3. *Summary of the mechanisms that underlie the pathophysiology that explains the diverse clinical presentations in some who received the COVID vaxgenes*

Component	Pathophysiology	Vaxgene
PEG	Anaphylaxis (severe allergy).	Pfizer Moderna
Polisorbate 80	Hypersensitivity, allergy and anaphylaxis.	AstraZeneca Janssen Sputnik Cansino
Synthetic mRNA	↑ expression of IFN-I leading to a proinflammatory antiviral state (this can cause systemic inflammatory conditions), ↑ expression of transcription factors for various immune molecules increasing the proinflammatory state, ↓↑ expression of microRNAs, ↑ expression of LINE-1 with the risk of integration, DNA strand breaks, genomic instability, altered ribosomal structure and cancer	Pfizer Moderna
AdV (vector)	Allergies, tumors, reversion to virulent wild type virus, ↑ coagulation (risk of thrombotic thrombocytopenia).	AstraZeneca Janssen Sputnik Cansino
Spike protein	Deregulation of the RAA axis (changes in blood pressure, endothelial damage, inflammation, reproductive cycle), autoimmunity due to molecular mimicry with human proteins, procoagulant effect, changes in CD147 expression, with harmful effects on the heart, binding to estrogen receptor alpha, with impact on the menstrual cycle.	Pfizer Moderna AstraZeneca Janssen Sputnik Cansino
Human cellular proteins (contaminants)	Risk of autoimmunity, with impact on the nervous and reproductive system.	AstraZeneca Janssen Sputnik Cansino
Double strand RNA (contaminant)	Sustained inflammation, risk of autoimmunity .	Pfizer Moderna
Plasmid with SV40 promoter (contaminant)	Risk of nuclear insertion, risk of chromosomal instability, risk of carcinogenic transformation.	Pfizer

Chapter 6. Main adverse effects associated to COVID vaxgenes

It is dangerous to be right when those in power are wrong.

Voltaire

In the previous chapter, I presented and explained the biological mechanisms through which COVID vaxgenes can cause molecular and cellular-level alterations, leading to various clinical conditions grouped into four categories: *i*) sustained inflammation and autoinflammation, *ii*) autoimmunity, *iii*) cell degeneration, and *iv*) genomic instability and uncontrolled cell proliferation (Fig. 22). Once this is understood, the high number of diverse types of adverse events occurring is no longer so mysterious. These can, in turn, be grouped by organs and systems, as I will do below. The clinical conditions I describe are not the only ones reported, but I selected the most relevant ones, either due to their frequency or severity. From my perspective, once the mechanisms by which COVID vaxgenes can contribute to these conditions are understood, there is no justification for a lack of knowledge in identifying these health issues.

In section 2.15, I described how regulatory agencies determined that COVID vaxgenes showed an adequate safety profile based on partial results presented by pharmaceutical companies. Reports did not find differences in adverse events recorded between the group that received vaxgenes and the placebo group (Baden et al., 2021; Falsey et al., 2021; Logunov et al., 2021; Sadoff et al., 2021; Polack et al., 2020). However, an independent analysis of the same data from studies of Pfizer's vaxgene (Polack et al., 2020) and Moderna's vaxgene (Baden et al., 2021) showed that if *the number of events* in each group is contrasted instead of *the number of people* who had adverse events in each group, the situation is very different, as the risk of adverse events in the vaccinated group was higher (Fraiman et al., 2023). It is the same data presented by the manufacturers of the vaxgenes to regulatory agencies; the only thing that changed is the factor for analysis, from the 'number of people who had adverse effects in each group' to the 'number of adverse effects reported in each group'. If regulatory agencies had conducted this numerical analysis before granting emergency authorization, they would have seen a concerning safety profile. Perhaps the story now unfolding would be very different.

In this chapter, I will present some of the health problems that have occurred in individuals who received one or more doses of COVID vaxgenes. It is not an exhaustive review; it simply provides an overview of the most relevant issues, grouped by physiological systems.

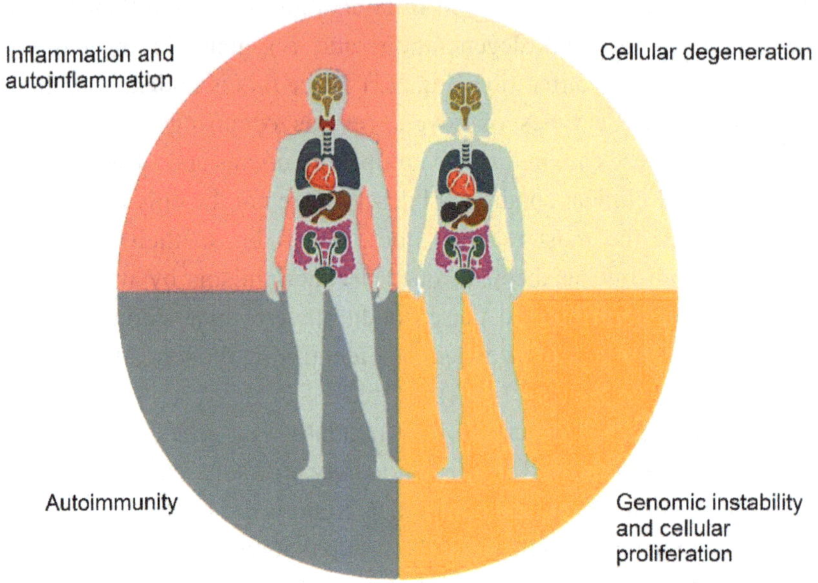

Figure 22. *Main mechanisms through which the molecular and cellular impact of COVID vaxgenes can lead to pathologies that affect all organs, generating a diversity of clinical conditions.*

6.1 Cardiovascular conditions

The regulatory agencies ruled that, based on the interim results of the COVID vaxgene clinical trials, there was no warning signal related to cardiovascular adverse events. However, a few months after granting emergency authorization to the two synthetic mRNA vaxgenes, the FDA issued an update for physicians and nurses regarding the administration of Pfizer and Moderna's products[263]. This update included a notice of the risk of myocarditis and pericarditis, particularly within seven days after receiving the second dose of the vaxgene. This risk was also included in the CDC's considerations on COVID vaccination[264].

The FDA and CDC updates are relevant because one of the adverse events of special interest that the Brighton Collaboration (a group of vaccine safety experts) indicated should be studied was those related to the cardiovascular system (see section 2.15). What is difficult to understand is why it took *six months* to update a risk they already knew about. I say this because the risk was detectable in the data that pharmaceutical companies provided to regulatory agencies, and on which they based the emergency authorization of COVID vaxgenes.

If you review the data found in the publications of Pfizer's phase 3 trials and compare them with what is in the reports submitted to the FDA in November 2020, there are inconsistencies (Michels et al., 2023): in the original data, deaths from cardiovascular events in those who received the synthetic mRNA vaxgene were 3.7 times higher than in the control group (Table 4).

---

[263] FDA News Release. Coronavirus (COVID) Update: June 25, 2021 [Internet]. Available at: https://www.fda.gov/news-events/press-announcements/coronavirus-COVID-update-june-25-2021

[264] CDC Clinical Considerations: Myocarditis and Pericarditis after Receipt of COVID Vaccines Among Adolescents and Young Adults [Internet]. Available at: https://www.cdc.gov/vaccines/COVID/clinical-considerations/myocarditis.html

Table 4. *Comparison of deaths in scientific publications of the Phase 3 clinical trials of Pfizer's vaxgene and the interim report, that was the basis for emergency authorization. The table shows the number of deaths and in parenthesis the number of deaths due to cardiovascular events (Based on Michels et al., 2023).*

<table>
<tr><th colspan="3">Data in scientific publications of clinical trial (Polack et al., 2020 y Thomas et al., 2021)</th><th colspan="3">Data in the interim evaluation of the clinical trial (VRBPAC Briefing Document 2020)</th></tr>
<tr><td colspan="6">Preliminary results of the trial (blinded and controlled) 27/07/20 – 14/11/20</td></tr>
<tr><td colspan="2">Vaxgene</td><td>Placebo</td><td colspan="2">Vaxgene</td><td>Placebo</td></tr>
<tr><td colspan="2">2 (1)</td><td>4 (2)</td><td colspan="2">6 (4)</td><td>5 (2)</td></tr>
<tr><td colspan="6">Preliminary results of the trial (blinded and controlled) before emergency authorization and after authorization 07/27/20 – 01/24/21</td></tr>
<tr><td colspan="2">Vaxgene</td><td>Placebo</td><td colspan="2">Vaxgene</td><td>Placebo</td></tr>
<tr><td colspan="2">15 (8)</td><td>14 (3)</td><td colspan="2">16 (10)</td><td>14 (3)</td></tr>
<tr><td colspan="3">They reported: There are no new signs with respect to the previous report.</td><td colspan="3">Analysis: Deaths from cardiovascular events differ between groups (Chi^2 = 5.13, p=0.02).</td></tr>
<tr><td colspan="6">Trial follow-up (unblinded, altered control group) 01/25/21-02/13/21</td></tr>
<tr><td>Vaxgene</td><td>Vaccinated placebo</td><td>Placebo</td><td>Vaxgene</td><td>Vaccinated placebo</td><td>Placebo</td></tr>
<tr><td>3(1)</td><td>2</td><td>0</td><td>5 (1)</td><td>3</td><td>0</td></tr>
<tr><td colspan="3">They reported: The causes of death are balanced between groups.</td><td colspan="3">Analysis: Deaths from cardiovascular events do not differ between groups</td></tr>
<tr><td colspan="6">Summary of deaths in the trial follow-up period 07/27/20-03/13/21</td></tr>
<tr><td>Vaxgene</td><td>Vaccinated placebo</td><td>Placebo</td><td>Vaxgene</td><td>Vaccinated placebo</td><td>Placebo</td></tr>
<tr><td>18 (9)</td><td>2</td><td>14 (3)</td><td>19 (9)</td><td>2 (2)</td><td>17 (3)</td></tr>
<tr><td colspan="3">They reported: 18 deaths occurred in vaccinated vs. 16 in unvaccinated.</td><td colspan="3">Analysis: They considered two deaths of vaccinated controls in the placebo group. They omitted one death in the vaccine group. Deaths due to cardiovascular events differ between groups (Chi2 = 4.87, p=0.02).</td></tr>
</table>

It seems that the UK Vaccine Advisory Committee (JCVI) also decided that the risk of myocarditis could not be ignored, as they announced that they would not recommend Pfizer's vaxgene for children aged 12 to 15 due to the risk of developing myocarditis[265]. In fact, they ruled that only children

[265] BBC Scientists not backing Covid jabs for 12 to 15-year-olds [Internet]. Available at: https://www.bbc.com/news/health-58438669

aged 12 to 17 with specific health conditions could receive the vaxgene, as the risk of developing myocarditis had to be weighed against the limited benefits of vaccination in this age group[266].

The JCVI's concern did not seem to last long because a couple of months later, in early August 2021, they ruled that all children aged 12 to 17 could receive Pfizer's COVID vaxgene[267]. However, the number of reported cases of myocarditis following synthetic mRNA vaxgenes grew to such an extent that it even made the news. At the end of 2021, The Wall Street Journal published an article discussing these cases and the need for scientists and doctors to study the phenomenon[268]. Just a few days after that news article, a research paper was presented at the 2021 American Heart Association (AHA) congress.

The study was conducted by Stephen Gundry, a Cardiovascular Surgeon and pioneer in heart transplants for children and adolescents. He raised concerns about the risk of COVID vaxgenes based on synthetic mRNA. Gundry (2021) observed cardiac abnormalities and an increased risk of developing acute coronary syndrome in most of his patients who received this type of vaxgene. In his presentation to fellow cardiologists, he proposed that the endogenous (self-produced) production of the Spike protein by the endothelial cells transfected with the synthetic mRNA triggers a cascade of events that leads to severe endothelial inflammation, with massive lymphocyte infiltration into the heart muscle. His argument was based on the measurement of nine proteins in patients' serum (MCP-3, FAS, Fas ligand, Eotaxin, CTACK, IL-16, HGT, HDL, and HdA1c). These proteins are considered biomarkers of cardiac and arterial damage and sustained

---

[266] Department of Health and Social Care. JCVI statement on COVID vaccination of children and young people aged 12 to 17 years: 15 July 2021 [Internet]. Available at: https://www.gov.uk/government/publications/COVID-vaccination-of-children-and-young-people-aged-12-to-17-years-jcvi-statement/jvci-statement-on-COVID-vaccination-of-children-and-young-people-aged-12-to-17-years-15-july-2021

[267] Department of Health and Social Care. JCVI statement on COVID vaccination of children and young people aged 12 to 17 years: 4 August 2021 [Internet]. Available at: https://www.gov.uk/government/publications/jcvi-statement-august-2021-COVID-vaccination-of-children-and-young-people-aged-12-to-17-years/jcvi-statement-on-COVID-vaccination-of-children-and-young-people-aged-12-to-17-years-4-august-2021

[268] The Wall Street Journal. Researchers probe link between COVID vaccines and myocarditis. November 7, 2021 [Internet]. Available at: https://www.wsj.com/articles/researchers-probe-link-between-COVID-vaccines-and-myocarditis-11636290002

inflammation (Ganz et al., 2016), and their presence at high concentrations indicates the formation of cardiac and endothelial lesions that become unstable and, if broken, cause an acute cardiac event (Gundry, 2021).

The relevance of Gundry's study (2021) lies in the fact that, as a clinical physician, he has determined the risk score for acute cardiac events for his patients every three to six months for the past eight years. This allowed him to detect changes when COVID vaxgenes began to be used in the United States. Gundry found that 566 of his patients showed an increase in biomarker concentration between two and 10 weeks after receiving the second dose of the synthetic mRNA vaxgene, compared to values they had before vaccination. The risk of developing acute coronary disease in the next 5 years increased from 11% to 25%, and this is not only in geriatric patients: the age range of his patients was 28 to 97 years. Additionally, the biomarkers remained high for at least two and a half months after the second dose of the COVID vaxgene, suggesting that they do indeed increase endothelial and cardiac muscle damage and inflammation (Gundry, 2021).

Despite the growing evidence of cardiovascular adverse events, authorizations for COVID vaxgenes continued to progress rapidly. By the end of 2021, the FDA had already authorized their use in children from the age of five[269], and shortly after, for babies as young as six months[270]. Since June 2022, in the United States, all citizens over six months of age were authorized to receive synthetic mRNA vaxgenes. The situation was similar in the United Kingdom, although it took a little longer for authorization. From December 9, 2022, onwards, all citizens aged six months and older were given the green light to receive Pfizer's vaxgene[271]. From that point on, like falling dominoes, COVID vaxgenes were authorized in most

[269] FDA News Release. Coronavirus (COVID) Update: FDA Authorizes Pfizer-BioNTech COVID Vaccine for Emergency Use in Children 5 through 11 Years of Age [Internet]. Available at: https://www.fda.gov/news-events/press-announcements/fda-authorizes-pfizer-biontech-COVID-vaccine-emergency-use-children-5-through-11-years-age

[270] FDA News Release. Coronavirus (COVID) Update: FDA Authorizes Moderna and Pfizer-BioNTech COVID Vaccines for Children Down to 6 Months of Age [Internet]. Available at: https://www.fda.gov/news-events/press-announcements/coronavirus-COVID-update-fda-authorizes-moderna-and-pfizer-biontech-COVID-vaccines-children

[271] Department of Health and Social Care COVID vaccination of children aged 6 months to 4 years: JCVI advice, 9 December 2022 (updated 26 April 2023) [Internet]. Available at: https://www.gov.uk/government/publications/COVID-vaccination-of-children-aged-6-months-to-4-years-jcvi-advice-9-december-2022

countries, including children, and in some cases, infants. To give you an idea of the magnitude of these authorizations, by the end of November 2021, 100 countries had already started administering synthetic mRNA COVID vaxgenes to children[272],. Currently, there are only a few countries that do not have a COVID vaccine or vaxgene available on a massive scale for their underage citizens (Fig. 23).

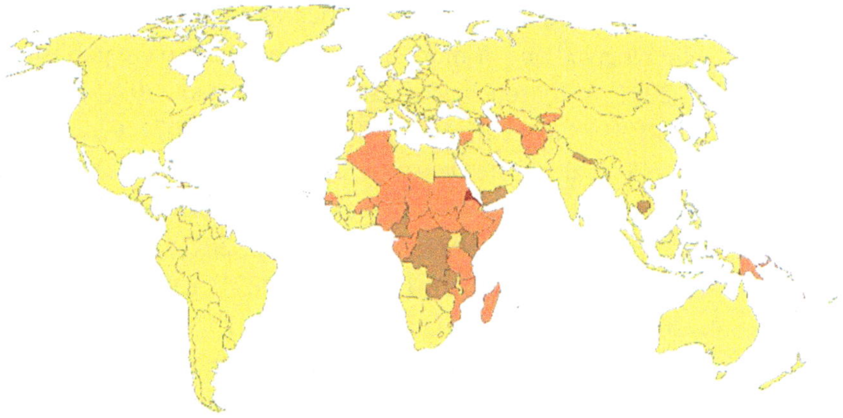

Figure 23. *Countries that have authorized a COVID vaccine or vaxgene for children[273]. Colour code: Red: none offered to children. Brown: Available for some over 16 years. Orange: Available to all over 16 years. Yellow: Available for everyone younger than 16 years. Lined: No data available. Data updated to July 24 2022. Source: Oxford COVID Government Response Tracker, Blavatnik School of Government, University of Oxford.*

To put this in context, as of May 2023, according to the CDC, 31.78 million children (ages 6 months to 17 years) in the United States had received at least one dose of the synthetic mRNA COVID vaxgene, and

[272] Al Jazeera. Infographic: Vaccinating children against COVID [Internet]. Available at: https://www.aljazeera.com/news/2021/11/24/infographic-which-countries-are-vaccinating-children
[273] Oxford COVID Government Response Tracker. Blavatnik School of Government. University of Oxford. Última actualización 24/07/2023 [Internet]. Available at: https://ourworldindata.org/grapher/covid-vaccine-age

26.2 million children had completed the full vaccination schedule[274]. This represents 36% of the child population in the country.

Now, let's look at what has been reported in the scientific literature regarding myocarditis following COVID vaxgenes, shall we?

In just the first six months of 2021, shortly after the mass vaccination campaign began worldwide and before emergency use was authorized to the vaxgenes to be used in adolescents and children, nearly 50 clinical cases of myocarditis, pericarditis, and myopericarditis, mostly in young individuals who received one or more doses of vaxgenes, were published. (Abbate et al., 2021; Abu Mouch et al., 2021; Albert et al., 2021; Bautista García et al., 2021; Bozkurt et al., 2021; Chamling et al., 2021; Cimaglia et al., 2021; D'Angelo et al., 2021; Deb et al., 2021; Díaz et al., 2021; Dionne et al., 2021; Hasnie et al., 2021; Hudson et al., 2021; Isaak et al., 2021; Jain S. S. et al., 2021; Kerbl et al., 2021; Kerneis et al., 2021; Khogali et al., 2021; Kim H. W. et al., 2021; Kim I. C. et al., 2021; King et al., 2021; Larson et al., 2021; Luk et al., 2021; Mansour et al., 2021; Marshall et al., 2021; McLean et al., 2021; Minocha et al., 2021; Montgomery et al., 2021; Muthukumar et al., 2021; Nassar et al., 2021; Navar et al., 2021; Nevet et al., 2021; Park et al., 2021a; Park et al., 2021b; Patel et al., 2021; Pepe et al., 2021; Rosner et al., 2021; Singer et al., 2021; Shaw et al., 2021; Sokolska et al., 2021; Starekova et al., 2021; Sulemankhil et al., 2021; Tano et al., 2021; Verma et al., 2021; Vidula et al., 2021; Viskin et al., 2021; Watkins et al., 2021). One of these cited studies reported two cases of fulminant myocarditis in healthy men after receiving the vaxgene. The first case occurred 10 days after the first dose, and the second case occurred 14 days after the second dose (Verma et al., 2021).

A few months later, Choi et al. (2021) reported autopsy findings in a healthy 22-year-old young man who experienced chest pain five days after receiving Pfizer's vaxgene. The young man was admitted to the hospital and died seven hours later, showing autopsy evidence of damage to the heart muscle cells. Infections and microthrombi, which could have caused

[274] Centres for Disease Control and Prevention. COVID Data Tracker. Atlanta, GA US. Department of Health and Human Services, CDC; 2023, July 11. [Internet]. Available at: https://covid.cdc.gov/covid-data-tracker

myocarditis and death without the vaccine's involvement, were ruled out. Therefore, Choi et al. (2021) concluded that the death was attributed to the vaxgene.

It is interesting and relevant to note that in August 2021, a team of four researchers (Tracy Beth Høeg, Allison Krug, Josh Stevenson, and John Mandrola) submitted a study[275] to a scientific repository regarding myocarditis associated with synthetic mRNA COVID vaxgenes in American children aged 12 to 17. The study's results are not trivial: they found that the risk of developing myocarditis or myopericarditis is significantly higher in boys than in girls. In children aged 12 to 15, the risk of this adverse effect is 3.7 to 6.1 times higher than their risk of being hospitalized for moderate or severe COVID. Unfortunately, this study, submitted for consideration before vaccination had begun in children in many countries, was not accepted until May 2022 (Krug et al., 2022)[276]. The authors concluded that further research was needed to investigate the severity and long-term consequences of adverse effects of COVID vaxgenes in children.

More recently, an analysis of the risk of developing myocarditis and pericarditis in individuals that were given synthetic mRNA vaxgenes was published (Kobayashi et al., 2023). Similar to the previous example, the study's results showed trends in cases of these cardiac conditions between the start of the vaccination campaign and November 2021. However, it was published 16 months later, making it unlikely to have been considered by health authorities when deciding whether to vaccinate minors or not. Kobayashi et al. (2023) compared the expected rates of myocarditis and pericarditis before the COVID pandemic with reports of myocarditis and pericarditis associated with synthetic mRNA vaxgenes from Pfizer and

---

[275] MedRxiv. The preprint server for Medical Sciences. Hoeg et al., 2021 "SARS-CoV-2 mRNA Vaccination-Associated Myocarditis in Children Ages 12-17: A Stratified National Database Analysis". Doi: https://doi.org/10.1101/2021.08.30.21262866 [Internet] Available at: https://www.medrxiv.org/content/10.1101/2021.08.30.21262866v1

[276] Es interesante notar que en la versión publicada, uno de los cuatro autores del artículo original (John Mandrola), ya no aparece como autor. Una de las fuentes de financiamiento de Mandrola es Medtronic (https://www.hrsonline.org/documents/hr16-faculty-disclosures/download), cuya directora ejecutiva es parte de la Junta Directiva de Moderna (https://www.medtronic.com/us-en/about/corporate-governance/board-directors.html). No es posible determinar que esa fue la causa, pero resulta curioso dado lo inusual del hecho.

Moderna. They found that the rate of myocarditis and pericarditis was significantly higher than expected for adolescent and young adult males after the second dose of the vaxgene, with a risk ranging from 1.13% up to 43,281.94% in males aged 10 to 19 who received two doses of Moderna's vaxgene. Therefore, they concluded that "*risks of myocarditis and pericarditis following SARS-CoV-2 mRNA vaccines in Japan seems to be significantly elevated for adolescent and young adult males*".

Their results align with a recent study conducted in New Zealand, which found a significant increase in myocarditis and myopericarditis in children and young adults who had received Pfizer's vaxgene, with a higher risk in children and young people aged 5 to 19, particularly after the second dose (Walton et al., 2023).

When reading the previous paragraphs, it might be understandable to conclude that the risk of myocarditis due to vaxgenes is only relevant for children and young people. However, scientific evidence shows otherwise. Let's look at the published studies:

1) Onishi et al., 2023: Case report of fulminant myocarditis in a 71-year-old man shortly after receiving the first dose of Pfizer's vaxgene. The cardiac condition worsened despite treatment, and the patient died three months later due to congestive heart failure caused by fulminant myocarditis leading to atrioventricular block.

2) Valore et al., 2023: A 70-year-old male patient developed acute myopericarditis after receiving the first dose of Moderna's vaxgene. He was treated with colchicine[277] to receive the second and third doses despite experiencing this adverse event.

3) Cueva-Recalde et al., 2023: Case report of myocarditis in a previously healthy 28-year-old man. Clinical signs, such as chest pain, abnormalities in the electrocardiogram, and biochemical evidence of cardiac damage, appeared four days after receiving the

[277] Medication that turns off the inflammasome, decreasing the activity of inflammatory cells.

second dose of Pfizer's synthetic mRNA vaxgene. After treatment, the symptoms decreased, and the patient was discharged.

4) Massari et al., 2022: Epidemiological study conducted with a large cohort (2,861,809 individuals aged 12 to 39 years who received Pfizer's or Moderna's mRNA vaxgenes). It was found that synthetic mRNA vaxgenes are associated with cardiac damage. While the risk was higher for young people, other age groups also had a higher risk than unvaccinated individuals. The risk was consistent with what other studies have found, higher for the second dose than the first. We are talking about risks up to 12 times higher than the control group, and those at higher risk are men aged 12 to 39 who have received two doses of Pfizer's vaxgene, as well as men and women aged 18 to 29 who have at least one dose of Moderna's vaxgene.

5) Oster et al., 2022: 1,626 cases of myocarditis were confirmed in individuals aged 16 to 31, mostly males, who had received one of the synthetic mRNA vaxgenes. The myocarditis rate was higher for males aged 16 to 17 (105.9 cases of myocarditis per million Pfizer doses administered), followed by children aged 12 to 15 (70.7 cases of myocarditis per million Pfizer doses administered). The rate was comparatively lower in males aged 18 to 24 (52.4 cases of myocarditis per million Pfizer doses administered and 56.3 cases of myocarditis per million Moderna doses administered). Even without applying a correction factor for underreporting (see Chapter 3), if we consider the number of doses that have been administered to these age groups worldwide it can be inferred that a high number of cases of myocarditis have occurred. It is worth noting that a more recent study (Rose et al., 2023), which has not yet been peer-reviewed, found that of almost a million reports of adverse events associated with synthetic mRNA vaxgenes registered in VAERS (see Chapter 3), more than five thousand were cases of myocarditis. This is more than three times the number of reports reported a year earlier by Oster et al. (2022). The cases affected almost exclusively men under 40, particularly after they received the second or third dose (Rose et al., 2023). Overall, all these studies demonstrate that the rate of myocarditis in individuals who received synthetic mRNA vaxgenes

is higher than expected in the population, and young men are more affected than other age groups, although myocarditis events also occur in older men and women.

6) Patrignani et al., 2021: They reported a case of myopericarditis in a 56-year-old man with no relevant medical history. The man presented with acute pain in the epigastrium[278], profuse sweating, tachycardia[279], and hypotension four days after receiving the first dose of Pfizer's mRNA vaxgene.

Before anyone might think that the presentation of these case reports and studies is a biased selection[280],, I assure you it's not. I am presenting cases that have demonstrated an association between synthetic mRNA COVID vaxgenes and the occurrence of myocarditis or myopericarditis. Science cannot prove that something does not happen. Therefore, those studies that reported not finding an association between the frequency of myocarditis cases and the administration of these synthetic mRNA vaxgenes can only say that they did not find it. In no way can this absence of evidence of an association be considered evidence of the absence of an association (Alderson, 2024; Altman and Bland, 1995). Those who do so, do not understand what hypothesis testing in science is, and I invite them to learn the basics of the scientific method as well as differentiate between type I and type II errors and the importance of statistical power. On the other hand, it has already been determined that the occurrence of myocarditis in individuals who received at least one synthetic mRNA vaxgene dose exceeds the expected rate of occurrence in individuals that have not been vaccinated against COVID (Nakahara et al., 2003), and that the occurrence rate, at least seven days after receiving the vaxgene, exceeds the normal rate in the population (Oster et al., 2022). Thus, persisting in looking the other way is an irresponsible decision.

---

278 Part of the abdomen that reaches from the tip of the sternum (breastbone) to the umbilicus (belly button).

279 Term used to refer to abnormally fast heart beats. In other words, it means that the heart rate is abnormally increased.

280 Commonly known as 'cherry picking'.

One of the reasons why regulatory agencies authorized synthetic mRNA COVID vaxgenes for minors was that they considered the risk of myocarditis from vaccination to be low, and that "most cases were mild, and resolved on their own"[281]. The problem with that assertion is that it is wrong on two counts. Let's take it step by step: first, the argument about the mildness of myocarditis. A case of myocarditis associated with synthetic mRNA COVID vaxgenes is not always a 'mild' condition. Specifically, a study that evaluated cases of myocarditis occurring within 30 days after receiving Pfizer's vaxgene in individuals under 21 reported that out of 136 cases of myocarditis unequivocally related to the vaxgene, 18% were severe enough to require admission to the Intensive Care Unit (Truong et al., 2022). Another study found that 96% of the cases of myocarditis associated with synthetic mRNA vaxgenes in individuals under 30 required hospitalization (Oster et al., 2022), and this study was conducted by CDC researchers, so it was not precisely carried out by 'anti-vaxxers'.

Secondly, let's examine the argument that myocarditis cases resolve on their own. Even though many cases of myocarditis can be managed conservatively, heart muscle cells do not have the ability to regenerate[282], and damaged myocardium turns into fibrotic tissue (Winkel and Carrillo, 2002). This has consequences for the affected patient's entire life (Frangogiannis, 2015), with a 50% chance of survival at five years post-occurrence (Kang & Chipa, 2022; Greulich et al., 2020). Furthermore, since damaged cardiac myocytes are replaced by fibrotic tissue, the heart's contraction ability can be impacted (Dumont et al., 2007). This means that myocarditis might not clinically manifest in a person until they need to increase their cardiac output. When engaging in demanding aerobic exercise, it might become impossible to meet the oxygen demand required by the body. Hence, many cases of myocarditis are 'silent', even though damage to cardiac cells is present (Truong et al., 2022).

---

[281] Infosalus. Miocarditis por la vacuna de la COVID, ¿cuál es el riesgo? [Internet; Spanish]. Available at: https://www.infosalus.com/farmacia/noticia-miocarditis-vacuna-COVID-cual-riesgo-20221110080049.html

[282] They only have the capacity to regenerate heart muscle cells in the embryonic stage and in the early neonatal stage.

A retrospective epidemiological study demonstrated that all individuals who had received a synthetic mRNA COVID vaxgene had evidence of myocardial damage[283], even without clinical symptoms, which was not observed in unvaccinated individuals included as controls in the study (Nakahara et al., 2023). The absence of clinical signs can be dangerous for someone with damage to the cardiac muscle. For example, two healthy adolescent males who died suddenly three and four days after receiving the second dose of Pfizer's synthetic mRNA COVID vaxgene had not reported any discomfort suggestive of a clinical picture of myocarditis. One of the patients had no symptoms before death, and the other only complained of a headache and stomach discomfort that began after the second dose (Gill et al., 2022). This is crucial to consider because both had myocarditis without any symptom that would allow prompt detection[284], and this led to sudden death. The cause of death was determined to be toxic myocarditis associated with Pfizer's synthetic mRNA vaxgene (Gill et al., 2022).

The above cases allow us to infer that it is likely that many more people who received these vaxgenes are affected by heart issues than those who exhibit clinical symptoms. Hence, the relevance of, in addition to measuring troponin levels in blood, conducting studies to detect heart damage in vaccinated individuals, such as electrocardiography, magnetic resonance imaging, and even positron emission tomography and computed tomography (PET/CT). Note that abnormalities in heart function are detectable in up to 72% of vaccinated individuals through electrocardiography and magnetic resonance imaging (Oster et al., 2022).

Perhaps some, while reading this, have wondered, '*How can one know that there is heart damage if there are no obvious signs that make me suspect it occurred?*'. It's an excellent and pertinent question, and the answer is that there are well-known diagnostic techniques to determine that there is damage to the heart. One of them is the measurement in blood of molecules that reliably indicate heart damage, such as troponin, a marker

---

[283] This was demonstrated by using positron emission tomography/computed tomography (PET/CT) to detect the incorporation of 18F-fluorodeoxyglucose (FDG) into swollen tissue cells. The amount of FDG detected in the hearts of vaccinated people up to 180 days after vaccination was higher than in unvaccinated people, regardless of sex or age.

[284] Such as chest pain, difficulty breathing, fever, fast heart beat.

known for decades, which rises when there is damage to heart cells (Coudrey, 1988). It was found that almost all patients with myocarditis after vaccination exhibit elevated levels of troponin in their blood (Oster et al., 2022) during the first days after receiving the mRNA vaxgene. Of course, as troponin only indicates acute damage, the values decrease after a week (Kohli et al., 2022; Salah and Mehta, 2021), but there are other ways to visualize heart damage, such as magnetic resonance imaging, radiology, and clinical examinations. These approaches have allowed us to understand that damage to the heart caused by synthetic mRNA vaxgene can be lasting, even up to a year later. This was reported by Shauer and colleagues (2022), finding that 68% of adolescents who received the synthetic mRNA COVID vaxgene still had radiological abnormalities, observed as the percentage of late gadolinium enhancement[285] (%LGE; Dumont et al., 2007) in addition to shortening of the heart muscle fibres up to four months after receiving the vaxgene (Schauer et al., 2022). It seems that this study fell short, as more recently, evidence has been found that cardiovascular damage associated with genetic vaccination can persist for up to six months in some who had myocarditis after receiving a dose (Patel Y. R. et al., 2022). It is likely that in some individuals, vaccine-associated cardiovascular damage may last even longer. For example, the evaluation of a small number (40) of adolescent males diagnosed with myocarditis after vaccination showed that even a year later, more than half of those examined still had cardiac abnormalities (Yu et al., 2023).

If you recall what I explained in Chapter 4 about causal inference, you will see that the criterion of temporality is met in all the clinical cases presented here, in addition to the criterion of the strength of the association (reported as a significantly higher risk in the vaccinated; for example, the studies by Krug et al., 2022; Oster et al., 2022), the criterion of the biological gradient (observed in studies showing that the risk of myocarditis is higher for the second dose than for the first; for example, Kobayashi et al., 2023; Yasmin et al., 2023; Massari et al., 2022), and the criterion of consistency (different studies using various diagnostic methods, from measuring troponin levels and other biomarkers to imaging evaluations and

[285] This is an important marker of cardiac damage and fibrosis, and is considered a sign of bad prognosis.

clinical evidence, have shown consistent results) are met. Now, a very important criterion is missing: Plausibility. That is, the mechanistic explanation of the association between synthetic mRNA vaxgenes and myocarditis, which I will address next.

It has been demonstrated that adolescents vaccinated with the synthetic mRNA vaxgene and who later developed myocarditis have high concentrations of free Spike in the blood (Yonker et al., 2023). If you read section 5.2 and section 5.5, you will recall that a portion of the Spike protein produced by the cells of those who received a synthetic mRNA vaxgene is released from cells in exosomes and distributed throughout the body (Yonker et al., 2023; Bansal et al., 2021). Therefore, it is necessary to consider the possibility that sustained Spike production and its release into the bloodstream may play a role in the pathophysiology of myocarditis and myopericarditis associated with these vaxgenes, given its known action on the vascular endothelium (Perico et al., 2022; Robles et al., 2022; Lei et al., 2021; Mosleh et al., 2020) and its pro-inflammatory action (Baumeier et al., 2022).

Additionally, it is known that synthetic mRNA from vaxgenes can be detected within cardiac cells for at least a month[286] after vaccination (Krauson et al., 2023), so it is plausible to consider that myocardial damage could also be due to the direct action of synthetic mRNA (see section 5.3) and not only by the action of the Spike protein.

It is noteworthy that atypical lesions have been detected in the myocardium of adolescents, such as fibrotic myocarditis and cardiac hypertrophy, and no cellular evidence of typical myocarditis, such as lymphocyte infiltration, was found. Instead, toxic myocarditis was found, which corresponds to a process triggered by a high presence of catecholamines (adrenaline) in response to cellular toxicity in the heart muscle cells (Gill et al., 2022). This condition, known as 'catecholamine-mediated cardiomyopathy', is characterized by the presence of necrotic cardiac myocytes, as well as inflammation derived from catecholamines.

[286] I do not mean that it stops being detected after one month. I mean that that was the follow up time of the study.

The two patients in the study by Gill and colleagues (2022) had visible contraction bands, and their cardiac muscle cells had a hyper-eosinophilic staining, which is very different from what is observed in a typical cardiac inflammation. Instead, it is like what is seen in patients with Takotsubo syndrome, also called broken heart syndrome (Nuñez-Gil et al., 2012).

The proposed mechanisms to explain catecholamine-mediated cardiomyopathy include, among other things, dysfunction of the blood vessels of the heart (Lyon et al., 2008). Given what is known about the pathogenic mechanisms of the Spike protein (see section 5.5), it is plausible that myocardial damage can be caused by the effect of synthetic mRNA and by the effects of the Spike protein on the vascular endothelium.

On the other hand, if we consider that the heart not only consists of muscle cells but also fibroblasts, endothelial cells, pericytes, and macrophages, among other cell types (Litviňuková et al., 2020), and that heart muscle cells express an important receptor for cardiac inflammatory responses (Toll-like receptor 4; Yang et al., 2016) activated by NF-κB, then it is not difficult to understand that if the Spike protein reaches the heart, it can initiate a localized inflammatory cascade (see section 5.5). Additionally, regardless of localized inflammation due to damage to heart cells, cardiac arrhythmias can occur due to the action of inflammatory molecules in the bloodstream, which, upon reaching the heart, affect the functioning of ion channels in the cell membrane (Lazzerini et al., 2019), impacting the heart's electrical potential (Pappano and Weir, 2019). Remember that synthetic mRNA induces a marked pro-inflammatory effect systemically (see section 5.3). This is not speculation. It was found that Moderna's vaxgene induced arrhythmias in addition to irregular heart contractions by altering calcium channels, while Pfizer's vaxgene increased heart contraction by increasing the activity of a cellular enzyme (protein kinase A) in the muscle cells of that organ (Schreckenberg et al., 2023). So, as you can see, there is no shortage of biological explanations for cardiac damage caused by the action of synthetic mRNA vaxgenes.

Perhaps some are thinking, '*But I (or my child, my nephew, my friend) was vaccinated with those products, and nothing happened to me*'. I'm glad that's the case, but it's important to remember that we are not mathematical equations that will react equally when exposed to the same thing. There are many intrinsic factors, such as age, nutritional status, immune function, as well as extrinsic factors, such as the amount of synthetic mRNA in the vials, the storage of ingredients, the presence of double-stranded RNA, etc. (see section 1.4) that influence the outcome. So, of course, not everyone who receives the synthetic mRNA vaxgene will develop myocarditis or pericarditis. There doesn't need to be mathematical determinism for us to recognize the contribution of a factor (the vaxgene) and an outcome (cardiac effects). Almost three years later, there is little chance of continuing to argue, as some do, that COVID vaxgene are not a risk factor for myocarditis, especially in children, adolescents, and young people.

Fortunately, authorities in some (few) countries have not completely ignored the evidence. For example, in Sweden, an indefinite suspension was imposed on Moderna's vaxgene for individuals under 31 years of age owing to the high number of cases of cardiac damage[287]. The holdup was specifically for this brand, not for the other synthetic mRNA vaxgene (Pfizer). This is because an analysis of adverse event data in Sweden showed that the risk of myocarditis or myopericarditis in people who had received a Moderna vaxgene was 13 times higher than that of those who received a Pfizer vaxgene.

It is possible that the difference in risk between both vaxgenes could be due to differences in the amount of synthetic mRNA between the brands (see section 1.1). Someone receiving a dose of Moderna receives three times more synthetic mRNA than someone receiving a dose of Pfizer (remember that the dose of Moderna's vaxgene is 0.5 mL of 200 µg/mL, while the dose of Pfizer's vaxgene is 0.3 mL of 100 µg/mL). It could also be due to differences in the cationic nanolipids used by each brand (Puranik et al., 2021). More importantly, Pfizer's vaxgenes contain a plasmid that includes the Spike gene sequence and a promoter for it to be expressed by

---

[287] Austin County News Online: International. Sweden Suspends Moderna Shot Indefinitely After Vaxxed Patients Develop Crippling Heart Condition [Internet]. Available at; https://austincountynewsonline.com/sweden-suspends-moderna-shot-indefinitely-after-vaxxed-patients-develop-crippling-heart-condition/

the human cells it enters, with a high chance of entering the nucleus and being integrated there (see section 5.6).

The differences between the two synthetic mRNA vaxgene brands are not trivial, as they determine the translation rate of the Spike protein and the persistence of synthetic mRNA in the cytoplasm before being degraded by cellular nucleases (Xia, 2021). The differences can even influence the possibility that Spike mRNA is constantly transcribed in heart cells if the plasmid from Pfizer's vaxgene enters the nucleus of these cells. Given these differences, the cellular and molecular interaction, as well as the protein translation rate in the vaccinated individuals, may not necessarily be the same for both vaxgene brands, and this could impact the occurrence rate of adverse events associated with these products. I clarify, however, that the study from Sweden is not evidence that Moderna's synthetic mRNA vaxgene is risky and that Pfizer's is not. The evidence I have shared here indicates that both brands are associated with a risk of myocarditis, and the effects do not depend on the age or sex of the vaccinated individual (Nakahara et al., 2023).

It is possible that some doctors may not be open to seeing this evidence that is published as epidemiological studies and case reports, and that they only take notice when a medical review or meta-analysis is published. If so, we are in luck because, after almost three years of the application of COVID vaxgenes, a systematic review has been published on cardiovascular complications, thrombosis, and thrombocytopenia occurring in people who received one or two doses of synthetic mRNA vaxgenes (Yasmin et al., 2023). This systematic review of medical and scientific literature covered publications from the beginning of vaccination until January 2022. The inclusion criteria for the review were observational studies and case reports on cardiovascular complications, studies including synthetic mRNA COVID vaxgenes, and studies in a language the authors could understand. I clarify that they excluded other reviews and meta-analyses, protocols, editorials, congress abstracts, and studies that included patients with pre-existing cardiovascular diseases. In other words, we cannot accuse the authors of the medical review of being lax.

Based on their review, they found 17,636 cardiovascular events associated with the first or second dose of synthetic mRNA COVID vaxgenes[288]. Of these events, those most frequently associated with receiving a dose were thrombosis (13,936 cases), stroke (758 cases), myocarditis (511 cases), heart attack (377 cases), pulmonary embolism (301 cases), and arrhythmias (254 cases), most of which were associated with Pfizer's vaxgenes. This could be because this brand has been more widely used than Moderna's. The authors concluded that since these vaxgenes were authorized so quickly, it was not possible to know the potential mechanisms of damage, and now, given the high number of cardiovascular adverse events, they should be studied, and caution is necessary in their use. Unfortunately, this recommendation comes 33 months after the start of inoculations and with approximately 13.5 billion doses administered to humanity.

As you can see, the most recent medical review identified other events that, due to their complexity, will be addressed in a separate section below. These include cases of stroke, intracranial haemorrhages, deep venous thrombosis, cerebral venous thrombosis, arterial thrombosis, portal vein thrombosis, coronary thrombosis, microvascular intestinal thrombosis, and pulmonary embolisms, which I will discuss along with other conditions in the next section, which I will call 'coagulopathies'.

I hope that what has been presented so far can help understand why so many cardiovascular events are occurring in people who received vaxgenes, including those events that caused sudden deaths in individuals with no medical history of cardiovascular problems (Cho et al., 2023), and even in high-performance athletes, especially considering that these events seem to be happening at a rate 20 times higher than in 2021 (Buergin et al., 2023).

6.2 Blood-clotting disorders

Since the COVID vaxgenes began to be administered to young people in the second half of 2021, news reports have been circulating about acute

[288] Distributed among 69 case series and case reports, four studies with data from hospital medical records or national databases, and eight prospective/retrospective observational studies.

myocardial infarctions and ischemic[289] stroke incidents (also known simply as strokes), especially in young people. All these cases are related to the formation of blood clots, also referred to as 'thrombi'. The main message of the news was to highlight that these events could occur randomly. However, a search on PubMed[290] regarding the topic, limited to publications before 2021, revealed that, for instance, "juvenile stroke" is defined in studies as the occurrence of strokes in individuals aged 18 to 55 years. In industrialized countries like Germany, it affects 30,000 people per year (Schöberl et al., 2017).

For practical purposes, this age range is too broad, especially considering that the risk increases with age. Therefore, it is not accurate to speak of "juvenile stroke" as if the risk were the same for all ages. If we break down age groups more finely, according to medical literature, the expected incidence for individuals aged 20 to 24 is 2.4 cases per 100,000; for those aged 35 to 44, it is 20 cases per 100,000, and for those aged 75 to 84, it is 1,200 cases per 100,000 (Putaala et al., 2009). On the other hand, children under 18 have an even lower risk (1.72 cases per 100,000, annually; De Veber et al., 2017). Of course, it is essential to consider factors that increase the risk, such as the use of oral contraceptives, hormone replacement therapy, pregnancy, migraines, and the use of illicit drugs like cocaine and amphetamines. However, undoubtedly, the incidence of strokes in individuals aged 20 to 24 has always been lower than in older individuals (Putaala et al., 2009).

In contrast to information published before 2021 (when COVID vaxgenes began to be used after emergency use authorization), a search on the VAERS (Vaccine Adverse Event Reporting System) website regarding strokes shows 13,205 reports in individuals who received a COVID vaxgene[291], with 348 reports pertaining to individuals under 29 years of age. Even if we consider that *all* cases that occurred were reported, these are concerning data, particularly noting that 71 of them occurred in individuals

---

[289] It refers to what happens when blood does not adequately reach a tissue or organ. One of the causes is that there is a clot that is blocking the flow in a blood vessel.
[290] National Library of Science. National Center for Biotechnology Information [Internet]. Search terms: "juvenile stroke". Searchable at: https://pubmed.ncbi.nlm.nih.gov/
[291] Open Vaers [Internet]. Available at: https://www.openvaers.com/vaersapp/reports.php Data updated to September 29 2023; Accessed October 19 2023.

under 18 years old. If this frequency of occurrence were expected normally in the young population, we would anticipate a similar number of events in the same period (33 months) for a vaccine that is also commonly administered among young people, such as the HPV (human papillomavirus) vaccine[292] or the flu vaccine. However, a search with those criteria shows only *eight* cases for the HPV vaccine (between 2017 and 2019) and *four* cases associated for the influenza vaccine in the same period. Furthermore, between 2008 (since the HPV vaccine started being used in the United States) and 2023, there are only 80 reports of strokes in individuals under 29 years old, and between 1990 and 2023, there are 44 reports of strokes in individuals under 29 years old who were vaccinated against influenza.

In Chapter 5, I presented information about the mechanisms that could explain the formation of clots in individuals who received COVID vaxgenes. These mechanisms focus on two things: the prothrombotic potential (clot-forming) of the Spike protein when it damages the endothelium of blood vessels (Trougakos et al., 2022a; Marino Gammazza et al., 2020; Paladino et al., 2020), and the prothrombotic potential of the adenovirus (AdV), which is the basis of vectorized vaxgenes (Marietta et al., 2022; Greinacher et al., 2021), as indicated in section 1.3.

Among the adverse events related to COVID vaxgenes that were attributed to clot formation, cases of immune thrombocytopenic thrombosis[293] stood out. These cases began to be observed with such high frequency that a new clinical entity was even coined, known as "Vaccine-Induced Immune Thrombotic Thrombocytopenia" or VITT (Dotan and Shoenfeld, 2021; Greinacher et al., 2021; Wiedmann et al., 2021). In Section 5.4, I attempted to describe the process by which components of vectorized vaxgenes can induce clot formation. Here, I am more interested

---

[292] Centers for Disease Control and Prevention. Understanding HPV Coverage [Internet]. Available at: https://www.cdc.gov/hpv/partners/outreach-hcp/hpv-coverage.html.

[293] Thrombocytopenia refers to an abnormal decrease in the number of platelets in the blood. Therefore, thrombotic thrombocytopenia is a condition characterized by a decrease in the number of platelets that coincides with the formation of many clots.

in making it clear how this alteration leads to VITT in susceptible individuals.

In 2021, a study was published demonstrating, through high-resolution microscopy, that some components of AstraZeneca's COVID vaxgene (based on recombinant adenoviruses, AdV) can induce the accumulation of immune complexes[294] formed by the interaction of anti-PF4 antibodies with PF4 molecules on the surface of platelets. The study also showed that when this vaxgene enters circulation, severe pro-inflammatory responses are stimulated, increasing the formation of these immune complexes, thus reinforcing the synthesis of high avidity[295] anti-PF4 antibodies, leading to a new activation of platelets (Greinacher et al., 2021). It becomes a vicious circle that is further complicated because anti-PF4 antibodies can induce the formation of neutrophil extracellular traps (NETs)[296], which, in themselves, further promote coagulation. This does not bode well for the normally carefully regulated coagulation process.

The findings led to the proposal of a mechanism explaining the condition. This mechanism is similar to what occurs during the clinical entity known as heparin-induced autoimmune thrombocytopenia (Lee and Arepally, 2013), although in the case of those receiving the vectorized COVID vectorized vaxgene, it has nothing to do with heparin (Datta et al., 2021). Essentially, the steps proposed by Greinacher and colleagues (2021) to explain what happens are as follows:

1) Early phase (lasting one to two days) in which complexes form between PF4 molecules and the AdV in the vaxgene. This triggers danger signals that initiate the inflammatory process.

2) Late phase (5 to 14 days) in which anti-PF4 antibodies are produced and accumulate at high levels in the blood. This amplifies clot

[294] Molecule that is formed by the union of several antigens with several antibodies.
[295] In Immunology it refers to the sum of the interaction strength at all related points between an antibody and an antigen. The greater the avidity, the stronger the union.
[296] Network that is formed by strands of DNA that come from neutrophils (one of the types of white blood cells) when they die. Its function is to trap bacteria, but it also promotes coagulation.

formation and platelet activation. In some individuals, NETs are formed.

It is also important to understand why blood clots persist in individuals who develop VITT. Normally, when coagulation occurs (such as when there is a bleeding wound), the formed clot is quickly dissolved after stopping the bleeding. However, when there is a disruption in the coagulation process, the formed clots do not dissolve easily. Having a high quantity of clots in the blood is a serious problem, as they can detach from the site where they were formed and travel through the bloodstream, causing obstruction in blood vessels that supply organs and tissues (Navarrete et al., 2023). This event is known as a thromboembolism and can affect any system of the body, depending on what it obstructs, such as the heart, lungs, kidneys, brain, abdomen, and limbs. It can also be widespread, with small clots throughout the body, and when it occurs, it is known as disseminated intravascular coagulation (Levi et al., 2018). The latter can also occur as a consequence of COVID vaxgenes (Yamada and Asakura, 2022).

Since the description of VITT as a specific clinical entity, clinical cases have been published describing this pathology in individuals who received COVID vaxgenes based on adenoviral vectors (e.g., Xie et al., 2023; Bangolo et al., 2022; Chen et al., 2022; Iba et al., 2022; Luciano et al., 2022; Wittstock et al., 2022; Ceschia et al., 2021; Sarifian-Dorche et al., 2021; See et al., 2021; Sánchez Van Kammen et al., 2021). Given the severity of VITT, most studies have concluded that any headache occurring after the administration of a COVID vaxgene justifies diagnostic testing to rule out other causes and initiate treatment, especially when the affected individual received a vectorized vaxgene that used AdV (such as AstraZeneca, Janssen, Canino, and Sputnik).

As mentioned earlier, VITT not only causes strokes but can also affect the limbs, leading to thrombophlebitis and deep vein thrombosis (Wali et al., 2023; Ikechi et al., 2022). These thrombotic conditions have required medical intervention with prolonged periods of anticoagulants, surgical interventions (Ceschia et al., 2021), and sometimes amputations (Roberge et al., 2022). This has been documented since the early months of 2021, shortly after the widespread initiation of COVID vaccination worldwide.

The risk of developing VITT or any other coagulopathy as a consequence of COVID vaxgenes led some countries, such as the United States[297], Denmark[298], Ireland, Sweden, Latvia, Germany, Italy, France, Spain, Norway, and the Netherlands[299], to temporarily or definitively halt the administration of vectorized vaxgenes in their young population. Good decision! Although it is regrettable that the decision was made after widespread application. However, what is interesting is that cases of VITT and other coagulopathies associated with the receipt of synthetic mRNA vaxgenes (e.g., Alhashim et al., 2022; Goh et al., 2022M; Kang, 2022; Ling et al., 2022; Syed et al., 2021) have also been reported without triggering an alert or restriction on their use. This is unfortunate and reinforces the importance of understanding the pathophysiology that the Spike protein of SARS-CoV-2 can trigger, and of the synthetic mRNA, which, as I explained in section 5.3, is inherently pro-inflammatory (Kannemeier et al., 2007) and can damage the vascular endothelium, causing, together with the Spike protein produced after vaccination, a cascade of prothrombotic events.

Specifically, when mRNA is outside the cells, it increases the activation of proteases factor XI and XII, both important for the coagulation cascade (Müller et al., 2011). This was seen in experimental studies, where extracellular RNA was found to provoke a strong procoagulant response in rabbits and was associated with the formation of fibrin-rich clots in mice (Kannemeier et al., 2007). It is not far-fetched to think that synthetic mRNA does the same, and the risk is even greater considering that vials may contain double-stranded RNA as a contaminant, in addition to degraded RNA, which may not be encapsulated in lipid nanoparticles (Tinari, 2021; Thacker, 2021). Perhaps this can explain why, until September 22, 2023,

---

[297] US Food and Drug Administration. FDA News Release [Internet]. Available at: https://www.fda.gov/news-events/press-announcements/coronavirus-COVID-update-fda-limits-use-janssen-COVID-vaccine-certain-individuals
[298] The New York Times [Internet]. Available at: https://www.nytimes.com/2021/04/14/world/europe/denmark-astrazeneca-vaccine.html
[299] Al Jazeera [Internet] Available at: https://www.aljazeera.com/news/2021/3/15/which-countries-have-halted-use-of-astrazenecas-covid-vaccine

26,918 cases of thrombosis and 12,871 cases of ischemia associated with synthetic mRNA vaxgenes (of Pfizer and Moderna) had been reported to VAERS[300]. Taking into account the underreporting factor of 31 (see Chapter 3), and the number of doses of each type of vaxgene administered in the United States, we can estimate an occurrence rate of thrombosis per dose of 0.13% for synthetic mRNA vaxgenes (13 cases per 10,000 doses administered) and an occurrence rate of thrombosis per dose of 0.48% for the vectorized vaxgene from Janssen (48 cases per 10,000 doses administered). The rate is higher for the vectorized vaxgene, undoubtedly, but it does not mean that it is not a risk of synthetic mRNA vaxgenes.

One of the first documented cases of deep vein thrombosis as a result of synthetic mRNA vaxgenes was that of a 59-year-old woman who experienced severe pain in her left leg that suddenly appeared seven days after receiving a dose of Pfizer's vaxgene (Al Maqbali et al., 2021). The patient had type 2 diabetes and osteoarthritis, both controlled, and had been diagnosed with non-severe COVID seven months earlier, without any complications from the disease. According to the authors of the case report, she had no medical condition that justified the condition, other than the Pfizer vaxgene (Al Maqbali et al., 2021). At the time of that case report being published, it was already known that some patients diagnosed with severe COVID could develop blood clots affecting the limbs. As I indicated in section 5.5, the Spike protein is one of the factors that can explain clot formation (Perico et al., 2022; Robles et al., 2022; Mosleh et al., 2020). This is because Spike can irreversibly deform platelets (Kuhn et al., 2023), promote blood clot formation by causing endothelial damage (Perico et al., 2022; Robles et al., 2022; Lei et al., 2021; Mosleh et al., 2020), and promote dysregulated immune responses in response to the presence of the virus (Barale et al., 2021). The prothrombotic effect of Spike on platelets depends on concentration: the higher the exposure to Spike, the greater platelet deformation and activation, resulting in many clots that are difficult to undo. This is because the Spike protein binds to integrin receptors on the surface of platelets, specifically integrin $\alpha v\beta 3$ (Kuhn et al., 2023). In that sense, it needs to be considered that receiving multiple doses of vaxgenes

[300] Open Vaers [Internet]. Available at: https://www.openvaers.com/vaersapp/reports.php. Accessed October 9 2023.

could increase the risk of coagulopathies, as well as other health issues that I will address in the following sections.

Knowing the mechanism of action of vaxgenes (see section 1.3) as well as the persistence of the Spike protein in people who received these gene-therapy products, it should not be surprising that clots could also form in the limbs in a person seven days after receiving Pfizer's vaxgene, as described in the Al Maqbali et al. (2021) case report. This case study is very relevant because, as explained before, the mechanism of action of vaxgenes is to make cells become 'factories' to produce a foreign protein (in the case of COVID vaxgenes, the protein is SARS-CoV-2 Spike), to induce a specific immune response against that protein in the vaccinated individual. The problem is, for synthetic mRNA vaxgenes at least, that synthetic mRNA remains viable within cells for months (Krausen et al., 2023; Röltgen et al., 2022), so the protein, Spike, is also produced for months in vaccinated individuals (Brogna et al., 2023; Samaniego-Castruita et al., 2023). A portion of the total Spike protein produced by vaccinated individuals remains attached to the cell membrane, turning that cell into a 'molecular target' for the immune system, but a portion of the Spike protein produced by cells of vaccinated individuals with this type of vaxgenes is released from cells in exosomes that circulate through the blood to various organs and tissues in the body (Bansal et al., 2021). This means that the Spike protein produced in the cells of vaccinated individuals has ample opportunities to interact with endothelial cells, increasing the risk of clot formation, causing thrombosis, including in the limbs.

Thrombosis associated with COVID vaxgenes can even occur in the cerebral venous sinus of young and healthy individuals, which, before 2021, was considered an unusual event (Mazzeo et al., 2021). An example is the case of a 28-year-old woman, without comorbidities or coagulopathy risk factors, who developed VITT after receiving the first dose of the synthetic mRNA vaxgene from Pfizer (Alhashim et al., 2022). According to the report's authors, the patient had persistent headaches for two weeks, which started four days after receiving the vaccine. The diagnosis of VITT was made through a brain computed tomography and venography[301], as she

[301] X-ray of the veins that uses a contrast media.

did not present any typical clinical markers suggestive of the condition. Her blood tests were normal, with a single anomaly: marked thrombocytopenia.

This clinical picture reminded me of one that I was informed of in February 2021, two months after the start of the COVID vaccination programme. I relate it here, respecting the identity of the patient and with great respect for her and her family. It involved a healthcare professional (initials A.C.) who, due to her work in the medical sector in England, had to be vaccinated against COVID. The first dose she received was of AstraZeneca's vaxgene on February 11, 2021. One day later, she began to feel unwell and fainted. Paramedics told her husband that it was "*a severe but normal reaction to the vaccine*" and that she would improve. That did not happen, and she continued to deteriorate. Unfortunately, she received no support from the emergency service, who asked her husband not to call again, although by the afternoon of the following day, A.C. was unresponsive. She was admitted to the hospital with a diagnosis of cerebellar ischemia. The family was told that it had no relation to the vaccine and that it was "a very unfortunate coincidence", even though A.C. had no prior history or predisposing factors to developing clots. The patient's husband tried to report the adverse event on official pages, but since they only accepted reports of adverse events that were recognized at that time, he could not do so. I do not know if A.C. survived cerebellar ischemia, as I lost contact with her husband, who had contacted me to tell me about the case[302]. I share it here because, among the many similar messages I have received since early 2021, A.C.'s case impacted me a lot and prompted me to continue with science communication activities regarding the lack of safety of COVID vaxgenes. That case is just one of the many that have occurred due to medical negligence, scientific ignorance, and the greed of the pharmaceutical industry. No one should have taken the risk of developing clots in the cerebellum (or anywhere else) because of being administered a product that has that inherent risk.

During the writing of this section, I have frequently asked myself if the paramedics and medics that stated, without evidence, that A.C.'s case was

[302] I was contacted by her husband a few weeks after the book was published and he has told me that although she is still not well, she survived.

"an unfortunate coincidence" are now familiarized with the many cases that are the same as hers. Do they still wave them away as coincidences?

Given the risk involved in the formation of a thrombotic condition for the patient's life, it is essential that doctors understand that it is one of the adverse events that COVID vaxgenes can cause, so they need to be able to identify these conditions and treat them promptly (Oldenburg et al., 2021). Certainly, some people will have a higher risk of thrombosis than others due to genetic, physiological factors (e.g., pregnancy), and related to their habits and lifestyle, such as obesity, smoking, contraceptive use, as well as certain medical conditions, and recent thromboembolic surgeries or traumas (McLendon et al., 2023). However, if a patient, with (or without) risk factors, complains of persistent headaches or pain in a limb after receiving the vaxgene, they do not need to be told that it is a coincidence. Their life may depend on diagnostic tests to rule out or confirm VITT. I am referring to the measurement of D-dimer in blood. This simple test, also called "D-dimer fragment test" or "fibrin degradation fragment test," is considered one of the most relevant for the detection of clots generated as a result of COVID vaxgenes. Ironically, the need to perform it in patients with severe COVID has been recognized (Miesbach and Makris, 2020), but if doctors are unaware that the vaxgenes carry a risk of serious coagulopathies, they are unlikely to request it for their vaccinated patients.

6.3 Neurological disorders

In section 5.5 I explained the known mechanisms by which the Spike protein can cause damage. If we consider that the COVID vaxgenes can cross the blood-brain barrier (see section 5.2), it becomes evident that their impact on the blood vessels, their pro-inflammatory activity and their potential to alter blood pressure can happen in the nervous system. Specifically, it has been proposed that, if the Spike protein is accumulated in the brain, it can accelerate or lead to the development of neurodegenerative diseases, in addition to depressive disorders and dementia (Sharma and Tan, 2021).

Remember that there are similarities between fragments of the Spike protein and fragments of proteins in the brain involved in myelin formation, the differentiation of support cells for neurons, and communication between neurons (see section 5.5). These similarities can lead to autoimmune responses against proteins of the nervous system (Cuspoca et al., 2022), and that is never a good idea. In addition, some parts of the Spike protein have prion-like amyloidogenic[303] behaviour. This is a risk factor for the development or exacerbation (Laudicella et al., 2021) of degenerative pathologies due to the accumulation of amyloid plaques, such as Alzheimer's disease (Murphy and LeVine, 2010), Lewy body dementia, and cerebral amyloid angiopathy (also called amyloid beta-related angiitis, or ABRA), as well as Creutzfeldt-Jakob disease (Chaudhuri and Paul, 2006).

If the above is clear, then it becomes evident why the Spike protein can be a factor that triggers clinical conditions resembling dementia (Hampel et al., 2021; Uttley et al., 2020) and other neurodegenerative pathologies (Fu et al., 2022).

In addition, the Spike protein alone induces the generation of exosomes that contain microRNAs. These induce severe pro-inflammatory responses in different organs, including the brain and spinal cord (Mishra and Banerjea, 2021). When microRNAs enter glial cells and activate the NF-κB factor, autoimmune conditions (Cuspoca et al., 2022), ischemia, and even triggering Alzheimer's disease (Kaltschmidt and Kaltschmidt, 2009) can be exacerbated or caused. This, in itself, could explain the neurological abnormalities observed in some patients with severe COVID (Merad et al., 2022; Melenotte et al., 2020), and also, for the same reasons, in some patients who received this genetic technology.

Remember that practically all the effects caused by the Spike protein of SARS-CoV-2 in patients diagnosed with COVID can be caused by the Spike protein produced by cells receiving COVID vaxgenes (Oldfield et al., 2021). However, vaxgenes can also cause damage independently of the Spike protein. On the one hand, AdV-based vaxgenes (AstraZeneca, Janssen, CanSino, Sputnik) can cause coagulopathies due to the prothrombotic action of the hexon protein of the adenovirus vector on

[303] I explained this in section 5.5. It means that the proteins aggregate and lead others to aggregate too, thus worsening the problem.

which they are based (see section 6.2). This means that if these vaxgenes enter the bloodstream and cross the blood-brain barrier, they can cause clots in the brain blood vessels, as explained in the previous section, causing various neurological clinical pictures due to lack of oxygen to the brain tissue or the spinal cord, where ischemia due to coagulopathies can also occur (Vargas et al., 2015).

All these mechanisms of damage, together, explain why in the pages of Eudravigilance there have been accumulated, at the time of writing this book, 428,776 reports of neurological problems in people who received Pfizer's vaxgene and 153,441 in people who received Moderna's vaxgene, while the vectorized vaxgenes from Janssen and AstraZeneca add up to 313,019 reports of neurological problems[304].

In 2022, a review was published on neurological adverse events associated with COVID vaccines and vaxgenes (Sriwastava et al., 2022). It is a systematic review of the literature on manifestations of conditions of the central nervous system and the peripheral nervous system that have occurred in vaccinated people who lacked a medical history that justified their occurrence. It is worth noting that their review covered publications between December 1, 2020, and October 10, 2021, so it is not updated. However, even in that 10-month period, Sriwastava and colleagues (2022) found that the most common adverse event of neurological manifestation of the central nervous system was cerebral venous sinus thrombosis (see section 6.2) but demyelinating conditions and encephalitis were also common, while at the level of the peripheral nervous system, the most common was the development of Guillain-Barré syndrome (GBS) and facial paralysis (also called Bell's palsy). However, more recently it has been found that COVID vaxgenes are also associated with neurological conditions such as convulsive disorder (Eslait-Olaciregui et al., 2023), and the review of adverse event monitoring systems suggests that they may also be associated with the development of amyloid neurodegenerative diseases.

[304] Eudravigilance. European Database of Suspected Adverse Drug Reaction Reports [Internet]. Available at: https://www.adrreports.eu/en/search_subst.html# Data updated to October 2 2023.

a) Neurodegenerative diseases

Neurodegenerative diseases are characterized by the progressive and irreversible loss of neurons, leading to serious impairments in the quality of life of patients due to the impact on movement, coordination, and cognitive abilities, often resulting in fatal outcomes (Checkoway et al., 2011). Generally, common neurodegenerative diseases such as Parkinson's, Alzheimer's, Huntington's, and Amyotrophic Lateral Sclerosis (ALS), also known as Lou Gehrig's or Charcot's disease (Ruiz-Rodríguez et al., 2008), are associated with amyloidosis, tauopathies, α-synucleinopathies, and TDP-43 proteinopathies (Dugger and Dickson, 2017). Beyond the complicated names, this means that they involve problems caused by proteins of the central nervous system when these proteins aggregate, forming clusters where they shouldn't be.

In healthy individuals, cellular proteins maintain a proper structure through interactions with various molecules that help them fold and aggregate correctly. However, these interactions can sometimes be disrupted, leading to the accumulation of misfolded protein clusters, forming fibrillar structures generically known as 'amyloid plaques' (Sengupta et al., 2022). Misfolded and aggregative proteins can spread, allowing damage to spread throughout the affected organism, leading to neurodegeneration.

Prions are a special type of amyloid protein. They are a subclass of the PrP protein that changes its folding (now known as PrPsc) and, when it begins to aggregate, induces other PrP proteins to become PrPsc like itself, achieving self-perpetuation. When this happens, it results in an irreversible and fatal neuronal pathology (Sigurdson et al., 2019) known as spongiform encephalopathy (which in simple terms means that the brain tissue becomes sponge-like, full of holes). The term 'spongiform' is used because when observing the affected tissue under the microscope, areas with no neurons are visible, resembling the holes in a sponge. This alteration does not cause inflammation or any other observable immune response since it is not something 'foreign' but rather something our body recognizes as its own, so it does not seek to control or destroy it. After all, if we encountered a friend hunched over after not seeing him for a few years, it is unlikely that we would not be able to recognize him just because he is hunched over, right? Our immune system works similarly. Thus, the brain slowly deteriorates due to these amyloid plaque formations, which do not induce inflammation, and the immune system is incapable of halting the process. That's why these are fatal diseases [and not referring to a 0.23% fatality rate as globally calculated for SARS-CoV-2 infections in 2021 (Ioannidis, 2021), but rather 100% lethality]. It's important to note that PrPsc is contagious, so if an individual is exposed to it through the bloodstream or orally (Huan and MacPherson, 2004), it can induce the same condition in the recipient.

Therefore, if we recall that the Spike protein has some regions similar to the prion protein that causes Creutzfeldt-Jakob disease, as well as Kuru, mad cow disease, and other similar neurodegenerative conditions in other animals (Zhao et al., 2022), we can understand that it is biologically possible for such events to occur in susceptible individuals as a consequence of vaccination.

As explained in section 5.5, the risk of prion diseases occurring due to the Spike protein in the brain was raised by Tetz and Tetz since 2021 when they submitted their study to a scientific server early that year. In that study, they reported finding a part (also called a domain) of the Spike protein of SARS-CoV-2 that was not present in the Spike protein of the first SARS-CoV (i.e., a very similar virus that appeared in 2002, Stadler et al., 2003). Now, published after the peer-review process, Tetz and Tetz (2022) suggested that part of the neuropathogenesis of SARS-CoV-2 could be due to this prion domain. On the other hand, the Spike protein binds to heparin in the brain (see section 6.2) and to heparin-binding proteins such as Aβ, α-synuclein, tau, PrP, and TDP-43 RRM (Idrees and Kumar, 2021). All these proteins have amyloid potential, and their binding to the Spike protein accelerates their aggregation in the brain, leading to neurodegeneration (Idrees and Kumar, 2021). Therefore, the risk of developing prion diseases as a result of exposure to the Spike protein was again highlighted in 2021 (Classen 2021a, 2021b) and reiterated in the review by Seneff and colleagues (2022).

At least two case reports have been published of individuals who developed Creutzfeldt-Jakob disease after being infected with SARS-CoV-2 before the COVID vaccination programme began, and these cases were attributed to the action of the Spike protein (Tayyebi et al., 2022; Young et al., 2020). There are also reports of prion diseases developed after the commencement of COVID vaccination (Alloush et al., 2023; Lecesse et al., 2023; Bernardini et al., 2022), and although they do not provide information about the vaccination status of the affected individuals, given the vaccination mandates in the countries of the patients, it is highly likely that they had been vaccinated.

In this sense, it is necessary to consider the possibility that COVID vaxgenes play a role in the development of prion-related neurodegenerative diseases. There is medical evidence of this, such as the case report of the onset of Creutzfeldt-Jakob disease in a 63-year-old man with a history of diabetes, dyslipidaemia, hypertension, and stroke, two weeks after receiving the second dose of Pfizer's vaxgene (Attia et al., 2023), as well as a spontaneous case of Creutzfeldt-Jakob disease in a healthy 68-year-old man after receiving Pfizer's vaxgene (Karabudak et al., 2023). There is also at least one case report presented at a medical conference indicating the occurrence of Creutzfeldt-Jakob disease in a healthy patient after receiving the second dose of Pfizer's vaxgene (Folds et al., 2022). We also cannot ignore its potential role in the worsening of pre-existing prion-related neurodegenerative diseases. There is at least one published case of the exacerbation of Creutzfeldt-Jakob disease in a 59-year-old man after receiving Pfizer's vaxgene (Doğru and Kehaya, 2022).

It is worth noting that this effect is not only associated with synthetic mRNA COVID vaxgenes but has also been linked to vectorized vaxgenes. For instance, a case report demonstrated the occurrence of progressive dementia with asymmetrical stiffness in a healthy 63-year-old woman after receiving the COVID vaxgene from AstraZeneca (Chakrabarti et al., 2022). The patient exhibited neurological symptoms (confusion, memory loss, hallucinations, difficulty walking, repetitive speech disorders, incoherence, and cervical and mandibular dystonia) consistent with a prion disease after the second dose, without experiencing any relevant symptoms after the first dose. No autoantibodies against the leucine-rich glioma inactivated protein

1 (LGI1), which can be associated with autoimmune encephalitis dementia (Lai et al., 2010), were found. Although confirmation through the detection of the 14-3-3 protein in the serum, considered a diagnostic indicator of rapid neuronal damage during Creutzfeldt-Jakob disease (Leitão et al., 2016), could not be obtained, radiological and electroencephalographic findings were suggestive of a prion disease. Given that she had no medical history that could explain the condition and considering the prion domains of the Spike protein, the most parsimonious explanation for the patient's rapid and fatal dementia in the clinical case is that it was an effect incited by the COVID vaxgene.

Compared to other clinical conditions associated with COVID vaxgenes presented gradually in this chapter, the occurrence of Creutzfeldt-Jakob is considerably lower. However, since it invariably leads to death, even a few cases should not be ignored. A review of the VAERS database shows that, at the time of writing this book, 30 reports of neurological abnormalities compatible with Creutzfeldt-Jakob disease have been accumulated in individuals who received a COVID vaxgene in the United States[305]. If we apply the underreporting correction factor (see Chapter 3), we would be talking about at least 930 cases. Comparatively, if we look for cases of Creutzfeldt-Jakob disease possibly associated with all flu vaccines since 1990, we have four cases (even with the correction factor, we would be talking about 124 cases in 33 years, which averages 3.76 cases per year), while for COVID vaxgenes, we are talking about 310 cases per year. That is an increase of 86 times. Furthermore, according to the CDC, the annual incidence of Creutzfeldt-Jakob disease is 350 cases, with the majority occurring in individuals over 60 years old[306]. This is relevant because at least four of the reports of Creutzfeldt-Jakob disease that occurred after receiving the COVID vaxgene were in individuals under that age, including the case of a 30-year-old woman (Table 5), and it is an irreversible, always fatal pathology, with death occurring within the first year from diagnosis in most cases (Uttley et al., 2020).

---

[305] Open Vaers [Internet]. Updated to September 22 2023. Searchable at: https://www.openvaers.com/vaersapp/reports.php

[306] National Institute of Neurological Disorders and Stroke [Internet]. Available at: https://www.ninds.nih.gov/health-information/disorders/creutzfeldt-jakob-disease.

Table 5. VAERS reports of neurological events compatible with Creutzfeldt-Jakob disease after receiving the COVID vaxgene. Data updated to October 2, 2023.

ID VAERS	Age (years)	Sex	Vaxgene
1244735	68	Man	Pfizer
1487386	60	Man	Moderna
1517906	62	Woman	Janssen
1535217	64	Woman	Pfizer
1700415	69	Woman	Moderna
1754973	60	Woman	Moderna
1828681	66	Man	Pfizer
2068888	30	Woman	Moderna
2109446	58	Man	Moderna
2165031	67	Woman	Moderna
2179519	49	Woman	Moderna
2223072	60	Woman	Pfizer
2251224	68	Woman	Pfizer
2256142	70	Woman	Moderna
2313180	72	Man	Pfizer
2326653	Not indicated	Woman	Pfizer
2326795	Not indicated	Woman	Pfizer
2361138	71	Man	Pfizer
2399087	72	Woman	Pfizer
2470430	Not indicated	Man	Pfizer
2471230	Not indicated	Man	Pfizer
2520446	Not indicated	Woman	Janssen
2538373	Not indicated	Not indicated	Pfizer
2549165	70	Man	Pfizer
2599818	Not indicated	Man	Pfizer
2608187	70	Woman	Moderna
2609742	67	Woman	Moderna
2609743	64	Woman	Pfizer
2615553	53	Man	Pfizer
2656416	82	Woman	Pfizer

In addition to cases of Creutzfeldt-Jakob disease, central nervous system amyloid pathologies have also begun to be reported as a possible consequence of COVID vaxgenes. For example, a case of cerebral amyloid angiopathy (ABRA) was reported in December 2022 in a 75-year-old patient two weeks after receiving the shot (Kizawa and Iwasaki, 2022). ABRA is associated with the accumulation of β-amyloid protein, leading to a dysregulated immune response against cerebral blood vessels (Salvarani et al., 2013).

In the clinical case, the patient developed severe headaches a few days after receiving the second dose of Pfizer's vaxgene, progressing to depression, aphasia[307], apraxia[308], limb weakness, and gait disturbances. Magnetic resonance imaging revealed evidence of cerebral infarctions in the occipital lobes and left parietal lobe. Brain tissue biopsy showed inflammation of blood vessels (granulomatous vasculitis), microhaemorrhages, and other features consistent with angiopathy, which, through immunohistochemistry, displayed deposits of β-amyloid protein. It is essential to mention that the patient had no medical conditions or family history that could explain the development of the condition (Salvarani et al., 2013).

We must also consider the onset and exacerbation of other progressive and irreversible neurodegenerative diseases, such as Parkinson's disease and Alzheimer's disease, as a possible consequence of the COVID vaxgenes. For instance, cases of symptom exacerbation have been reported in at least six patients with Parkinson's disease (Imbalzano et al., 2022; Mörz et al., 2022; Russell and Quinn, 2022; Erro et al., 2021). The population-level relevance of post-vaccination exacerbations of Parkinson's disease is still uncertain. For example, a study that followed 177 vaccinated patients for two months with two doses of Pfizer's vaxgene found evidence of post-vaccination exacerbation in 1.1% of patients (Cosentino et al., 2022). However, a more recent study found that nearly 40% of 34 Parkinson's disease patients experienced an exacerbation of their symptoms after receiving the vaxgene, with a duration of up to two weeks (Sabat et

[307] Speech disorder that affects a person's ability to communicate.
[308] Difficulty to perform coordinated movements.

al., 2023). These contrasting results may reflect differences in the sampled population, particularly regarding the time elapsed since the administration of the vaxgene until patients were diagnosed with Parkinson's disease, as well as their age and the duration of symptom monitoring.

In the case of Alzheimer's disease, case reports of delirium after receiving the COVID vaxgene have been published (Naharci and Tasci, 2021; Zavala-Jonguitud and Pérez-García, 2021). Since cases of symptom exacerbation have also been reported in Alzheimer's patients infected with SARS-CoV-2 (Nuovo et al., 2022), it is plausible that the pathophysiology may be due to the effects of the Spike protein or to an uncontrolled inflammatory process (Hromić-Jahjefendić et al., 2023).

On the other hand, post-vaccination onset of amyotrophic lateral sclerosis (ALS) [309], also known as Lou Gehrig's or Charcot's disease, a condition affecting motor neurons, has also been reported (Feldman et al., 2022). ALS progresses rapidly, leading to muscle weakness, limb paralysis, and ultimately paralysis of the respiratory muscles within two to five years of symptom onset (van Es et al., 2017). One of the most recent cases involved a previously healthy 47-year-old male who developed weakness on the left side of his body, falls, speech impairments, and dysphagia. His symptoms developed over seven days after receiving Janssen's COVID vaxgene and worsened over several months, eventually leading to an ALS diagnosis. The authors of the case proposed the case be due to an exacerbated inflammatory response caused by the vaxgene that caused neuroinflammation (Feghali et al., 2023). The patient likely had a genetic predisposition, as indicated by the case authors, given that his grandmother had the same disease.

These reports are concerning, especially considering the accumulated reports in adverse event monitoring systems. For example, in the United States adverse event monitoring system, 5,944 cases of ALS possibly

---

[309] It is a disease that affects motor neurons, that is, those that allow movement, and is characterized by a fatal progressive arrest. It is also known as Lou Gehrig's disease.

associated with COVID vaxgenes have been reported, in contrast to the 1,050 reports of ALS possibly associated with all flu vaccines since 1990[310].

Many neurodegenerative diseases can lead to dementia (Gale et al., 2018). Therefore, it is relevant that, to date, 1,037 cases of dementia in individuals who received a COVID vaxgene have been reported in the U.S. adverse event monitoring system, with 185 occurring in individuals under 70 years old (71 in individuals under 60 and 41 in individuals under 50). Applying the correction factor (see Chapter 3), we would be talking about 32,147 possible cases so far, with 1,271 in individuals under 50. Again, comparing this with the 62 cases of dementia possibly associated with any flu vaccine administered since 1990 it is clear there is a potential problem. Furthermore, unlike with COVID vaxgenes, of these 62 cases associated with the flu vaccine, only two have occurred in individuals under 50. Applying the same correction factor to these reports, we see that annual cases of dementia associated with COVID vaxgenes are 183 times more frequent than annual cases of dementia associated with all flu vaccines. In Europe, similar data have been recorded; in Eudravigilance[311] the following cases of dementia associated with different COVID vaxgenes have been reported:

- Pfizer original and Pfizer bivalent vaxgenes - 381 (of which 9% were reported in individuals under 64 years).

- Moderna original and Moderna bivalent vaxgenes - 192 (of which 18% were reported in individuals under 64 years).

- AstraZeneca vaxgene - 103 (of which 29% were reported in individuals under 64 years).

---

[310] Open Vaers [Internet]. Data updated to September 29 2023. Searchable at: https://www.openvaers.com/

[311] European database of suspected adverse drug reaction reports [Internet]. Data updated to October 2 2023. The count includes cases of dementia, Alzheimer's dementia, dementia with delirium, dementia with depression and dementia with Lewy bodies. Searchable at: https://www.adrreports.eu/en/search_subst.html#

- Janssen vaxgene - 16 (of which 50% were reported in individuals under 64 years).

There is already evidence that dementia associated with COVID vaxgenes goes far beyond sporadic clinical cases and reports on adverse event monitoring pages. A review of official data from the Australian Government by Andrew Madry[312] found a marked increase in dementia-associated mortality compared to previous annual averages. This increase coincides with the start of COVID vaccination in Australia's elderly care facilities (Fig. 24). The observed increase represents 800 excess deaths due to dementia. Obviously, with this data, it is not possible to attribute causality of dementia to the vaxgenes, but given that there is biological plausibility, it should be considered that there may be an association between COVID vaxgenes and the increase in dementia-related deaths.

Regrettably, as I have written before, COVID vaxgenes were administered widely, with no studies on the risks they could represent for people with a family history that could suggest predisposition to this and other neurodegenerative diseases. Given the severity of some conditions, such as Creutzfeldt-Jakob disease and dementia, induced by autoimmune encephalitis, even if there are relatively few cases reported, these should be considered as a risk by the doctors who are recommending these vaxgenes to their patients, and by the patients themselves. It should certainly be part of the information given to patients before they consent to receiving one or more doses.

[312] https://andrewmadry.substack.com/p/excess-dementia-deaths-in-australia. Accessed October 9, 2023.

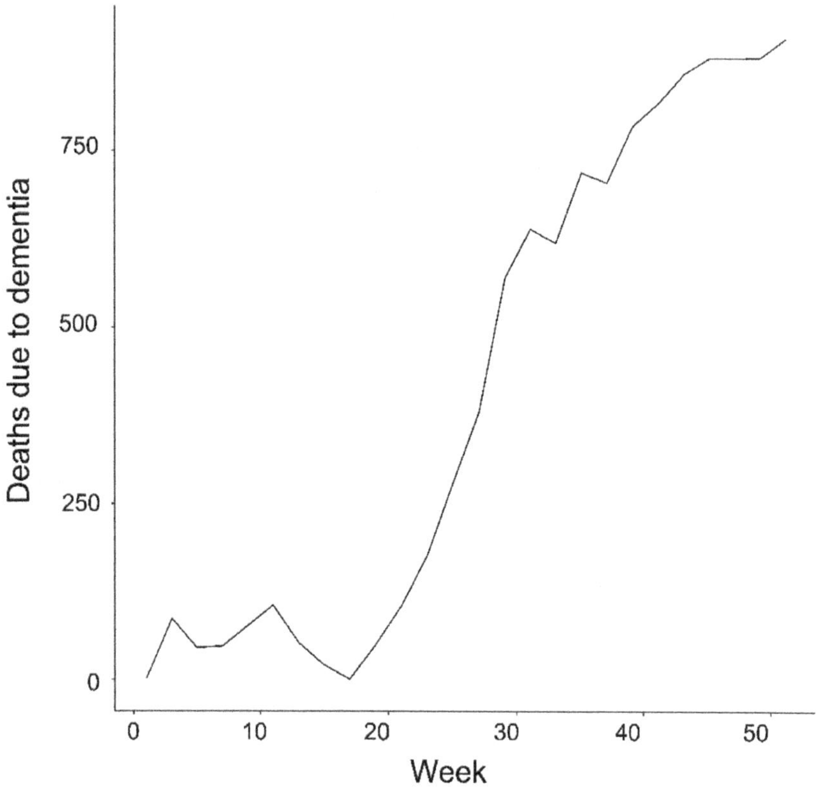

Figure 24. *Deaths due to dementia in Australia during 2021. The graph shows the deaths due to dementia that accumulated weekly during 2021 minus the deaths due to dementia that accumulated weekly in 2020. Graph drawn using data from Andrew Madry (2023) Source: https://andrewmadry.substack.com/p/excess-dementia-deaths-in-australia.*

b) Demyelinating diseases and myelopathies

In September 2021, an article was published online that analysed clinical cases of inflammation of the central nervous system in individuals who had received an mRNA-based COVID vaxgene (Khayat-Khoei et al., 2022). The article reported seven cases of demyelination (loss of myelin) in individuals aged 24 to 64, occurring within 21 days after vaccination with Pfizer or Moderna vaxgenes. The affected patients exhibited neurological symptoms and signs, and magnetic resonance imaging revealed changes consistent with active demyelination of the optic nerve, brain, and spinal cord. These changes led to conditions such as blindness, optic dysmetria (differences in vision between the eyes), walking instability, paraesthesia, loss of sphincter control, and muscle weakness (Khayat-Khoei et al., 2022). Two of the demyelination-related conditions most commonly associated with mRNA-based COVID vaxgenes are Guillain-Barré Syndrome (GBS) and multiple sclerosis.

GBS is characterized by acute involvement of peripheral nerves[313], leading to muscle weakness that progresses ascendingly[314] over days or weeks and may result in paralysis (Dash et al., 2015). It is termed a 'syndrome' because its origin is multifactorial, although increasing research points to an autoimmune origin following various infections (Kuwabara, 2004). This is due to the resemblance of some proteins from bacteria (such as *Campylobacter jejuni* or *Mycoplasma pneumoniae*) or viruses (such as human herpesvirus 4, also called Epstein-Barr virus, or Cytomegalovirus) to cellular components (Jasti et al., 2016), such as gangliosides, which are essential glycolipids for maintaining myelin[315] stability (Schnaar, 2010).

The evidence of the relationship between GBS and autoimmune responses caused by the similarity of proteins in some bacteria and viruses to gangliosides is compelling (Laman et al., 2022). For example, around 30% of GBS cases are associated with prior *Campylobacter jejuni* infections. The mechanism also helps explain why GBS cases can occur

---

[313] The nerves of the extremities and body trunk.

[314] That advances from bottom to top in the body.

[315] Layer of lipids, water and associated proteins that covers the neurons of the central and peripheral nervous system.

after receiving certain vaccines (Shoenfeld and Aron-Maor, 2000; Stratton et al., 1994), although the risk of occurrence also depends on genetic susceptibility (Dutta et al., 2022; Khanmohammadi et al., 2021), which influences the regulation of inflammatory processes.

The annual incidence[316] of Guillain-Barré Syndrome (GBS) is 1.3 cases per 100,000 people, and it is generally more common in men than in women (1.5 cases in women per case in men), regardless of age (Dash et al., 2015; Kuwabara, 2004). While a high percentage of people recover (sometimes without sequelae), it can be fatal in 9-17% of cases (Jasti et al., 2016), because it can weaken the diaphragm and intercostal muscles, making breathing impossible (Orlikowski et al., 2004).

A particular type of GBS, less common, is known as Miller Fisher Syndrome. The mechanisms by which this syndrome occurs are similar to those of GBS but typically do not manifest as lower limb weakness. Instead, it presents as incoordination (ataxia), absence of reflexes (areflexia), and ocular paralysis (ophthalmoplegia), which has been proposed to result from a direct action of anti-ganglioside antibodies on the neuromuscular junctions between cranial nerves and ocular muscles (Rocha Cabrero and Morrison, 2023).

The potentially causal association between COVID vaxgenes and the development of GBS has been known since July 2021, eight months after the initiation of the vaccination campaign in most countries, when the FDA issued a warning about the risk after recording 100 cases of post-vaxgene GBS[317]. These reports had occurred after receiving the COVID vaxgene from Janssen. Ninety-five of the 100 cases were critical, requiring hospitalization, and one case resulted in death. Due to the risk, the CDC added Guillain-Barré Syndrome to the list of adverse events that could occur in individuals who received Janssen's COVID vaxgene[318]. However, in its recommendations, the FDA downplayed its own warning, stating that

---

[316] Number of new cases in a given population at a given time. It is normally expressed as cases per 100,000 people in a year.
[317] Food and Drug Administration. Coronavirus Update. [Internet]. Available at: https://www.fda.gov/news-events/press-announcements/coronavirus-COVID-update-july-13-2021
[318] Centres for Disease Control and Prevention [Document]. Available at: https://stacks.cdc.gov/view/cdc/108880

the number of cases was low, given that "*of 12.5 million doses administered, only these 100 cases have been reported*", and they indicated that "*although the available evidence suggests an association between the Janssen [Johnson & Johnson] vaccine and increased risk of GBS, it is insufficient to establish a causal relationship*" [297].

It's interesting that despite the FDA stating in July 2021 that a similar signal had not been identified with the synthetic mRNA vaxgenes from Moderna and Pfizer, out of the 385 reports of GBS in individuals who had received any mRNA-based COVID vaxgene registered in the United States, 157 were associated with Pfizer's, and 145 with Moderna's, while Janssen's vaxgene was linked to 76 cases (representing 20% of the total). A more recent search shows that as of September 29, 2023, 4,231 reports have been registered, with 617 associated with Janssen and 3,564 associated with synthetic mRNA vaxgenes (84% of all cases registered up to the time of writing this book)[319]. According to Statista, by April 2023, 19,003,955 doses of Janssen's COVID vaxgene had been administered in the United States, while 655,377,391 doses of Moderna's and Pfizer's synthetic mRNA vaxgenes had been administered[320]. This means that if we consider that the vaccination rate in the United States has remained almost stable between April and October 2023, the reported cases of GBS associated with Janssen occur at a rate of 0.00032% per dose, while GBS cases associated with synthetic mRNA vaxgenes occur at a rate of 0.00054%. In other words, despite the FDA's statement in July 2021 warning of this risk for that particular vaxgene, the synthetic mRNA vaxgenes from Moderna and Pfizer are associated with an equivalent or slightly higher risk of GBS.

Should the occurrence of GBS cases among those vaccinated against SARS-CoV-2 surprise us? Not really, considering that during 2020, at the beginning of the COVID pandemic, cases of GBS were reported in individuals diagnosed with COVID (e.g., Dufour et al., 2021; Filosto et al., 2021; Fragiel et al., 2021; Abu-Rumeileh et al., 2020; Lucchese and Flöel,

---

[319] Open Vaers [Internet]. Data updated to September 29 2023. Searchable at: https://www.openvaers.com/

[320] Statista. Number of COVID vaccine doses administered in the United States as of April 26, 2023, by vaccine manufacturer [Internet]. Available at: https://www.statista.com/statistics/1198516/COVID-vaccinations-administered-us-by-company/

2020). This suggests that something in the pathogenic process, either due to the action of the SARS-CoV-2 virus or due to dysregulated immune responses to the virus, may explain the association. It's unlikely to be a linear and direct causal relationship, as not all studies found evidence of an association between GBS cases and COVID at the population level (Keddie et al., 2021). However, the presence of anti-ganglioside antibodies has been reported in some individuals diagnosed with COVID who developed GBS (Butler et al., 2022; Dufour et al., 2021). This is relevant because, regardless of the initial promoting factor, anti-ganglioside antibodies are detected in up to 50% of GBS cases (Cutillo et al., 2020) and are often associated with an unfavourable prognosis for the condition (Thomma et al., 2023). On the other hand, the occurrence of GBS with synthetic mRNA vaxgenes may be associated with immune dysregulation due to the excessive synthesis of pro-inflammatory cytokines (see section 5.3) or a "bystander effect" in which self-reactive lymphocytes activated by the presence of antigens similar to self-antigens trigger a severe inflammatory response (Eslait-Olaciregui et al., 2023; Wan et al., 2022; Shemer et al., 2021).

Since the beginning of the vaccination campaign, reports have been accumulating of individuals developing Guillain-Barré Syndrome (GBS) from days to months after receiving a COVID vaxgene. It's noteworthy that these cases occurred in individuals with no history of neurological or autoimmune disorders and no comorbidities. The cases were associated with both vectorized and synthetic mRNA vaxgenes. At the time of writing this book, there are 374 scientific publications in the PubMed scientific library discussing GBS related to COVID vaxgenes, and 73 of these publications are clinical case reports that occurred in individuals after being vaccinated with COVID vaxgenes[321]. I want to clarify that I've excluded from the list cases reported in individuals vaccinated with inactivated or protein-based vaccines since the focus of this book is on vaxgenes. I've also excluded cases where individuals developed GBS and were diagnosed with COVID despite being vaccinated, to avoid attributing the case to the virus rather than the vaxgene.

[321] National Library of Medicine. National Center for Biotechnology Information [Internet]. Search conducted October 22 2023. Searchable at: https://pubmed.ncbi.nlm.nih.gov/

If you take the time to read the published clinical cases (Acharya et al., 2023; Algahtani et al., 2023; Berrim et al., 2023; Do et al., 2023; Donaldson and Margolin, 2023; Lee and Lien, 2023; Mufti et al., 2023; Ogunjimi et al., 2023; Sii et al., 2023; Soh et al., 2023; Sukockienė et al., 2023; Anjum et al., 2022; Bazrafshan et al., 2022; Bellucci et al., 2022; Biswas and Pandey, 2022; Bonifacio et al., 2022; Bouattour et al., 2022; Chang and Chang, 2022; Eren et al., 2022; Fakhari et al., 2022; Fukushima et al., 2022; Gunawan et al., 2022; Hilts et al., 2022; Hwang and Bong, 2022; Ilyas et al., 2022; Khan et al., 2022; Kim J. W. et al., 2022; Kim N. et al., 2022; Lanman et al., 2022; Lázaro et al., 2022; Liang et al., 2022; Malamud et al., 2022; Masuccio et al., 2022; Nagalli et al., 2022; Nanatsue et al., 2022; Onoda et al., 2022; Pegat et al., 2022; Pirola et al., 2022; Prado et al., 2022; Richardson-May et al., 2022; Siddiqi et al., 2022; Sosa-Hernández et al., 2022; Su et al., 2022; Thant et al., 2022; Zubair et al., 2022; Allen et al., 2021; Aomar-Millán et al., 2021; Badoiu et al., 2021; Čenščák et al., 2021; Christensen et al., 2021; Dalwadi et al., 2021; Dang and Bryson, 2021; Finsterer et al., 2021a; Introna et al., 2021; Jain E. et al., 2021; James et al., 2021; Kanabar and Wilkinson, 2021; Kripalani et al., 2021; Ling et al., 2021; Maramattom et al., 2021; Matarneh et al., 2021; Min et al., 2021; Morehouse et al., 2021; Nasuelli et al., 2021; Ogbebor et al., 2021; Oo et al., 2021; Osowicki et al., 2021; Prasad et al., 2021; Rao et al., 2021; Rossetti et al., 2021; Szewczyk et al., 2021; Theuriet et al., 2021; Trimboli et al., 2021; Waheed et al., 2021), you will see that there is no clear relationship between the presentation of GBS and the patient's age, the type of vaxgene they received, or the dose after which the event occurs. Additionally, the presence of anti-ganglioside antibodies among those affected is not consistent. This suggests that the molecular mimicry mechanism of the Spike protein, which would be expected to explain the clinical picture, does not necessarily involve gangliosides but may be directed towards other cellular carbohydrates important for the interaction of neurons with myelin in the peripheral nervous system (Mufti et al., 2023; Butler et al., 2022; Finsterer 2021b; Lucchese and Flöel, 2020) or neuroinvasion of inflammatory cells (Rzymski, 2023), as warned about in 2021 as a potential risk for COVID vaccination (Dufour et al., 2021).

Beyond the clinical case reports, which involve more than 73 affected individuals since some reports detail cases of more than one person, studies have been conducted to investigate if there is evidence of a population-level association between COVID vaccination and the frequency of GBS. In general, the conclusions of these studies suggest that COVID vaxgenes may be associated with GBS (Berrim et al., 2023; Shapiro Ben David et al., 2021), and these reactions are common (Chalela et al., 2023), although it remains unclear whether synthetic mRNA vaxgenes pose the same risk as vectorized ones (Abara et al., 2023). More importantly, in nearly half of the cases, patients do not experience recovery and are left with permanent disability (Chalela et al., 2023; Reddy et al., 2023). Additionally, the effects could be even worse for those who have had GBS in the past or if they receive another dose of the vaxgene after experiencing GBS as an adverse reaction to the first dose (Finisterer, 2021).

The finding that there may be other mechanisms, different from the generation of anti-ganglioside antibodies, to explain the occurrence of GBS cases in individuals vaccinated against COVID is highly relevant. This is also important for understanding reports of other conditions that may be related to demyelination processes, such as transverse myelitis, multiple sclerosis, and myelopathies[322] in some individuals who received COVID vaxgenes. Literature reviews have found that the most common clinical cases of myelopathies associated with COVID vaxgenes are transverse myelitis, multiple sclerosis, acute disseminated encephalomyelitis, and neuromyelitis optica spectrum disorder (briefly described below). These conditions mostly occur in women and typically present around nine days after receiving the first vaxgene dose (Garg and Paliwal, 2023; Garg and Paliwal, 2022; Ismail and Salama, 2022). In many cases, these conditions seem to be related to the production of antibodies against myelin oligodendrocyte glycoprotein (MOG), and demyelinating tumefactive lesions have been observed in some patients (Salunkhe et al., 2023).

Transverse myelitis results from inflammation of the spinal cord and is associated with back or neck pain, depending on where the inflammation occurs, and can cause weakness in the limbs or even loss of sphincter control (Beh et al., 2013). Transverse myelitis doesn't necessarily involve

[322] Myelopathy refers to diseases of the spinal cord, while myelitis is a type of myelopathy and refers to an inflammatory disease of the spinal cord.

demyelination; other factors can increase the risk of this condition, including infections, certain drugs, and systemic autoimmune conditions (Beh et al., 2013). Acute transverse myelitis is considered a rare disease, with an expected frequency of 1.34 to 4.6 cases per million people per year (Borchers and Gershwin, 2012). Therefore, it was alarming that during the phase 3 clinical trials of AstraZeneca's COVID vaxgene, three people who were vaccinated developed transverse myelitis (Voysey et al., 2021). Of these, at least one was determined to have been caused by the vaxgene. This fact alone should have alerted regulators, given that the number of people in the clinical trial exposed to AstraZeneca's vaxgene at the time of developing transverse myelitis during the trial was 12,021 (Voysey et al., 2021). If AstraZeneca's vaxgene could not directly or indirectly cause this condition, not a single case would have been expected in the clinical trial, considering the common occurrence rate of less than 5 per million people in the population (Borchers and Gershwin, 2012). This led to the suspension of AstraZeneca's COVID vaxgene clinical trials[323], although they were resumed shortly after, despite expressions of concern from some in the medical and scientific community (Mallapaty and Ledford, 2020).

Multiple sclerosis is a debilitating autoimmune disease against myelin that typically manifests between the ages of 20 and 40 (West et al., 2012). As myelin becomes the target of reactive lymphocytes, neuronal axons in the brain and spinal cord, as well as brain bodies, are affected (Liu R. et al., 2022; Lemus et al., 2018). The disease is characterized by the formation of plaques or lesions of fibrous tissue in the areas where the immune system destroyed myelin. The clinical presentation of multiple sclerosis includes blurry or double vision, pain on eye movement due to optic neuritis, rapid loss of vision, muscle weakness in limbs, muscle spasms, tingling or pain in limbs, trunk, or face, dizziness, balance impairment, loss of sphincter control, fatigue, and cognitive dysfunction (Garg and Smith, 2015).

Acute disseminated encephalomyelitis is caused by inflammation of the brain and spinal cord that results in damage to myelin. Unlike multiple sclerosis, it is more common in children (Wang, 2021; Cole et al., 2019).

---

[323] CNN. "Internal AstraZeneca safety report sheds light on neurological condition suffered by vaccine trial participant" [Internet. Available at: https://edition.cnn.com/2020/09/17/health/astrazeneca-vaccine-trial-document/index.html

The onset of symptoms (loss of vision, muscle weakness, and incoordination) can be confused with multiple sclerosis and other myelopathies, but an important characteristic is that it is associated with a rapid high fever and loss of consciousness (Paolilo et al., 2020).

Neuromyelitis optica spectrum disorder is an autoimmune disease generally mediated by antibodies against aquaporin 4 (Jarius and Wildemann, 2013), a water channel protein in astrocytes[324], affecting the central nervous system (Huda et al., 2019). The condition is characterized by inflammation of the spinal cord, severe involvement of the optic nerve and the area postrema[325] of the brain, leading to uncontrollable vomiting and hiccups. It is a serious condition that, without treatment, leaves half of the patients blind and without mobility in the limbs, with a mortality rate of 5% (Huda et al., 2019).

A literature search shows that cases of myelopathies do occur after COVID vaccination, affecting people of all sexes, ages, including young individuals, and many have no medical history that would attribute the cause to factors other than the COVID vaxgene (e.g., Madike and Lee, 2023; Mahajan et al., 2023; Anamnart et al., 2022; Finsterer 2022; Ismail and Salama, 2022; Shetty et al., 2022; Tan et al., 2022; Badrawi et al., 2021; Fujikawa et al., 2021; Notghi et al., 2021; Pagenkopf and Südmeyer, 2021; Román et al., 2021). It has also been reported that receiving a COVID vaxgene in people who already suffer from myelopathies can worsen their condition (Cai et al., 2022; Nabizadeh et al., 2022; Dinoto et al., 2021).

In general, literature reviews that are published conclude that despite the occurrence of various myelopathies as neurological adverse events of COVID vaccination, the benefits outweigh the risks (e.g., Eslait-Olaciregui et al., 2023; Ghaderi et al., 2023). It is not the goal of this book to discuss the expected, observed, and modelled benefits of COVD vaxgenes, so I will not comment on that conclusion. However, what is relevant is the fact that,

[324] Cell of the nervous system that is star-shaped and whose function is to support neurons to develop and function properly and stay in place.
[325] Anatomical region located outside the blood-brain barrier on each side of the fourth cerebral ventricle, which receives neurons from the brain, spinal cord, and medulla oblongata. It functions as a receptor for chemical signals that activate the vomiting reflex (emesis).

nearly three years after the start of the global vaccination campaign, it is now starting to be acknowledged that there is a risk of developing demyelinating diseases and other myelopathies that are not mild conditions, rarely self-limiting, and if not fatal or disabling, diminish the quality of life of affected individuals (Rosa Silva et al., 2020; Højsgaard et al., 2018).

I do not want to end this section without mentioning the cases of facial nerve paralysis that have also been associated with the COVID vaxgenes. Facial nerve paralysis, an impairment of the facial motor nerve, is more common in people aged 15 to 45 and can occur because of various conditions such as infections, traumas, tumours, and autoimmune conditions (Zhang W. et al., 2020). In addition, people with diabetes, hypertension, chronic respiratory illnesses (Baugh et al., 2013) and during pregnancy (Hussain et al., 2017). There are different types of facial nerve paralysis, with idiopathic facial nerve paralysis, also known as Bell's palsy, being the most common. This form is associated with the reactivation of herpesviruses (Gilbert 2002), with herpes simplex virus, varicella-zoster virus, and human herpesvirus 6 being the most common (Freire de Castro et al., 2022). The clinical presentation is usually unilateral and includes symptoms such as decreased tearing, increased salivation, and dysgeusia. This reflects the spectrum of the nerve damage. When incomplete, it can result in paresis[326], and when complete, it presents itself as paralysis (George et al., 2020). In many cases, facial nerve paralysis has spontaneous resolution, even without treatment (McCaul et al., 2014).

In December 2020, the FDA conducted a review of preliminary data from clinical trials of Pfizer's vaxgene as part of the emergency authorization process. They mentioned that there had been four cases of Bell's palsy in the vaccinated group and none in the control group[327]. A similar thing happened for Moderna's vaxgene, with three cases of Bell's palsy in the vaccinated group versus one in the control group (Baden et al., 2021). The regulatory agency did not consider these results as a reason to

---

[326] Mild to moderate muscular weakness.

[327] US Food and Drug Administration. Vaccines and related biological products advisory committee December 10, 2020 meeting briefing document – FDA, 2020 [Internet]. Available at: https://www.fda.gov/advisory-committees/advisory-committee-calendar/vaccines-and-related-biological-products-advisory-committee-december-10-2020-meeting-announcement

alert about the risk, arguing that the observed incidence was not higher than expected in the general population [11.5 to 53.3 per 100,000 people per year (Baugh et al., 2013)]. However, if you remember the chapter on causal inference (see Chapter 4), you know that this is not a criterium to negate causality.

Given the idiopathic behaviour of facial nerve palsy, establishing causality with a particular factor is complex. Before establishing that it is an adverse event to something, all pre-existing conditions that could increase the risk need to be taken into account (Baugh et al., 2013). This criterion has led medical reviews of cases of Bell's palsy after vaccination to frequently ignore reports, considering only a fraction of the cases that have been published in the literature (see reviews in Soltanzadi et al., 2023; Shahsavarinia et al. al., 2022; Shemer et al., 2021).

The medical review of Bell's palsy cases after vaccination has often been selective, considering only a fraction of the cases published in the literature and overlooking other risk factors that could have contributed. However, as I have explained earlier (see Chapter 4), causality is rarely linear, and facial nerve paralysis would not occur simply due to pre-existing risk factors without exposure to the COVID vaxgene (Eslait-Olaciregui et al., 2023).

At the population level, the initial epidemiological study published did not find an increase in hospital admissions due to Bell's palsy after the start of COVID vaccination in Israel (e.g., Shemer et al., 2021). However, it's crucial to note that this study involved only 37 patients. Subsequent studies with larger sample sizes indicated a significant difference in the incidence between those vaccinated against COVID and the general population. For example, Wan et al. (2022) identified 16 clinically confirmed cases of Bell's palsy after the first dose of Pfizer's vaxgene within 42 days, with an age-adjusted incidence of 42.8 per 100,000 person-years, representing 2 additional cases per 100,000 persons above the expected incidence in the general population. Another more recent study found 54 cases of Bell's palsy associated with the second dose of Pfizer's vaxgene, with an incidence of 1.58 per 100,000 doses administered and an increased risk compared to being unvaccinated, particularly during the first two weeks (Wan et al., 2023).

Wan and colleagues' (2023) findings imply that an additional 1.12 cases of Bell's palsy would be expected per 100,000 individuals receiving two doses of Pfizer's vaxgene above what is expected in the normal population. Regarding Moderna's vaxgene, while cases of Bell's palsy following vaccination have been reported (Poudel et al., 2022; Pothiawala et al., 2021), an equivalent case-control epidemiological study does not appear to have been conducted. Still, it is reasonable to consider that the risk would be similar to what has been observed for Pfizer's vaxgene.

While the potential risk may seem low at just two additional cases of Bell's palsy per 100,000 individuals receiving synthetic mRNA vaxgenes, when considering the 653.54 million doses of this type of vaxgene administered in the United States at the time of writing this book[328], and the fact that most individuals in the country have received at least two doses of vaxgenes, it implies an expectation of at least 6,535 additional cases of Bell's palsy due to these products.

It is plausible that this calculation is a reliable representation of the problem, if not an underestimation, as a search in the US adverse event monitoring system shows that as of September 29, 17,285 cases of Bell's palsy associated with COVID vaxgenes have been reported. Of these, 16,501 are attributed to the synthetic mRNA vaxgenes from Pfizer and Moderna, and 763 to the vectorized vaxgene from Janssen[329].

Although a fraction of the total reports might be cases not caused by COVID vaxgenes but by other factors, comparing these numbers with the overall reports of facial paralysis in the adverse event monitoring system indicates that COVID vaxgenes account for 38% of the total number of reports of Bell's Palsy. Let me write it again, as the percentage is very important: Over 34 months of using these vaxgenes, 38% of the 45,654 reports of facial paralysis recorded since 1990 have accumulated. Based on this, we can calculate that monthly reports of Bell's palsy associated with

---

[328] According to the WHO, at least 1,557.45 million doses of Pfizer's vaxgene have been administered in the world. The data does not reflect the doses applied in all countries. Source: https://ourworldindata.org/covid-vaccinations Accessed October 22 2023.
[329] Open Vaers [Internet]. Data updated to September 29 2023. Searchable at: https://www.openvaers.com/

COVID vaxgenes in the United States are seven times more frequent than those that have accumulated each month for all other vaccines combined, without taking into account the correction factor for underreporting (see Chapter 3).

c) Psychoneurological alterations

The COVID vaxgenes have also been associated with behavioural alterations, such as suicidal thoughts, psychotic episodes, clinical depression, etc. Case reports and series analyses on this topic have been published. One of the early articles on the subject was published in October 2021. In this case report, psychotic symptoms were described in a 31-year-old patient with no physical or mental health issues. Days after receiving a dose of the synthetic mRNA vaxgene, the patient exhibited 'erratic and strange' behaviour, including the belief that he was clairvoyant, that he could communicate with the deceased, claims that he heard people playing a drum outside his house (which was not real), and believing to be in a romantic relationship with a colleague. His symptoms worsened after the second dose of the vaxgene, to the point where police intervention was required, and he was taken to the emergency room (Reinfeld et al., 2021). Shortly afterward, two case reports were published on psychotic alterations with acute mania in healthy patients who received Pfizer's vaxgene (Yesilkaya et al., 2021). An additional case involved a 20-year-old woman who, after receiving Pfizer's vaxgene, exhibited symptoms of anxiety and hypochondriac delusions that progressed to psychosis and catatonia caused by encephalitis triggered by autoimmune responses against N-methyl-D-aspartate (NMDA) receptors induced by the vaxgene (Flannery et al., 2021).

Following these initial reports, in February 2022, another case report was published describing a psychosis associated with Pfizer's COVID vaxgene (Aljeshi et al., 2022). The case involved a 20-year-old woman with no relevant psychiatric or medical history and no family history of psychiatric problems. She was admitted to the emergency room after experiencing a seizure episode four weeks after anxiety, altered sleep patterns, and behavioural changes that began a few days after receiving the second dose of the synthetic mRNA vaxgene. In the emergency room, the patient reported anxiety, restlessness, decreased appetite, hearing voices, and feeling that people were staring at her. Her sleep was interrupted by nightmares and night terror. All physical examination data, imaging studies of the brain, pelvis, and abdomen, electroencephalography, and neurological examination were normal. She remained hospitalized for a week to determine if she had more epilepsy-like episodes, which did not occur; however, during that time, the patient showed disorientation and visual and auditory hallucinations, as well as speech and aggression alterations. She was treated with antipsychotics and transferred to the psychiatric unit, where she stayed for a month (Aljeshi et al., 2022).

A month later, in March 2022, a case of post-vaccination psychosis with a vectorized vaxgene (AstraZeneca) was published. The patient was an 18-year-old female who, like previous cases, had no physical or mental medical history and did not use recreational drugs. The patient presented with irrelevant speech and strange behaviour that prompted her family to take her to the emergency unit. Her symptoms began days after receiving the first COVID vaxgene dose and included episodes of irritation, attempts to escape from her home, a feeling of being pursued, and visual hallucinations of God and demons. Physical and neurological examinations found nothing relevant, and autoimmune causes, delirium, and others, were ruled out. The diagnosis was psychosis associated with vaccination (Grover et al., 2022). The described case was similar to another case involving a healthy 25-year-old man, who developed psychosis after the second dose of a synthetic mRNA COVID vaxgene (Renemane et al., 2022). The patient experienced insomnia, anxiety and tremors immediately after receiving the vaxgene. The condition progressed to episodes of persecution delusions, thoughts he did not identify as his own, suicidal ideas, and attempted suicide, requiring the use of antipsychotic drugs. The authors concluded that there was strong evidence of causality between the psychotic condition and the mRNA vaxgene (Renemane et al., 2022). On the other hand, cases of exacerbation of bipolar disorder after receiving synthetic mRNA COVID vaxgene doses have also been reported (Guina et al., 2022).

Since then, case reports of nearly 20 patients who experienced psychotic episodes after receiving COVID vaxgenes have been published (Siao et al., 2023; Balasubramanian et al., 2022), including paediatric patients (Lien et al., 2023). In most cases, these are individuals without a psychiatric history. While these events are not very common, it is relevant to note that some cases have occurred after receiving the third dose of synthetic mRNA vaxgenes, without noticeable adverse events occurring after the first two doses (Imbalzano et al., 2022). It has even been advised to consider vaxgene-induced psychosis as a relevant aetiology to consider (Alphonso et al., 2022).

It is surprising to read the results of a recent study that, despite detecting neuropsychological and neurological symptoms (including cognitive impairment in 36% of cases, as well as attention, executive function, and memory deficits) in a high proportion of patients who received Pfizer's COVID vaxgene, the authors concluded that "*as no pathological findings were obtained in routine diagnostics, uncertainty remains about the underlying pathophysiological mechanisms ...*" (Gerhard et al., 2023). It is surprising because they did not perform any of the analyses that would allow them to understand the pathophysiology by which the synthetic mRNA vaxgene could have caused these events, such as searching for autoantibodies, measuring Spike protein levels in cerebrospinal fluid, among others.

According to Mopuru and Menon (2023), the mechanisms that can explain the causal relationship between COVID vaxgenes and the presentation of psychoneurological conditions include:

1) Proinflammatory events due to uncontrolled cytokine synthesis that can lead to a reduction in NMDA receptor function, decreasing inhibitory control of dopaminergic neurons. Indeed, alterations in the concentration of pro-inflammatory cytokines are known to cause schizophrenia, bipolar disorder, and depressive states (Goldsmith et al., 2016).
2) Autoimmunity caused by the similarity between peptides of the Spike protein and cellular proteins of the nervous system, such as NMDA receptors or leucine-rich glioma-inactivated protein 1 (LGI1). There is evidence that some cases of encephalitis occurring in individuals after receiving COVID vaxgenes may be due to autoimmunity (Deniz et al., 2023; Grover et al., 2022; Zlotnik et al.,

2022; Flannery et al., 2021; Roberts et al., 2021). Post-vaccination psychotic symptoms may be due to autoimmune encephalitis, as reported for some vaccines in the past (Kayser and Dalmau, 2016).

3) Changes in neuronal metabolism. Since it is known that COVID vaxgenes cause sustained inflammation and that such inflammation can suppress the metabolism of molecules metabolized by cytochrome P450 (White, 2022), it is possible that in vaccinated people medicated with drugs like clozapine, the metabolism of these drugs is reduced, leading to various mental disturbances.

4) Vaccine stress caused by fear of the risks of COVID vaxgenes and vaccines. This was proposed by Ransing and colleagues (2021), who argued that concerns about the vaccine's safety could cause high stress, which could promote psychiatric reactions. However, although this is a possible mechanism, it is unlikely that reports of psychosis after receiving the COVID shot are due to this mechanism, as it cannot explain the presence of anti-NMDA receptor and anti-leucine-rich glioma-inactivated protein 1 (LGI1) antibodies detected in some patients who developed these psychoneurological conditions after vaccination (Deniz et al., 2023; Grover et al., 2022; Zlotnik et al., 2022; Flannery et al., 2021; Roberts et al., 2021).

To understand why COVID vaxgenes might cause autoimmune and autoinflammatory pathologies in the brain, it is necessary to remember that the Spike protein of SARS-CoV-2 shares similarity in many of its regions with fragments of human proteins (see section 4.5 in Chapter 4) and that the persistence of synthetic mRNA in the cytoplasm of transfected cells activates immune responses that can lead to autoinflammatory states (see section 4.3 in Chapter 4). On the other hand, the Spike protein of SARS-CoV-2 can also induce inflammatory states, including cytokine storms (see section 4.5). If an autoimmune reaction occurs against an essential protein of neurons, or if these proteins are damaged by sustained inflammatory action, psychoneurological alterations may occur. Remember that neurons communicate with each other through synapses, which are connections between cell membranes where molecules called neurotransmitters are released, exciting or calming the cells they act upon. Glutamic acid, or glutamate, is the main neurotransmitter with an excitatory postsynaptic effect in the brain and is related to different types of receptors in the cells of the nervous system, including NMDA receptors (Paoletti et al., 2013). These have been implicated in various psychoneurological alterations following reception of a COVID vaxgene. NMDA receptors are proteins expressed in the membrane of postsynaptic neurons that, when activated, allow cations to pass through ion channels (Vyklicky et al., 2014). Under normal conditions, the functioning of NMDA receptors is strictly regulated. It is so controlled that the ion channel only opens if the postsynaptic neuron is depolarized when glutamate touches the synapse, achieving a gradual response to a given stimulus (Kandel et al., 2014). So, when activated, many brain processes are impacted, such as memory, especially episodic or experiential memory, and learning, which are based on neuronal plasticity, as it is essential to maintain functional connections between neurons. Therefore, NMDA receptors are related to some neurodegenerative pathologies such as Alzheimer's disease, Parkinson's disease, and Huntington's disease, as well as schizophrenia and epilepsy (Jewett et al., 2022; Wang et al., 2015).

Thus, if NMDA receptors in the brain are damaged, the synapses of neurons that use glutamate as a neurotransmitter will be affected (Dalmau et al., 2008). This can cause various psychiatric symptoms, prompted by a mechanism known as the glutamatergic model of schizophrenia. In this model, dysfunction of NMDA receptors would cause a reduction in glutamate transmission, which in some individuals can induce states of inactivity, catatonia, or autism, while in others it can cause a reduction in GABA transmission, increasing dopaminergic transmission, resulting in symptoms of schizophrenia or psychosis, with delirium and hallucinations (Tsutsui et al., 2017; Gordon, 2010). On the other hand, the occurrence of autoimmune encephalitis due to antibodies against the leucine-rich glioma-inactivated protein 1 (LGI1) has also been reported after the second dose of Pfizer's vaxgene (Zlotnik et al., 2022). This pathology leads to rapid progressive dementia and cognitive impairments, among other clinical manifestations (Li et al., 2019).

Anti-NMDA receptor antibody encephalitis is the second most common immune encephalopathy (Dalmau et al., 2011), and there are reports of its occurrence following some infections with certain herpesviruses, such as herpes simplex virus 1 (Nosadini et al., 2017), Epstein-Barr virus (Hou et al., 2019), Japanese encephalitis virus (Ma et al., 2020), and SARS-CoV-2 (Valadez-Calderon et al., 2022; Sarigecili et al., 2021; Paterson et al., 2020). This encephalitis has also been reported after vaccination against yellow fever, H1N1 influenza, Japanese encephalitis, and more recently, with COVID vaxgenes and vaccines (Deniz et al., 2023; Etemadifar et al., 2022; Flannery et al., 2021). The most parsimonious explanation for this pathology is the similarity of some virus proteins to NMDA receptors (Vasilevska et al., 2021). The fact that it has occurred in some people who were infected with SARS-CoV-2, as well as in at least one case in a patient vaccinated with a traditional COVID vaccine (inactivated, Sinovac brand; Etemadifar et al., 2022), and in a patient that received a COVID vaxgene (Pfizer brand) suggests that the effect is, indeed, due to similarities between the Spike protein of SARS-CoV-2 and the NMDA receptor protein.

An additional, not mutually exclusive, mechanism that could help understand the relationship between psychoneurological alterations and COVID vaxgenes is that cholesterol present in these products can directly interact with dopamine transporters (Jones et al., 2012). This could explain the involuntary movements (known as dyskinesia) observed in some individuals with or without previous neurological conditions who have received the inoculation (Batot et al., 2022; Cincotta et al., 2022; Cosentino et al., 2022; Ryu et al., 2022; Erro et al., 2021; Matar et al., 2021).

Beyond the mechanisms that may explain the occurrence of psychoneurological alterations, it is particularly relevant in the context of COVID vaccination that these are not isolated cases (Abdelhady et al., 2023; Finsterer, 2023). In the European Union adverse event reporting system, Eudravigilance, there are, at the time of writing this book, 121,859 reports of psychiatric events after receiving a COVID vaxgene, including hundreds to thousands of cases of hallucinations, delirium, and suicidal ideation[330]. The occurrence of these psychoneurological alterations is likely

[330] Eudravigilance. European Database of Suspected Adverse Drug Reactions [Internet]. Data updated to October 2 2023. The value considers what has been reported for all COVID vaxgenes and vaccines used in the European Union. Available at: https://www.adrreports.eu/en/search_subst.html#

determined by susceptibility factors in vaccinated individuals, which have not yet been systematically identified.

It is important to note that these reports in adverse event monitoring systems, as well as published case reports, cannot be taken as evidence that everyone who received the vaxgenes will develop psychotic disorders after receiving a dose, nor does it mean that all psychotic episodes occurring since December 2020 are due to the vaxgenes. However, considering that, according to the WHO[331], 5,630,000,000 people have received at least one COVID vaccine, and that authorities in various countries are recommending booster doses (see section 6.7), the risk of psychotic episodes associated with these vaxgenes should not be ignored. Unfortunately, it adds to the list of events that were not identified in the short phase 3 studies that led to the authorization of these products.

Another one of the many things that was not studied prior to the authorization of COVID vaxgenes was the possibility of negative interactions between vaccine components and various drugs. In other words, it was not known, before authorizing them, whether these vaxgenes could interfere, enhance, or suppress other drugs, or vice versa (Sfera et al., 2022). Despite that, administration was prioritized for people with a wide range of comorbidities, including severe psychiatric illnesses (Mazereel et al., 2021). This recommendation was made even though there were no studies on the efficacy and safety of COVID vaxgenes in patients being treated with psychotropic drugs.

To understand why a person taking psychotropic drugs might have a negative interaction when given a vaxgene, or a reduction in the protection it could confer, it is necessary to understand that various psychotropic drugs, such as haloperidol, clozapine, olanzapine, and imipramine, increase the expression of a cholesterol transporter, ApoE, which is often affected in people with severe psychiatric illness. This implies potential interference with the transfection rate (cell entry) of vaccine nanolipids. On the other hand, psychotropic drugs also increase the expression of the ATP-binding

[331] Our World in Data [Internet]. Data updated to October 23 2023. Available at; https://ourworldindata.org/explorers/coronavirus-data-explorer

cassette transporter (ABCA1), which increases cholesterol efflux from cells, and this can also alter the effectiveness of vaxgenes by expelling the nanolipids from the cells (Sfera et al., 2022).

In terms of adverse effects, many anaesthetics interact with NMDA receptors (Dalmau et al., 2011) and can, therefore, worsen a case of encephalitis caused by anti-NMDA receptor antibodies (Pascual-Ramírez et al., 2011). This occurs because anti-NMDA receptor antibodies bind to a receptor subunit and disrupt the communication between its substrate (NMDA) and ephrin-B2 receptor, causing synaptic receptor displacement and a decrease in NMDA receptor density (Mikasova et al., 2012). Inhibitory GABA-dependent interneurons may also be inactivated, as they express high concentrations of NMDA receptors, contributing to the pathophysiology of anti-NMDA receptor antibody encephalitis (Mikasova et al., 2012), leading to a hyperglutamatergic state, clinically manifested with confusion, memory loss, personality changes, depression, and, in later stages, hallucinations, seizures, coma, and autonomic instability (Dalmau et al., 2011). Since many anaesthetics act by inhibiting NMDA receptors, they can induce the same symptoms as those observed in anti-NMDA receptor antibody encephalitis and exacerbate existing symptoms in people suffering from this pathology (Lapébie et al., 2014; Kawano et al., 2011; Pascual-Ramírez et al., 2011). Given that, despite isolated cases of anti-NMDA receptor antibody encephalitis being reported, the number of people who have developed anti-NMDA receptor antibodies as a result of COVID vaxgenes is unknown, systematic epidemiological monitoring at the neuropsychiatric level would be imperative to identify vaccinated individuals who might experience symptom aggravation if administered any anaesthetic that inhibits NMDA receptors, including nitric oxide, xenon (Jevtović-Todorović et al., 1998), propofol, and sevoflurane (Lapébie et al., 2014).

It is worth noting that, in addition to their action on calcium, potassium, and sodium channels in neurons, local anaesthetics also operate on anti-NMDA receptors (Dingledine et al., 1999). This is relevant because it means that even common local anaesthetics (bupivacaine, lidocaine, procaine, and tetracaine), when applied to the spinal cord, whose neurons also express NMDA receptors (Woolf and Salter, 2000), inhibit the function of NMDA receptors. This inhibition is more potent with ester-type local anaesthetics, such as procaine, than with amide-type local anaesthetics, such as bupivacaine (Sugimoto et al., 2003). This means that, after epidural administration, local anaesthetics can inhibit NMDA receptors since they reach high concentrations in the spinal cord (Sugimoto et al., 2003). Therefore, it is not unreasonable to consider the possibility that individuals that received a COVID vaxgene and who developed anti-NMDA receptor antibodies may have exacerbated clinical symptoms associated with that autoimmune process if they are administered local anaesthetics for a surgical intervention.

Almost two years after the start of inoculations, evidence is beginning to emerge that could be explained by interactions between COVID vaxgenes and psychotropic drugs. Specifically, a study reported that out of nearly 270,000 vaccinated war veterans, 15% developed COVID after being vaccinated (Nishimi et al., 2022). If a vaccine is effective, the disease it aims to prevent should not occur. So, when it does, it could be due to vaccine failures, issues with the immune systems of the recipients, or the vaccine itself causing the disease. Considering what has been explained in previous chapters, where it was highlighted that different components of COVID vaxgenes cause pro-inflammatory and autoinflammatory effects, along with prothrombotic conditions, as seen in some people infected with SARS-CoV-2, it cannot be ruled out that what is being diagnosed as COVID is actually a pathological condition with clinical signs indistinguishable from COVID but caused by the vaxgene itself (Parry et al., 2023).

In the study by Nishimi and colleagues (2022), vaccinated individuals that had a psychiatric disorder had a higher risk of developing COVID, even when accounting for confounding factors and adjusting for comorbidities, smokers, and age. Among these patients, the greatest risk was for those addicted to drugs and those with an adaptive disorder, although there was a significantly higher risk for those with various psychiatric conditions such as depression, schizophrenia, bipolar disorder, psychotic episodes, post-traumatic stress, anxiety, and dissociative disorders, among others. This is relevant as psychiatric disorders, common among veterans, are sometimes treated with psychotropic medications, including benzodiazepines. While the authors of the mentioned study do not discuss this possibility and rather focus on the idea that psychiatric disorders may be associated with a lower competence of cellular immune responses (Kiecolt-Glaser and Glaser, 2002), this reduced immune ability could explain their observations (Nishimi et al., 2022). However, another, not mutually exclusive, possibility, would be a drug interaction between the nanolipids in synthetic mRNA vaxgenes and psychotropic drugs. As I mentioned, the possibility of drug interactions was not addressed by any study prior to the authorization of COVID vaxgenes. Given the adverse reports of neuropsychiatric disturbances, controlled studies will be needed to investigate whether there might be an increased risk of exacerbation of these conditions in medicated patients.

6.4 Reproductive anomalies

Before delving into this section, it is essential to clarify the key points about the physiological control of reproduction. In mammals, reproduction depends on the proper functioning of different hormones that are controlled by the nervous system and the gonads (ovaries and testicles), known as the hypothalamic-pituitary-gonadal axis (Kaprara and Huhtaniemi, 2018). The hypothalamus, a specialized structure located in the centre of the brain, responds to various physical and chemical stimuli, and in response to these stimuli, it secretes the gonadotropin-releasing hormone (GnRH). This hormone acts on the pituitary gland (also called the pituitary), which is below the hypothalamus, and it consequently produces three hormones known as 'gonadotropins': luteinizing hormone (LH), follicle-stimulating hormone (FSH), and human chorionic gonadotropin (HCG), which is essential for the formation of the placenta (Herkert et al., 2022). These gonadotropins travel through the blood and in women reach the ovaries and, if pregnant, the embryo, while in men they reach the testicles (Casati et al., 2023). In the gonads, gonadotropins have various actions, such as facilitating spermatogenesis, facilitating the formation of ovarian follicles, ovulation, the growth of the uterine endometrium, and, during pregnancy, the formation and maintenance of the placenta (Mota-Mena and Puts, 2017). The secretion of GnRH is regulated by testosterone (in men) and by oestradiol, inhibin, and progesterone in women, according to the stage of the reproductive cycle. In this way, hormonal control through positive or negative feedback of the reproductive cycle is achieved.

This hormonal control adds to other factors that determine the fertility of the species, such as the viability of gametes (i.e., ovules and sperm), hormones of local action (activin, follistatin, and anti-Müllerian hormone; Ando, 2021), and the health, nutritional status, and bioenergetic status of the individual (Dupont et al., 2014).

If the above description is clear, then it should not be surprising that anything that impacts the hypothalamic-pituitary-gonadal axis or the gonads directly can affect reproduction, a process that is key for the species' continuity. In other words, a species with sexual reproduction that fails to reproduce properly would experience demographic effects and, if it continues that trend, may increase the risks of extinction. This is well understood for populations of wildlife (Harvey et al., 2022; Brook et al., 2008) or for laboratory animal lineages (Shorter et al., 2017), and given the size of the human population, it is unlikely that a decline in the reproductive rate would lead to the extinction of the human species in the near future. However, for at least the past five years, there have been discussions about the risk of a drastic decrease in fertility parameters, such as human sperm count[332], especially considering that it seems to have decreased by 50% in the last 40 years (Levine et al., 2017).

When the COVID vaxgenes were granted emergency authorization to be used widely, no studies on their safety and potential impact on reproduction had been conducted, nor had clinical trials on their safety and efficacy on pregnant women, nursing babies or on people with reproductive problems (see Chapter 2). This means that there was no way to ensure, when they began to be used outside of clinical trials, that there was certainty of safety for their use in those groups. However, 34 months after being authorized, many reports of reproductive adverse events have accumulated on the adverse event monitoring pages, as well as clinical case reports and epidemiological studies that suggest that reproduction may be being affected, directly or indirectly, by the COVID vaxgenes. We can group

---

[332] BBC "Sperm count drop 'could make humans extinct'" [Internet]. Available at: https://www.bbc.com/news/health-40719743

adverse reproductive events into three: alterations in menstruation, alterations in pregnancy and alterations in sperm parameters.

a) Menstrual alterations

Menstruation is a physiological process in primates, where reproductive-age females experience cyclic shedding of the first layer of the uterus. For this to occur in an orderly manner, it is necessary for the hormones produced by the hypothalamic-pituitary-gonadal axis to interact with each other and regulate. The follicular phase of menstruation is proliferative, while the luteal phase is the secretory phase where bleeding occurs (Reed and Carr, 2018). Irregularities in menstruation can have various causes, including pregnancy, hormonal imbalance (such as high levels of prolactin or thyroid hormone alteration), trauma, infections, certain diseases (such as polycystic ovary syndrome, diabetes, Cushing's disease, and congenital adrenal hyperplasia), and some medications (Foster and Al-Zubeidi, 2018).

Since a proper menstrual cycle is central to reproduction, it was concerning that shortly after the initiation of administration of COVID vaxgenes, numerous cases of menstrual adverse events began to be reported in adverse event monitoring systems. In just the first year of administering these products, 432 reports of menstrual irregularities had accumulated in the United States, of which 76 corresponded to reports of these alterations in women over 50 years old[333]. The same pattern was observed in other monitoring systems, including the Yellow Card system in England, and it even made international news[334]. However, the note indicated that "*women should feel confident in getting the vaccine, and reports of* [menstrual] *changes are not unexpected, as similar reactions have been observed with the influenza vaccine*"[335].

---

[333] OpenVaers. Search terms: "menstrual disorder" OR "intermenstrual bleeding" OR amenorrhea OR dysmenorrhea. Data reported 2021. [Internet]. Searchable at: https://www.openvaers.com/

[334] Sky News "COVID: More than 13,000 women report changes to periods after having vaccine, but experts say fertility not affected" [Internet]. Available at: https://news.sky.com/story/COVID-more-than-13-000-women-report-changes-to-periods-after-having-vaccine-but-experts-say-fertility-not-affected-12350899

[335] Dr. Vicky Male. Reproductive Immunologist at Imperial College London, cited by Sky News [Internet]. Available at: https://news.sky.com/story/COVID-more-than-13-000-women-report-changes-to-periods-after-having-vaccine-but-experts-say-fertility-not-affected-12350899

Let's take a moment to see if this is true. How about we compare the 423 cases of menstrual alterations associated with the COVID vaxgenes reported in 2021 with the cases of menstrual alterations associated with any flu vaccine reported in 2021? We can see that in the US adverse event monitoring system menstrual alterations associated with flu vaccines in 2021 were zero (0).

Could it be that not many flu vaccine doses were administered in 2021? If you came up with that valid question after reading the last paragraph, the answer to your question is no. According to the CDC, 198 million flu vaccine doses were distributed in 2021 in the US [336], so at least we know that it is unlikely that few doses were administered that year. Of course, 581 million doses of COVID vaxgenes were administered that year, but people were given two doses that year (at least), so if we consider the number of people who were immunized with each product (198 million people with flu vaccines vs. 210 million people with COVID vaxgenes) it is pretty equitable.

OK. But, and the reports of menstrual alterations associated with flu vaccines in prior year? Let´s see: 2017: zero reports, 2018: one report, 2019: two reports, 2020: two reports[337]. I don´t know about you, but I see a consistent pattern here. There does not appear to be an excess of menstrual alterations being reported in association with flu vaccines. How about in a year when people were afraid of the flu? I mean 2009, the year of the near pandemic of HIN1 flu. Surely many people were vaccinated against the flu that year because that is what the health authorities recommended[338]. Let's do the search, shall we?

Yes, that year was definitely much worse: there were three reported cases of menstrual alterations.

---

336 Centres for Disease Control and Prevention "2020-2021 Seasonal Influenza Vaccine Total Doses Distributed" [Internet]. Available at: https://www.cdc.gov/flu/prevent/vaccinesupply-2020.htm

337 Open Vaers. Search terms: "menstrual disorder" OR "intermenstrual bleeding" OR amenorrhea OR dysmenorrhea. Only data that were associated with any flu vaccine were included. [Internet]. Searchable at: https://www.openvaers.com/

338 Centres for Disease Control and Prevention "2009 H1N1 Vaccination Recommendations" [Internet]. Available at: https://www.cdc.gov/h1n1flu/vaccination/acip.htm

In 2022, Thorp and collaborators published a study on the number of reports of menstrual adverse events in women that had received a vaxgene. They found that the number of reports of menstrual alterations plausibly associated with COVID vaxgenes was 1,060 per billion doses compared to 0.985 per billion doses of the flu vaccines (Thorp et al., 2022). The number of reports has continued to increase. Until September 29 2023 1,009 cases of menstrual alterations had been reported to VAERS[339]. An identical search on menstrual alterations in women that were vaccinated against the flu since they started using this vaccine in the US reveals 24 reports. In other words, in the 33 years (1990 to 2022) of using attenuated and inactivated flu vaccines only 24 cases of menstrual alterations in vaccinated women have been reported. This can be translated to a rate of 0.727 reports per year and 0.06 reports per month, while the 1,009 reports that were accumulated in 34 months (between December 2021 and October 2023) since the authorization of the vaxgenes represents 29.68 reports per month. This means that menstrual alterations associated with COVID vaxgenes are 495 times more frequent than reports associated with flu vaccines. Furthermore, if we get really crazy and review the reports of menstrual disorders that have occurred against *all* vaccines (not only flu) administered from 1990 to date, we can see that 1,428 reports have accumulated in this time. This means that 71% of *all* cases of menstrual alterations reported to VAERS are associated with COVID vaxgenes.

Furthermore, of the 1,009 reports of menstrual alterations registered to date, 119 occurred in women of over 50 years, while none of the reports associated with any other vaccine occurred in women of this age group. None! This means that COVID vaxgenes can reactivate bleeding in women that had stopped menstruating. This point is very important, because although menstrual alterations and changes to the reproductive cycle could be seen as "*mild adverse events*", "*small changes*" or that "*variations are occasional, they are not dangerous and are associated with certain triggering factors*"[340], the only way in which COVID vaxgenes can be

[339] Open Vaers. Search terms: "menstrual disorder" OR "intermenstrual bleeding" OR amenorrhea OR dysmenorrhea. Data updated to September 29 2023 [Internet]. Searchable at: https://www.openvaers.com/

[340] Textual quote of the Sinc Agency. Science told in Spanish [Internet]. Available at: https://www.agenciasinc.es/Noticias/Cambios-en-la-regla-tras-la-vacuna-de-la-covid-leves-y-temporales-pero-dignos-de-estudio

associated with a resumption of bleeding in women who have already gone through menopause is that they induce hormonal alterations, either locally (in the ovary or uterus) or in the brain (impacting the hypothalamic-pituitary-gonadal axis). That is why it was so important that the basic explanation of the physiology of the reproductive cycle that I presented at the beginning of this section be clear.

Based on what we know of the biodistribution of vaxgenes (see section 5.2) and the molecular impacts of the active compounds of the vaxgenes within the cells (see section 5.3 and section 5.4), is it so complicated to understand that the alteration of the reproductive cycle due to these vaxgenes is biologically plausible?

Now, let's see what has been published about this topic. At the beginning of 2022, an epidemiological study was published that evaluated, with data collected between April and October 2021, the relationship between COVID vaxgenes and menstrual disorders (Lee et al., 2022). The authors investigated changes in menstrual bleeding among women of reproductive age and post menopause. For this, they included almost 40,000 participants between 18 and 80 years old (the average age was 33 years) who had received the complete vaccination schedule and who had not contracted COVID previously. More than half had received Pfizer vaxgenes (21,620 participants), followed by Moderna (13,001 participants), Janssen (3,469 participants), and AstraZeneca (751 participants) vaxgenes, the protein-based Novavax vaccine was received by 61 participants and 'other' vaccines by 204 participants. It was found that among women who received vaxgenes or vaccines, 42% of those who had regular menstrual cycles suffered heavier bleeding than usual. In particular, the alteration was more common among women who used long-acting contraceptives, since 71% of them reported atypical bleeding. More worrying was that menstrual bleeding was observed in 66% of postmenopausal women who had been vaccinated. The increase in blood flow and unexpected bleeding were associated with age and having other adverse effects after vaccination. No differences in menstruation disorders were found between different brands of vaxgenes (Lee et al., 2022).

Some researchers from the University of Granada carried out a cross-sectional epidemiological study between June and September 2021 on the effect of COVID vaxgenes on the menstrual cycle of Spanish women (Baena-García et al., 2022). According to this study, of the 14,153 vaccinated women who participated in the study, 78% (11,017) reported changes in their menstrual cycle after receiving the vaxgene. The most common premenstrual changes were increased fatigue (43%), abdominal bloating (37%), irritability (29%), sadness (28%), and headache (28%). The most common menstrual changes were heavier bleeding (43%), dysmenorrhea (41%), delay in menstruation (38%), shortening of bleeding days (34.5%), and shortening of the cycle (32%). The probability of changes occurring in the reproductive cycle increased with increasing age (Baena-García et al., 2022).

Another retrospective epidemiological study investigated menstrual cycle disturbances after COVID vaccination in Colombian women aged 18 to 41 years with a complete vaccination schedule[341]. These women had no reproductive or menstrual problems, were not lactating or pregnant, had no diseases associated with menstrual irregularities, and were not high-performance athletes (Rodríguez Quejada et al., 2022). Out of the 408 women included in the study, almost half (184 women) experienced menstrual disturbances after receiving the shots. The disturbances included changes in menstrual regularity (irregularity or amenorrhea[342]), changes in bleeding duration, and changes in bleeding volume. The synthetic mRNA vaxgene from Pfizer and the inactivated vaccine from Sinovac were more frequently associated with alterations in cycle regularity, but with dissimilar effects: while Pfizer's was associated with lighter bleeding, Sinovac's and other brands were associated with very heavy bleeding. It is relevant to note that of the 184 women who experienced menstrual disturbances, 56% reported a deterioration in their quality of life after being vaccinated (criteria included perception of physical and mental health, pain, and wealth) (Rodríguez Quejada et al., 2022).

[341] Perhaps you don't remember, given that in some countries they are already on the sixth booster, but in 2021 the 'full' vaccination schedule consisted of two doses, except for Janssen, which consisted of a single dose.
[342] Lack of menstruation.

More recently, a cross-sectional study conducted on adult Lebanese women who had been vaccinated against COVID showed evidence that vaxgenes were associated with changes in bleeding volume, decreased regular cycles, increased premenstrual syndromes, and that the effects were worse in women using hormonal contraception methods, those with osteoporosis, or coagulation problems (Dabbousi et al., 2023). These results were consistent with another study involving 7,904 premenopausal Israeli women over 18 years old who found that 48% experienced changes in the menstrual cycle after receiving the synthetic mRNA COVID vaxgene from Pfizer, with the most common alterations being excessive bleeding, prolonged bleeding, and intermenstrual bleeding (Issakov et al., 2023).

For those who only give value to meta-analyses, i.e., the analysis of data from all publications on the same topic to detect robust trends, I can suggest the study by Al Kadri and colleagues (2023), which, after analysing 16 studies that were valid for their methodology and experimental design, concluded that menorrhagia[343], oligomenorrhea[344], and polymenorrhea[345] are common menstrual disturbances after COVID vaccination, and the frequency of events is high (Al Kadri et al., 2023). It was also observed that some specific menstrual disturbances, such as pain, fatigue, and headache associated with menstruation, were more frequent in women with endometriosis who had received the synthetic mRNA vaxgene than in women without endometriosis that received the same shot (Martínez-Zamora et al., 2023).

The studies I mention are not the only ones that found evidence that COVID vaxgenes can alter the menstrual cycle. The list of case reports and epidemiological studies shows clear trends in women from different countries. Although most studies focused on women who received the synthetic mRNA vaxgene from Pfizer, effects have been reported for different vaxgenes (e.g., Farland et al., 2023; Lessans et al., 2023; Rastegar et al., 2023; Gibson et al., 2022; Laganà et al., 2022; M M Al-Mehaisen et al., 2022; Muhaidat et al., 2022; Sarfraz et al., 2022). It is interesting that the same authors often downplay their results, saying that although

[343] Excessively heavy or prolonged vaginal bleeding.
[344] Infrequent menstruation with abnormally long menstrual cycles.
[345] Menstrual bleeding between menstrual periods.

vaxgenes are associated with menstrual disturbances, "*changes to the menstrual cycle that occur after COVID vaccination are small and temporary and should not discourage individuals from getting vaccinated*" (Gibson et al., 2022).

It is true that the observed changes seem to be transient, at least after one or two vaxgene doses (at the time of writing this book, no study had been published on menstrual disturbances in women who had received more than two doses). However, it implies two things: 1) These studies should have been conducted before authorizing these products, and 2) COVID vaxgenes do have an impact on the menstrual cycle, which is greater than what can be caused by more commonly used inactivated or attenuated vaccines. The obligatory question to ask is, why? Although it might be a transient and mild effect, why do vaxgenes impact the menstrual cycle when inactivated and attenuated vaccines from the past do not seem to have an impact?

Now, based on the knowledge about the menstrual cycle, and what is known about the biodistribution and molecular and cellular consequences of vaxgenes (see Chapter 5), the alterations to menstruation observed could be explained by the following five mechanisms, which are not mutually exclusive:

1) Action of the Spike Protein on the Renin-Angiotensin-Aldosterone Axis: A portion of the Spike protein produced in the cells of those vaccinated with synthetic mRNA vaxgenes is released from the cell. In fact, the Spike protein has been detected in high amounts in the blood, unbound to antibodies (Yonker et al., 2023). Considering that the cellular receptor to which the Spike protein binds is angiotensin-converting enzyme 2 (ACE2), which is expressed in the ovaries, uterus, vagina, and placenta (Wu et al., 2021; Domińska 2020; Reis et al., 2011; Pereira et al., 2009), it is reasonable to suggest that Spike may interact with ACE2 on the membrane of ovarian cells. The renin-angiotensin-aldosterone axis is dysregulated once Spike binds to ACE2, and this controls the development of follicles and ovulation, modulates the formation of blood vessels supplying nutrients to the *corpus luteum*, influences its degeneration, and affects endometrial tissue and embryo

development (Jing et al., 2020). It is precisely this axis that is dysregulated by the Spike protein when it interacts with ACE2 (Dettlaff-Pokora and Swierczynski, 2021).

2) Binding to the oestrogen receptor (ER alpha): Recall that the Spike protein can bind to ER alpha (Solis et al., 2022), a protein expressed in the mammary gland, uterus, ovaries, testicles, epididymis, and prostate, among other organs (Paterni et al., 2014). Therefore, it can cause menstrual disturbances (Laganá et al., 2022) by disrupting the oestrogen signalling pathway.

3) Coagulation Abnormalities: Another plausible explanation for changes in menstrual bleeding could be coagulation abnormalities caused by mRNA and vectorized vaxgenes (see section 5.3 and section 5.5), which could lead to heavy bleeding by impacting the ability to repair endometrial bleeding (Deligeoroglou and Karountzos, 2018). Heavy menstrual bleeding can occur in women with platelet disorders (Rajpurkar et al., 2016). In line with this, in April 2021, it was proposed that, given that out of 958 cases of menstrual irregularities in vaccinated women in England, more than twice as many cases were associated with AstraZeneca's vaxgene than Pfizer's vaxgene, this could be a sign that the prothrombotic potential of the vectorized vaxgene could explain this phenomenon (Merchant 2021)[346]. It is a plausible mechanism; however, it would not explain the reactivation of bleeding in postmenopausal women, which is better explained by the alteration of hormonal pathways.

4) Disruption of the Hypothalamic-Pituitary-Gonadal Axis: For a normal menstrual cycle to occur, it is necessary for the hormone GnRH to be released appropriately and in pulses. Any condition that prevents or interferes with this cyclical pulsation would affect the menstrual cycle. This has been observed in Kallmann syndrome, a clinical condition characterized by a defect in neurons

[346] Merchant H. BMJ "COVID post-vaccine menorrhagia, metrorrhagia or postmenopausal bleeding and potential risk of vaccine-induced thrombocytopenia in women". Rapid response to BMJ 2021;373:n958 [Internet]. Available at: https://www.bmj.com/content/373/bmj.n958/rr-2

that produce GnRH (Sonne and Lopez-Ojeda, 2023), causing a delay in puberty and hypogonadism, as well as anosmia (Stamou and Georgopoulos, 2018). Stress, whether psychogenic[347], dietary, or caused by intense physical exercise, can itself affect the hypothalamic-pituitary-gonadal axis, leading to hypothalamic amenorrhea due to a reduction in GnRH pulses (Berga et al., 1989) and can also result in anovulation (Filicori et al., 1993). Depending on the stressor, the degree and duration of menstrual cycle disruption will vary; usually, if the stressor is eliminated, the condition is reversible (Ryterska et al., 2021). On the other hand, experimental studies in non-human primates have shown evidence that stress affects hypothalamic function, causing hypothalamic amenorrhea (Ferin, 1999), and even disruptions at the level of the cortex of the adrenal gland can affect pulsatile secretion of the hormone LH, also disrupting menstruation (Phumsatitpong et al., 2021).

Some may ask, *is there evidence that COVID vaxgenes impact the hypothalamic-pituitary-gonadal axis?* Directly, no, but it has been observed that the Spike protein of SARS-CoV-2 suppresses the secretion of gonadotropins from the anterior pituitary (Abdillah et al., 2022), and in some patients diagnosed with COVID, neuroendocrine problems occur due to autoimmunity against proteins in the hypothalamus or pituitary gland (Artamonova et al., 2022; Gonen et al., 2022). Therefore, it is not unreasonable to consider the possibility that it may occur due to the action of the Spike protein produced in those who receive COVID vaxgenes.

5) Ovarian Dysfunction: It is known that the synthetic mRNA of Pfizer's and Moderna's vaxgene reaches the ovaries (see section 5.2), and this is important because its presence in ovarian or endometrial cells may trigger pro-inflammatory events in the reproductive tract (e.g., Azlan et al., 2020; Berbic and Fraser, 2013;

[347] When a disease or pathological alteration has something psychological as its cause, and not something physiological.

Evans and Salamonsen, 2012; Oertelt-Prigione, 2011) that could result in menstrual cycle disturbances.

Well, – some may ask – *is there experimental or epidemiological evidence that ovarian dysfunction is occurring that could explain the menstrual cycle alterations in some vaccinated women?* The short answer is no. But there is also no definitive evidence that gives us confidence that ovarian dysfunction is not occurring. I will try to explain why: It is true that to date, there is no published evidence demonstrating ovarian dysfunction in women who received COVID vaxgenes. On the contrary, published studies have not found differences in ovarian function parameters in women who received a vaxgene. However, most of these studies suffer from several shortcomings, including lack of statistical power[348], the use of study subjects who were undergoing fertility treatments instead of studying ovarian dysfunction in women who had no fertility problems, making comparisons between vaccinated and unvaccinated women who had been infected with SARS-CoV-2 instead of having unvaccinated, uninfected controls, and the conclusions that they reach are not supported. For example, one study recruited 60 reproductive-age women, 30 of whom had received the synthetic mRNA COVID vaxgene, and 30 who had not. Since they found no evidence of differences in anti-Müllerian hormone levels between the groups, they concluded that synthetic mRNA COVID vaxgenes do not cause ovarian dysfunction (Soysal and Yılmaz, 2022). This conclusion was drawn despite the lack of consensus on the clinical utility of this hormone (Dewailly et al., 2014), and even *in vitro* fertilization centres do not consider it useful as a reliable indicator of fertility[349].

Another interesting example of a study with methodological errors or impressions is one that analysed several reproductive parameters, including the number of oocytes collected, the number of mature

[348] The statistical power of a study refers to the probability that the hypothesis to be challenged will be accepted as true. It depends on several things, including the number of samples. If it is not enough, there may be low statistical power in the analysis, and we may not detect a difference when it is real.
[349] IVF Australia [Internet]. Available at: https://www.ivf.com.au/blog/is-the-amh-test-reliable

oocytes, fertilization rate, and HCG level in 37 women who received the synthetic mRNA vaxgene and 22 who did not receive it. However, all the women in the study were undergoing treatment for *in vitro* fertilization (thus, they do not represent the normal population). The most incomprehensible thing is that they did not make comparisons of the parameters between vaccinated women, women who had been infected and women who were neither vaccinated nor infected. Instead, they analysed the data regarding the women's anti-Spike and anti-Nucleocapsid antibody levels (Odeh-Natour et al., 2022). In order to analyse the data this way, it must be assumed that all women who received the vaxgenes will generate antibodies against the Spike protein, that all people who had previously been diagnosed as COVID cases and who were not vaccinated will generate antibodies against Spike and Nucleocapsid, and that all people who have not been diagnosed as COVID cases do not have antibodies. There are many sources of potential error in that assumption. Without going any further, anti-Nucleocapsid antibodies have been detected in human blood collected in 2018! (Burbelo et al., 2020). However, the authors of the aforementioned study concluded that not having found differences in the number of oocytes collected, fertilization rate and pregnancy "*supports the belief that the vaccines did not alter the fertility potentials of the patients*".

So, in summary, perhaps the alterations to the menstrual cycle of some women who received one or more COVID vaxgenes are not due to ovarian dysfunction, but to alterations, caused by the Spike protein, to the renin-angiotensin-aldosterone axis, to the hypothalamus-pituitary-gonadal or coagulation. However, it is not only alterations in the menstrual cycle that have been observed, but alterations in pregnancy, which also need to be addressed.

b) Pregnancy alterations

The potential impact of COVID vaxgenes is not only in terms of menstrual alterations. They can also affect fertility and pregnancy.

In May 2021, an article was published and widely interpreted as evidence that synthetic mRNA vaxgenes were safe for use in pregnant women. This interpretation was based on an article that reported data from a clinical trial on the safety and efficacy of the vaccine in pregnant women. The article stated, "*Preliminary findings from their study did not show obvious signals of [lack of] safety among pregnant women who received mRNA vaccines against COVID*" (Shimabukuro et al., 2021). However, the article had to be corrected[350] after a critical analysis found errors and omissions. A serious error was the misinterpretation and omission of results by the authors, as according to the clinical trial results, one in eight pregnant women had experienced a miscarriage after receiving the vaxgene[351]. Independent researchers (Brock and Thornley, 2021) reached the same conclusion and raised concerns about the errors, omissions, and incorrect conclusions of the study by Shimabukuro and colleagues (2021). This study was being used by medical societies for obstetrics and gynaecology worldwide as justification for the safety of these synthetic mRNA vaxgenes in pregnant women and their foetuses. This led the authors of the initial article to write an erratum, acknowledging the errors identified by the researchers. Specifically, Shimabakuro and colleagues had to admit that "*There was no denominator available to calculate the risk estimate for spontaneous abortions because at the time of this report, follow-up at 20 weeks was not available for 905 of the 1,224 participants who were vaccinated within 30 days before the last menstrual period or during the first trimester* [of gestation]. *Moreover, any risk estimate would need to take into account the specific risk by gestational week for spontaneous abortion*". The issue was deemed so relevant that a year later, Bartoszek and Okrój (2022) revisited controversies regarding data presentation concerning the safety of synthetic mRNA COVID vaxgenes in women. In that article, they highlighted serious statistical errors made by the authors of the original study and called for caution in publishing partial results.

A review of reports recorded in the US adverse event monitoring system found that the proportional reporting rate of reproductive adverse events associated with COVID vaxgenes with respect to those related to flu

---

[350] See errata in: https://www.nejm.org/doi/10.1056/NEJMx210016

[351] Ciencia y Salud Natural [Internet; Spanish] Available at: https://cienciaysaludnatural.com/1-de-cada-8-mujeres-embarazadas-pierden-a-su-bebe-despues-de-recibir-la-inyeccion-k0-b1t.

vaccines is at least twice as high, both for menstrual abnormalities (see previous subsection), and for abortions, stillbirths[352] and foetal deaths, placental thrombosis, low level of amniotic fluid, preeclampsia, premature births, premature rupture of membrane, foetal abnormalities among which highlight chromosomal anomalies, malformations, cystic hygromas, growth problems, as well as foetal cardiac disorders such as cardiac arrest, arrhythmias, poor vascular perfusion, and premature death of the baby (Thorpe et al., 2022). In fact, that same study calculated that the relative risk of suffering a miscarriage if pregnant women had been vaccinated against COVID was 15 times the risk associated with flu vaccines.

As with alterations in the menstrual cycle, studies have been published that indicate that they have found no differences in the initial implantation rates, sustained implantation rate and abortion rate associated with COVID vaxgenes. As discussed before, the studies have several problems. For instance, a study published in 2021 examined the pregnancy success rate in a group of women that received the COVID vaxgene. All women were undergoing fertility treatments. Twenty-six women had received at least one dose of any of the two synthetic mRNA vaxgenes and 91 women had not received any dose (of any type of vaxgene or vaccine against COVID) nor had they been infected with SARS-CoV-2 (Morris and Morris, 2021). The authors of the study concluded that embryos that were produced by women who had been exposed to synthetic mRNA vaxgenes were just as likely to reach term successfully as non-vaccinated women. They also concluded that their results "*refute the rumours that COVID vaccines are 'toxic' to the ovaries*" and that their study "*contributes to the growing body of evidence that the vaccines do not cause infertility*" (Morris and Morris, 2021). However, that and many other studies do *not* show this. What they show is that in that group of studied women, who are not representative of the normal population (given that they were undergoing treatments for fertility problems) they did not find any difference between groups. Unfortunately, those who have conducted reviews of published studies have ignored this point.

Other studies have used surrogate indicators of pregnancy success, such as the amount of beta-human chorionic gonadotropin (β-hCG) present 12

[352] The term refers to babies who are stillborn, while foetal death occurs inside the uterus before birth.

days after embryo transfer or whether a foetal heartbeat was visible on examination. by ultrasound after seven weeks of gestation, not the successful term of gestation.

It is necessary to carry out more studies with sufficient statistical power, that focus on a valid population for what is intended to be studied, and that the duration of the study allows for a reliable determination of the possible alteration in fertility. However, the biological plausibility of COVID vaxgenes causing adverse reproductive events is clear: the same mechanisms that can explain menstrual alterations could explain problems in pregnancy. Given that the cells of the pituitary gland express the protein ACE2, which is a receptor for the Spike protein, it is understood that if vaxgene-produced Spike protein reaches the pituitary after crossing the blood-brain barrier or after the vaxgenes reach that organ and endogenous production of the Spike protein begins, it can bind to these cells. If this union occurs, the levels of GnRH, LH and FSG could be affected. This was demonstrated experimentally using cell cultures, which showed that the secretion of LH and FSH from bovine pituitary cells that had been exposed to biologically relevant concentrations of the full-length Spike protein (as well as that produced by COVID vaxgenes) for 3.5 days was suppressed (Abdillah et al., 2022). Of course, these results must be considered for what they are: *in vitro* experimental studies. However, they show a biologically plausible mechanism that, if it occurs in people that received these products, could have severe consequences, even at the population level.

c) Alterations in sperm parameters

During the second year of the COVID immunization campaign, a study was published reporting that the synthetic mRNA vaxgene from Pfizer affected semen concentration and sperm motility (Gat et al., 2022). This retrospective epidemiological study included 220 semen samples from different sperm banks in Israel. Samples were taken at three times after the second dose in 32 donors, the last one up to 150 days later. They reported a significant reduction of 15.4% in sperm concentration and a 22.1% reduction in total motile sperm count compared to the parameters before vaccination in the same donors. The parameters recovered after 150 days.

The results of Gat and colleagues' study (2022) contrast with those published a year earlier in a study that reported no reduction in any sperm parameter after the second dose of the mRNA vaxgene and, on the contrary, observed a slight increase in all parameters (González et al., 2021). They also contrast with what was reported in a more recent study that found no evidence of semen quality impairment during a follow-up of 6 to 14 months in men who received the synthetic mRNA vaxgene (Karavani et al., 2022). To understand the differences in results between studies, we need to understand the following. To make reading easier, I will refer to Gat and colleagues' study (2022) as the Gat study, González and colleagues' study (2021) as the González study, and Karavani and colleagues' study (2022) as the Karavani study:

1) The Gat study was conducted on healthy semen donors, with an average age of 26.1 (± 4.2 years). In contrast, the Karavani and González studies included men from a wider age range (from 32 to 42 in the former and from 18 to 50 years in the latter). This age difference is important because it implies that there will be more variation in semen parameters in the samples, as men between 41 and 50 years are three times more likely to have a reduction in motility and count (Pino et al., 2020).

2) The follow-up period: The Gat study followed participants for more than 150 days, while the González study followed participants for half of that period. The Karavani study did follow participants for a longer time (between 6 and 14 months).

3) The Gat study included repeated samples (i.e., had replicates) to reduce parameter variation in each individual. The González and Karavani studies did not.

4) The Gat study included healthy men, while the González study included samples from men who already had low initial counts (i.e., oligospermia: less than 15 million sperm/mL), and the Karavani study mixed healthy men with men with abnormal semen characteristics.

5) The way the studies present the results does not allow for a comparison of values between studies, nor the baseline values (prior to inoculations) of healthy participants in Israel and those in the United States. This value would be important to know because there may be differences in semen parameters between countries due to other factors.

Based on the González study, the official narrative from health agencies[353] and the media[354] was that '*the COVID vaxgene does not affect male fertility*'. This is even though the authors of the González study clarified that the parameters they measured are not the sole determinants of fertility.

It is certainly reassuring that the Gat study reported that sperm parameters normalized after five months of receiving the second dose, but since they did not include anyone with additional booster doses, we cannot know what the administration of repeated doses will cause. However, a reduction of the magnitude detected in sperm concentration and total motile count for five months after vaccination should not be ignored. We will have to see the impact on birth rates. It is complex to do so because birth rates are affected by many factors, from biological to economic and cultural. However, it is inaccurate and incorrect to say that "*mRNA inoculations do not impact the quantity and parameters of sperm motility*". Perhaps we need to start fact-checking the fact-checkers to avoid the dissemination of inaccurate or misinterpreted information.

On the other hand, it is important to remember that proteins from cellular debris were found in the vials of AstraZeneca's vaxgene (Krutzke et al., 2022). One of the detected proteins is the nuclear autoantigenic sperm protein (NASP; see section 1.4). The NASP protein detected was the testicular isoform (NASPt), which is normally expressed by testicular cells

---

353 CDC. [Internet]. Available at: https://espanol.cdc.gov/coronavirus/2019-ncov/vaccines/planning-for-pregnancy.html. Medium "¿La vacuna contra el COVID afecta la fertilidad en los hombres?" [Internet]. (Spanish) Available at: https://medium.com/bienestarwa/la-vacuna-contra-el-COVID-afecta-la-fertilidad-en-los-hombres-c6f0f8716a02.

354 The Conversation "El COVID puede causar infertilidad masculina y disfunción eréctil. Las vacunas, en cambio, no" [Internet; Spanish]. Available at: https://theconversation.com/el-COVID-puede-causar-infertilidad-masculina-y-disfuncion-erectil-las-vacunas-en-cambio-no-165291

during spermatogenesis and remains in the periacrosomal membrane of mature sperm (Richardson et al., 2000).

As explained in section 5.7, the problem with the presence of NASP in the vials analysed by Krutzke and colleagues (2022) is that if autoantibodies are generated against the testicular isoform of NASP, it can lead to male infertility (Chereshnev et al., 2021; Lu et al., 2008). This is why the idea of creating 'infertility vaccines' by inducing autoimmunity to the NASP protein was born (Alexander, 1989), as autoantibodies against this protein can be generated due to testicular infection or trauma, or after vasectomy (Batova et al., 2000). Furthermore, anti-NASPt antibodies are associated with infertility due to autoimmunity (Chereshnev et al., 2021), so it is not unreasonable to postulate the possibility that the presence of the NASP protein (testicular isoform) in AstraZeneca's vaxgene represents a risk to the fertility of those who received this product. To date, it does not seem that a single study has been conducted to investigate whether men who received AstraZeneca's vaxgene, have fertility impairments.

Let us consider that, according to the WHO, at the time of writing this book, at least 5,630,000,000 people (70.54% of the world's population) have received at least one (and some up to four or more) doses of COVID vaccines or vaxgenes[355], with an important percentage of these being the latter. As I explained in Chapter 2, none of the clinical studies that led to emergency authorization of these products addressed the potential impact on fertility, but if the results observed by Abdillah and collaborators (2022) can also occur in vaccinated people, then there could soon be a notable impact on the human fertility rate due to these "immunizations". This scenario would be worrying since fertility rates have declined since 1950 from 5 births per women on average, to 2.3 births per women in 2021. This has led to global fertility being projected to be equal or less than 2.1 births

---

[355] Our World in Data [Internet]. Data updated to October 23 2023. Available at: https://ourworldindata.org/explorers/

per women in 2050. Furthermore, live birth rates in 2021 were 16.94 per 100,000 inhabitants, which is a 65% decline since 1990[356].

There is no evidence that the COVID vaxgenes will contribute more to this decline. However, a recent study estimated the rates of reproductive adverse events affecting pregnancy and menstruation in sexually mature women that received vaxgenes. They used data from the US reporting system (VAERS) and designed a retrospective cohort study. Data from January 1 1998 to June 30 2022 were included, as they wished to have data from before the vaxgenes were used, as they wished to compare reports associated with flu vaccines, also commonly offered to adult women (Thorp et al., 2023). The authors of the study reported that the COVID vaxgenes are associated with a significant increase of reproductive adverse effects compared to prior vaccines, with reporting rates >2.0 (with a significance of <0.05) for menstrual anomalies, abortions, foetal chromosomal abnormalities, malformations, foetal cystic hygromas, foetal heart problems, foetal vascular problems, growth abnormalities, foetal thrombosis, low amniotic fluid and foetal death. Differences in the number of doses, lapse between doses, and number of vaccinated women were accounted for. They found that the signal of adverse events from these vaxgenes exceeds all previously recognized thresholds. This is why they concluded that the menstrual and reproductive anomalies are more frequent in women that have received one or more COVID vaxgenes that in women that have received flu vaccines (Thorp et al., 2023).

To summarize, there are reports in the adverse event monitoring systems, case reports, and scientific evidence that has been analysed in an epidemiological context, that suggest an association between COVID vaxgenes and reproductive disorders, ranging from menstrual alterations to pregnancy issues. The biological mechanism that would explain this association has already been proposed and is biologically plausible. This is why it would not be correct to underestimate this association. On the

---

[356] Statista [Internet]. Available at: https://www.statista.com/statistics/1328270/crude-birth-rate-worldwide/. Worldometers [Internet]. Available at: https://www.worldometers.info/demographics/world-demographics/#tfr

contrary, we should explore the relationship in more depth (Zeginiadou et al., 2023).

6.5 Autoinflammatory and autoimmune conditions

In section 6.3 I described some neurological clinical conditions that can be associated with autoinflammatory and autoimmune problems. However, given the distribution of vaxgenes in the body (see section 5.2), their molecular interactions within the cell, and the impacts outside the cell, which induce sustained inflammation, it is expected that autoinflammatory and autoimmunity processes occur in different organs and tissues of the body.

The number of case reports that describe these pathological conditions in vaccinated people has increased significantly since mid-2021, with, at the time of writing this book, 191 published clinical cases that refer to autoinflammation and autoimmunity[357]. Accordingly, there are a high number of reports of these conditions associated with COVID vaxgenes on the VAERS pages. Reports are 100 times more numerous than those reported for other vaccines in more than 30 years since the creation of that monitoring system. Below I will describe some of the clinical conditions associated with autoinflammation and autoimmunity in people who received the vaxgenes.

a) Skin conditions

Some of the clinical presentations indicative of autoinflammation that have been reported in people that received an COVID vaxgene are skin conditions. In early 2022, a literature review worldwide was published on skin manifestations post-COVID vaccination (Gambichler et al., 2022). It was found that the most common adverse effects on the skin range from nonspecific, local, and self-limiting reactions to immediate or near-immediate type I hypersensitivity reactions (allergies, which can be severe), triggered by nanolipids (allergies to PEG or polysorbate 80 contained in

[357] National Library of Medicine. National Center for Biotechnology Information [Internet]. Search terms: (autoimmune OR autoinflammatory) AND (Pfizer OR Moderna OR AstraZeneca OR Janssen) AND vaccine AND "case report". Searchable at: https://pubmed.ncbi.nlm.nih.gov

synthetic mRNA and adenoviral vector vaxgenes). These reactions, when promptly addressed, are not fatal and leave no lasting effects. However, type IV hypersensitivity reactions were also identified, characterized by delayed cellular immune reactions that can cause large and painful lesions, known as "COVID arm," as well as morbilliform or erythematous eruptions (Ujiie et al., 2022). Type IV hypersensitivity reactions are considered serious clinical conditions.

Much more serious, however, are post-vaccination autoimmune reactions, including leukocytoclastic vasculitis, lupus erythematosus, and immune thrombocytopenia, which have also been described as adverse events to COVID vaxgenes and vaccines (e.g., Magnaterra et al., 2023; Wang Y. J. et al., 2023; Ball-Burak et al., 2022; Carrillo-García et al., 2022; Fiorillo et al., 2022; Khanna et al., 2022; Wollina et al., 2022; Sandhu et al., 2021).

The fact that these clinical manifestations have also been observed in some patients infected with SARS-CoV-2 suggests that their cause may be attributed to the action of viral Spike proteins as well as exacerbated immune responses against them. Since almost all vaccines and vaxgenes that have been granted emergency use authorization or approval to prevent COVID are based on the viral Spike protein, it is prudent and valid to propose that the immune response to the Spike protein is the cause of the dermal manifestations following vaccination.

Other dermatological conditions observed and described in individuals vaccinated against COVID include effects on the blood vessels of the skin leading to chilblains (known as chilblain-type lesions), both on the fingers and knees (e.g., Bassi et al., 2022; Mungmunpuntipantip and Wiwanitkit, 2022), rashes like pityriasis rosea, and reactivation of herpetic lesions (Gambichler et al., 2022).

A study of dermal adverse effects in Spain revealed that over a three-month period (February to May 2021), there were 405 reactions to COVID vaxgenes (Català et al., 2022). They were more frequent in individuals who had received Pfizer's vaxgene, followed by Moderna's vaxgene, and fewer in those who received AstraZeneca's vaxgene. Beyond severe persistent inflammation at the injection site (known as 'COVID arm'), cases of urticaria, reactivations of varicella-zoster and herpes simplex, as well as morbilliform, papulovesicular, pityriasis rosea-like, and purpuric reactions were relatively common. It's noteworthy that the vast majority (over 90%) of dermal adverse events occurred in women. This suggests an inflammatory or autoimmune mechanism in response to the vaxgene, as these reactions tend to be more frequent in women than in men (Gee et al., 2021; Kronzer et al., 2020). The most alarming aspect of the Català et al. (2022) study is that 21% of the reactions were severe or very severe, and 81% required medical treatment.

There are various mechanisms by which COVID vaxgenes can cause dermal injuries in some vaccinated individuals. One mechanism involves molecular mimicry due to the similarity between the amino acid sequences of the Spike protein and some human proteins (see section 5.5), which can generate antibodies against the Spike protein of SARS-CoV-2 with cross-reactivity against human tissue proteins (Kim et al., 2023). This explains the occurrence of some autoimmune diseases with cutaneous manifestations in individuals who received one or more COVID vaxgenes.

One of the autoimmune conditions that has been reported is vitiligo. To date, there are 26 published case reports in scientific journals documenting the onset of vitiligo or exacerbation of stable vitiligo following vaccination (Mancha et al., 2023; Tsai and Ng, 2023; Aktas and Ertuğrul, 2022; Abdullah et al., 2022; Bukhari 2022; Bularca et al., 2022; Carbone et al., 2022; Caroppo et al., 2022; Ciccarese et al., 2022; De Domingo et al., 2022; Flores-Terry et al., 2022; Gamonal et al., 2022; Herzum et al., 2022; Kaminetsky and Rudikoff, 2022; Koç Yıldırım, 2022; López Riquelme et al., 2022; Macca et al., 2022; Magen and Landman, 2022; Militello et al., 2022; Okan and Vural, 2022; Piccolo et al., 2022; Patrizio et al., 2021; Singh, 2022; Tatu et al., 2022; Uğurer et al., 2022; Ujiie et al., 2022). In VAERS, there are 352 reports of vitiligo in Americans who were vaccinated against COVID from December 2020 to August 11, 2023 (32 months) [358], whereas, in comparison, there are 437 reports of vitiligo associated with the

[358] Open Vaers [Internet]. Data updated to September 29 2023. Searchable at: https://www.openvaers.com/vaersapp/reports.php

rest of the routine vaccines administered since their creation in 1990. This means that considering an equal rate per month, COVID vaxgenes have been associated with 10.63 monthly cases of vitiligo that appeared or worsened in individuals after receiving the vaxgene, while the rest of the routine vaccines were associated with 0.25 reports of vitiligo that appeared or worsened in individuals after receiving any of those vaccines. In other words, COVID vaxgenes represent 77.8% of the total reports of vitiligo in VAERS since the monitoring system started.

b) Hepatic conditions

In section 5.2, I presented evidence regarding the biodistribution of vaxgene components in the body following intramuscular administration. The organ that receives 80% of nanolipids within a few hours of application is the liver. Therefore, it's not surprising that one in every 2,600 people who received the COVID vaxgene developed acute liver damage, with no noticeable differences in risk between mRNA-based and adenoviral vector-based vaxgenes (Guardiola et al., 2022). Liver damage appears to be more common and severe after the administration of the second dose (86% of hepatic adverse events occurred after the second dose; Guardiola et al., 2022). This is significant, as from the perspective of causality in Epidemiology, it suggests a biological gradient, which is expected for a cause-and-effect relationship (Hill 2015). From a medical standpoint, it implies that liver damage is cumulative and suggests autoinflammatory and autoimmune damage (Acevedo-Whitehouse and Bruno, 2023). In this regard, the risk of developing severe hepatitis is likely to increase with each additional dose received.

Among the published reports, cases of severe acute autoimmune hepatitis in vaccinated patients without a prior history of liver disease have been described. An example is the case of a 65-year-old patient who experienced a fulminant autoimmune hepatitis two weeks after receiving the first dose of Moderna's synthetic mRNA vaxgene (Garrido et al., 2021). Histological analysis of the liver biopsy showed confluent foci of necrosis[359] and severe lymphocytic inflammation[360]. As other causes of acute hepatitis were ruled out, the vaxgene was considered the cause of her condition (Garrido et al., 2021).

Autoimmune hepatitis as an adverse event of COVID vaxgenes doesn't only occur in older individuals. For example, a case occurred in a 27-year-old individual with no previous diseases who developed a clinical picture consistent with autoimmune hepatitis two weeks after receiving one dose of Pfizer's vaxgene (Kim et al., 2023). The young person experienced sweating, a febrile sensation, and weakness, with elevated liver enzymes. A liver biopsy confirmed lymphocytic inflammation and histiocytosis with rosette formation and interface hepatitis, in addition to plasma cells, eosinophils, and hepatocyte necrosis (Kim et al., 2023). Since the patient had elevated liver enzymes for two months after vaccination, the authors considered the possibility of vaccine-induced autoimmune hepatitis. This concurs with other observations on autoimmune hepatitis and pancreatitis that have occurred in people that received synthetic mRNA vaxgene (Patel A. H. et al., 2022).

This is not an isolated case: of 15 additional cases of autoimmune hepatitis that occurred in individuals who received COVID vaxgenes, 12 had no autoimmune conditions or previous liver medical history (Kim et al., 2023). Furthermore, scientific literature has published, at the time of writing this book, at least 40 studies describing the occurrence of autoimmune hepatitis associated with COVID vaxgenes[361]. In the adverse event monitoring system of the United States in the 34 months since their authorization, 11,407 reports of autoimmune hepatitis have been recorded after receiving either of the two COVID vaccines (the original and the bivalent)[362]. In comparison, since January 1990, 25,570 reports of

---

[359] Cell death.
[360] Inflammation can be acute, and neutrophils would net he most commonly infiltrating cells in an infected tissue. If there are lymphocytes it means that the inflammation is chronic and there is a higher risk that it reveals an autoinflammatory or autoimmune process.
[361] National Library of Medicine. National Center for Biotechnology Information [Internet]. Search term: (autoimmune AND hepatitis) AND (COVID vaccine) AND (Pfizer OR Moderna OR AstraZeneca OR Janssen OR BNT162b2)". Search done October 23 2023. Searchable at: https://pubmed.ncbi.nlm.nih.gov/
[362] Open Vaers [Internet]. Data updated to September 29 2023. Searchable at: https://www.openvaers.com/vaersapp/reports.php

autoimmune hepatitis associated with all other vaccines (i.e., the 101 vaccines administered in the United States that are not against COVID) have been received. This means that common vaccines that are not COVID vaxgenes have accumulated 62.67 reports of autoimmune hepatitis per month associated with all other vaccines, while COVID vaxgenes are associated with 335.5 reports of autoimmune hepatitis per month per dose, which is a rate almost 5.5 times higher.

Clearly, extrapolating the results of Guardiola et al. (2022) to the general population is subject to many other variables and risk determinants. Still, it cannot be ignored that there is a possibility that a considerable number of people are experiencing liver problems after vaccination, nor can the possibility be dismissed that individuals with pre-existing liver problems may experience an aggravation of their symptoms, especially considering that liver diseases currently cause up to 2 million annual deaths, representing 4% of all deaths globally (Devarbhavi et al., 2023).

c) Renal problems

Adverse events following COVID vaccination also include kidney-related complications. One of the most serious conditions is nephrotic syndrome, which can occur concurrently with acute kidney injury, a clinical condition known as 'minimal change disease' (see Vivarelli et al., 2017). These cases of new-onset or reactivation of conditions that had been silent for decades (Komaba et al., 2021; Mancianti et al., 2021; Morlidge et al., 2021) have been observed mainly after receiving the first or second dose of mRNA-based vaxgenes (D'Agati et al., 2021; Holzworth et al., 2021; Kervella et al., 2021; Lebedev et al., 2021; Leclerc et al., 2021; Maas et al., 2021; Mancianti et al., 2021; Morlidge et al., 2021; Salem et al., 2021; Weijers et al., 2021). However, they have also been reported after receiving AdV vectorized vaxgenes (Lim et al., 2021; Morlidge et al., 2021) and inactivated vaccines (Özkan et al., 2022).

Additionally, cases of glomerulonephritis (Fernández et al., 2023; Jefferies et al., 2022; Hakroush and Tampe, 2021) and nephropathies associated with immunoglobulins produced by vaccination have been reported, causing severe conditions that may include haematuria[363] (Negrea et al., 2021). The increasing number of new cases or recurrences of kidney disease led Sugita and colleagues (2022) to state that "*within the context of mass vaccination against COVID, cases of new or recurrent kidney disease and vasculitis, including minimal change nephrotic syndrome, nephropathy, immunoglobulin A-associated nephropathy, and immunoglobulin A-associated vasculitis, developed after receiving COVID vaccines are increasing*".

The trend of adverse events following immunization (ESAVI) associated with renal complications due to COVID vaxgenes has continued. In the recent review by Vudathaneni and colleagues (2023), the main renal complications that have arisen because of their administration are highlighted:

- Acute interstitial nephritis
- Acute kidney injury (AKI)
- Acute renal failure associated with anti-neutrophil cytoplasmic antibody (ANCA) vasculitis
- Acute tubular necrosis (ATN)
- Acute tubulointerstitial nephritis
- AKI pre-renal (pre-renal acute kidney injury)
- ANCA-associated glomerulonephritis
- ANCA-associated vasculitis
- ANCA-associated vasculitis with rhabdomyolysis and pauciimmune glomerulonephritis
- Anti-glomerular basement membrane antibody disease (Anti-GBM)
- De novo or exacerbation of necrotizing vasculitis
- Focal segmental glomerulosclerosis
- Glomerular disease associated with the COVID vaccine
- Glomerulonephritis
- IgG4-associated disease
- Immunoglobulin A nephropathy
- Immunoglobulin A vasculitis with severe glomerulonephritis

---

[363] Haematuria is the presence of blood in the urine.

- Lupus nephritis
- Membranous nephropathy
- Minimal change disease
- Minimal change disease with anti-nuclear autoantibodies
- Minimal change disease with severe acute renal damage
- Minimal change glomerulonephritis
- Myeloperoxidase-ANCA-associated vasculitis (MPO-ANCA)
- Nephrotic syndrome
- Paediatric nephrotic syndrome
- Renal scleroderma crisis
- Renal thrombotic microangiopathy

The occurrence of renal conditions as a consequence of COVID vaxgenes reflects, as mentioned throughout this document, the lack of complete safety data since they were authorized for emergency use with only a few months of information. Additionally, phase 3 trials excluded individuals with chronic health issues (including renal problems[364]), so the risk of exacerbation and/or new renal disease in susceptible individuals could not have been determined. Considering that chronic kidney disease affects more than 10% of the global population (estimated at 800,000,000 people) and is considered a major cause of mortality worldwide (Kovesdy, 2022), it should be a public health priority to monitor the impacts that COVID vaxgenes may be causing in this group.

The clinical trial initiated after emergency use authorization to investigate safety and efficacy in renal patients[365] is analysing the effects of the vaxgene in 350 renal patients, 300 transplant patients, and 200 controls. However, it only examines adverse effects reported within seven days after vaccination, which, given the findings reported in the publications mentioned above, is too short a time to observe the occurrence of renal problems associated with COVID vaxgenes. Furthermore, in the

---

[364] National Library of Medicine. National Center for Biotechnology Information. Clinical Trials [Internet]. Each clinical trial mentioned is available at: https://clinicaltrials.gov/ct2/show/NCT04368728, https://clinicaltrials.gov/ct2/show/NCT04470427, https://clinicaltrials.gov/ct2/show/NCT04516746, https://www.clinicaltrials.gov/ct2/show/NCT04526990, https://clinicaltrials.gov/ct2/show/NCT04505722, https://clinicaltrials.gov/ct2/show/NCT04587219

[365] https://www.clinicaltrials.gov/ct2/show/NCT04741386

supplementary information of that clinical trial (Kho et al., 2021), it is indicated that renal patients who are recipients of multiple transplants, those with hematologic oncologic processes, immune disorders, HIV infection, and blood diathesis were excluded, as well as those who had previously been diagnosed with COVID[366]. This makes it impossible to have accurate data on the potential consequences that the vaxgenes may have on the health of renal patients, most of whom have likely already had COVID, according to CDC data for the United States (Clarke et al., 2022).

One of the mechanisms by which COVID vaxgenes can cause renal conditions is through damage to the vascular endothelium that the Spike protein can generate, in addition to its dysregulating action on the renin-angiotensin-aldosterone axis (see section 5.5), which could impact renal pathogenesis, as previously described for COVID (Ahmadian et al., 2021). Since December 2021, one year after the emergency authorization of COVID vaxgenes, cases of necrotizing vasculitis in previously healthy individuals, as well as a resurgence of necrotizing vasculitis in individuals with controlled conditions, were reported after vaccination. Of the patients who presented it, 50% of those affected with this condition subsequently experienced renal dysfunction (Fillon et al., 2021). Another mechanism of renal damage leading to glomerulonephritis and nephrotic syndrome is the dysregulation of T lymphocytes (Hashimura et al., 2019), a well-known cause of these renal conditions, which is known to be a consequence of COVID vaxgenes (Seneff et al., 2022).

Beyond the published case reports mentioned above, a search in the U.S. adverse event monitoring system shows that between December 2020 and August 2023, 610 reports of glomerulonephritis and acute renal damage associated with COVID vaxgenes have accumulated, while reports of glomerulonephritis and acute renal damage associated with all vaccines since 1990 are 859[367]. In other words, COVID vaxgenes, within just 33 months since their emergency authorization, are associated with 71% of all

[366] Kho et al., 2021. The RECOVAC IR study: the immune response and safety of the mRNA-1273 COVID vaccine in patients with chronic kidney disease, on dialysis or living with a kidney transplant. Supplementary material [Internet]. Available at:
https://www.ncbi.nlm.nih.gov/labs/pmc/articles/PMC8241423/#sup1

[367] Open Vaers [Internet]. Data updated to August 23 2023. Searchable at:
https://www.openvaers.com/vaersapp/reports.php

serious renal adverse event reports accumulated in 589 months since the adverse event monitoring system was implemented in that country.

d) Pancreatitis and gallstones

Cases of pancreatitis and pancreatic cancer have been reported in previously healthy individuals who received COVID vaxgenes. It is known that acute pancreatitis can occur almost spontaneously in people with no history of pancreatic issues, and this has been happening before the administration of COVID vaxgenes: the annual incidence of acute pancreatitis in the United States ranges from 4.9 to 35 cases per 100,000 inhabitants[368] and is considered a significant cause of mortality globally, with varying rates between countries (Li et al., 2022).

There are various causes of acute pancreatitis, including autoimmune reactions, alcoholism, gallstones[369], certain drugs (including tetracycline, sulphonamides, didanosine), metabolic disorders, abdominal trauma, iatrogenic damage during surgeries, and viral infections (Mederos et al., 2021). Cases of acute pancreatitis have also been reported in individuals infected with SARS-CoV-2, although they are infrequent as this virus does not damage pancreatic cells (van der Heide et al., 2022).

Acute pancreatic issues are considered serious clinical conditions, with a mortality rate that can be as high as 20% (Popa et al., 2016). Therefore, it is concerning that cases of pancreatitis following immunization have been reported in association with COVID vaxgenes. A literature review reveals that in the 33 months since the authorization of the first COVID vaxgene, at least 22 case reports of acute pancreatitis following COVID vaxgene administration have been published (Allen et al., 2023; Aochi et al., 2023; Becker et al., 2023; Bangolo et al., 2023; Boskabadi et al., 2023; Chahed et al., 2023; Gamonal et al., 2023; Stöllberger et al., 2023; Cacdac et al., 2022; Chue et al., 2022; Consolini et al., 2022; Dey et al., 2022; Kalra et al., 2022; Mousa et al., 2022; N et al., 2022; Ozaka et al., 2022; Patel A. H. et al., 2022; Taieb and Mounira, 2022; Walter et al., 2022; Cieślewicz et al., 2021;

[368] Up to date. Etiology of Acute Pancreatitis. Autor: Santhi Swaroop Vege, MD [Internet]- Available at: https://www.uptodate.com/contents/etiology-of-acute-pancreatitis.
[369] Calculi ('stones') that are formed in the gallbladder.

Kantar et al., 2021; Parkash et al., 2021). These cases have occurred even in a pregnant woman who was vaccinated (Dey et al., 2022) and in vaccinated adolescents. Some of the cases showed an autoimmune component driven by the presence of IgG4 antibodies produced in response to COVID vaxgenes (e.g., Aochi et al., 2023; Patel A. H. et al., 2022).

Almost all case reports of acute pancreatitis are associated with the synthetic mRNA COVID vaxgenes. If we conduct an identical search regarding a traditional vaccine, such as the influenza vaccine, there are zero (0) published case reports from 1970 to the present[370]. On the other hand, a search in the United States adverse event monitoring system reveals 1,698 cases of pancreatitis associated with mRNA (Pfizer and Moderna) and vectorized vaccines in the United States up to September 29, 2023[371]. The same search for influenza vaccines, applied for over four decades, reveals a total of 10 cases of pancreatitis.

e) Ocular issues

The ocular adverse events associated with COVID vaxgenes are also being reported at a high rate. One of the early case reports, published in 2021, involves a healthy 41-year-old man who experienced progressive vision loss and ocular floaters that appeared 48 hours after COVID vaccination. Ophthalmological examination revealed bilateral anterior uveitis, progressing to panuveitis with occlusive vasculitis that persisted despite topical cortisone treatment (Hebert et al., 2021). Physicians could not find any other cause, concluding that it is plausible to consider the COVID vaccination as the cause of panuveitis, and clinicians should be aware of this possibility.

This case of uveitis is the result of uncontrolled inflammatory processes, which may be associated with autoimmunity. In addition to Hebert and

---

[370] National Library of Medicine. National Center for Biotechnology Information [Internet]. Search terms: https://pubmed.ncbi.nlm.nih.gov/?term=pancreatitis+AND+%28influenza+OR+flu%29+AND+vaccine+AND+%22case+report% Search done August 24 2023.

[371] Open Vaers [Internet]. Data updated to September 29 2023. Searchable at: https://www.openvaers.com/vaersapp/reports.php

colleagues' case report (2021), many published clinical cases[372] describe uveitis following COVID vaccination (e.g., Habot-Wilner et al., 2023; Li S. et al., 2023; Ogino et al., 2023; Lin and Chien, 2023; Dutta Majumder et al., 2023; Sadeghi et al., 2023; Sanjay et al., 2023a; Sanjay et al., 2023b; Chew et al., 2022; Fei et al., 2022; Li et al., 2022; Mahendradas et al., 2022; Murgova and Balchev, 2022; Nanji and Fraunfelder, 2022; Ortiz-Egea et al., 2022; Patel K. G. et al., 2022; Sangoram et al., 2022; Sanjay et al., 2022a; Sanjay et al., 2022b; Sanjay et al., 2022c; Sanjay et al., 2022d; Sanjay et al., 2022e; Bolleta et al., 2021). However, uveitis is not the only type of ocular adverse event associated with COVID vaxgenes. Retinitis (e.g., Kawali et al., 2023) and activations of herpesviruses leading to ocular issues (e.g., Mahendradas et al., 2023; Mishra et al., 2023; Sangoram et al., 2022) have also been reported, affecting not only older individuals but also healthy adults and even children.

A recent article (Joo et al., 2022) describes a case of Vogt-Koyanagi-Harada syndrome (VKH) following the administration of Moderna's mRNA vaxgene. The patient was a 50-year-old woman who experienced bilateral serous retinal detachment 35 days after receiving the first dose. The symptoms she initially experienced were typical local and immediate vaccine reactions (redness, pain in the arm, headache, muscle pain, and allergy symptoms). However, more than a month later, she developed VKH. This autoimmune condition involves uveomeningeal inflammation affecting the retina and the nervous system (Ortiz-Balbuena et al., 2015). According to the authors, the clinical condition was likely triggered by the COVID vaxgene due to its ingredients or by the Spike protein produced after vaccination, which activated the inflammatory process and induced VKH (Joo et al., 2022).

There has also been an emerging understanding of the risk of retinal vascular occlusion as a consequence of COVID vaccination (Li J. X. et al., 2023). It is worth noting that retinal vascular occlusion is the second most common cause of visual loss, occurring when a blood vessel experiences blockage due to external compression or microclots, spasm of the vessel

---

[372] https://pubmed.ncbi.nlm.nih.gov/?term=%E2%80%9Cuveitis+AND+%22COVID+vaccine%22 Search done August 24 2023.

fibres, or alteration of the inner wall of blood vessels, either due to degeneration or vasculitis. Regardless of the mechanism, the result is reduced blood flow, leading to decreased oxygen reaching the retina, causing cell death. This, in turn, results in loss of visual acuity and, in some cases, blindness in the affected eye[373]. Retinal vascular occlusion had been observed in some patients diagnosed as positive for SARS-CoV-2. One explanation is that severe COVID is a predominantly pro-inflammatory and thromboembolic disease, and its effects can be observed, in susceptible individuals, in various organs, including the eyes (Yener, 2021). Therefore, given the known impact of the Spike protein (both viral and endogenously produced after COVID vaccination) and the interaction between synthetic mRNA and the cells and organs of the recipient (see section 5.3), two potential mechanisms explaining an association between COVID vaxgenes and retinal vascular occlusion become apparent.

Li and colleagues (2023) acknowledge in the introduction of their published study that there is an increasing number of reports of retinal vascular occlusion in individuals who were vaccinated with synthetic mRNA vaxgenes (Pfizer and Moderna) and AdV based vaxgenes (AstraZeneca, Janssen, CanSino, and Sputnik). To justify their study, the authors cite 10 peer-reviewed scientific studies and clinical cases. They aimed to investigate whether COVID vaxgenes are associated with a higher risk of developing retinal vascular occlusion than the 'normal' risk in unvaccinated individuals. For this, they conducted a retrospective epidemiological cohort study, including individuals that received at least one dose of Pfizer, Moderna, or AstraZeneca between January 2020 and December 2022, as well as an unvaccinated cohort. They evaluated the risk of developing retinal vessel occlusion in both groups. It is important to note that, in both cohorts, they excluded individuals with a previous history of retinal vascular occlusion or those taking medications that could promote intravascular coagulation before the study period (Li J. X. et al., 2023).

---

373 Centro Oftalmológico de Barcelona (Ophtalmological Centre of Barcelona). "Occlusions and obstructions of the retinal veins and arteries" [Internet]. Searchable at: https://icrcat.com/enfermedades-oculares/oclusiones-u-obstrucciones-las-venas-y-arterias-retina

For Li and colleagues' study, a database of 95 million individuals in the US Collaborative Network in the United States was used. From this database, they studied 739,090 vaccinated individuals and an equal number of unvaccinated individuals matched by age, religion, ethnic group, comorbidities, etc. The study reports that the occurrence of retinal vascular occlusion significantly increased after the first and second doses of synthetic mRNA-based vaxgenes over the two years of the study. The risk was similar between both synthetic mRNA brands (Pfizer and Moderna). For AstraZeneca's vaxgene, no increased risk was found. The risk of developing retinal vascular occlusion in vaccinated individuals was 2.19 times higher than that in the unvaccinated cohort after 2 years (95% confidence interval: 2.00–2.39), with a higher risk at 12 weeks. Subsequently, they investigated the biweekly incidence of this pathology in both cohorts 12 weeks after vaccination. They found that the risk significantly increased in vaccinated individuals in those 12 weeks starting from two weeks after receiving the vaccine, with sustained risk throughout the period. Additionally, the cumulative incidence of retinal vascular occlusion significantly increased in the vaccinated group but not in the unvaccinated group (Li J. X. et al., 2023).

Given the increasing number of case reports and adverse events following immunization in international monitoring systems related to ocular damage associated with COVID vaxgenes, a cohort study was conducted to investigate the retinal and optic disc vascular structures before and after the administration of synthetic mRNA COVID vaxgenes in healthy individuals without ocular pathologies, including diabetic retinopathies, uveitis, glaucoma, as well as myopia with a refractive error greater than 6 and an axial length greater than 26 mm, or those who had undergone eye surgery or had systemic disease (Gedik et al., 2023). Using optical coherence tomography angiography (OCTA), they examined retinal and vascular structures before and after vaccination in 40 people meeting the study criteria. They found that after receiving Pfizer's COVID vaxgene, there was a significant decrease in total irrigation, indicated by a reduction in the density of the foveal, parafoveal, and perifoveal superficial capillary plexus, as well as the density of the perifoveal deep capillary plexus vasculature. They also observed a significant increase in foveal and parafoveal retinal thickness. Based on their results, the authors concluded that the decrease in retinal vascular density may be due to damage to vascular endothelium and inflammation leading to reduced irrigation of ocular structures (Gedik et al., 2023). It is worth noting that the reduction in ocular irrigation can be associated with retinopathies, which is particularly relevant in people with diabetes (Czakó et al., 2019). In other words, receiving synthetic mRNA vaccines increases the risk of developing retinopathies due to reduced blood perfusion and may consequently increase the risk of blindness.

The results of Gedik and colleagues' study (2023) mirror those found a year earlier in a study that focused on structural changes associated with the inactivated COVID vaccine (Sinovac) (Gedik et al., 2022). Although that study and another independent one (Yorgun et al., 2023) found no evidence of changes in retinal vasculature density, both determined that retrobulbar blood flow was decreased by the action of the vaccine. These results imply that the observed effect on retinal vasculature density and foveal and parafoveal retinal thickness is due to the effects of synthetic mRNA and not to the Spike protein produced endogenously or received with the inactivated vaccine. Meanwhile, changes in irrigation may be due to a vaccine-induced inflammatory response regardless of the platform or the molecular similarity between various peptides of the SARS-CoV-2 Spike protein and human somatic antigens, which can lead to an autoimmune and autoinflammatory response (see section 5.5).

Taking into account the quantity of published case reports, it should not be surprising that to date, 3,952 reports of blindness[374] (in some cases, transient) have been recorded in association with Pfizer's and Moderna's vaxgenes (both made with synthetic mRNA) in the adverse event monitoring system of the United States. Additionally, there are 347 reports of blindness associated with Janssen's vaxgene (based on an adenoviral vector). As I have done for other adverse events, to provide a point of comparison between blindness events associated with the COVID vaxgenes and those associated with the flu vaccine, there have been 411 reports

[374] Open Vaers [Internet]. Data updated to September 29 2023. Searchable at: https://www.openvaers.com/vaersapp/reports.php

(recorded in the 392 months from 1990 to the present)[375]. Adjusting for months allows us to see that monthly reports of blindness associated with the flu vaccine accumulate at a rate of 1.05 reports per month, while the monthly rate of reports of blindness associated with COVID vaxgenes is 126.44, meaning it is 120 times higher.

This high number of reports of blindness, as well as other ocular problems, should not be too surprising. Since 2021, it has been known that there is similarity between SARS-CoV-2 proteins and human retinal proteins (MRP-4, MRP-5, RFC1, SNAT7, TAUT, and MATE) that could cause autoimmune ocular reactions (Karagöz et al., 2021). Although the similarity between retinal proteins and the virus's envelope protein (E protein) was greater, the Spike protein also had regions of high similarity (Karagöz et al., 2021). This led the authors to call for caution in the use of vaccines and vaxgenes due to the risk they would pose in generating autoimmune retinopathies since the role of retinal proteins is well identified in the pathogenesis of this disease (Morohoshi et al., 2009).

Understanding the occurrence of ocular adverse events associated with COVID vaxgenes is essential for problems to be precisely diagnosed, treated promptly and effectively, and to avoid recommending new doses of the product that caused the harm. Undoubtedly, correct early treatment is the foundation for a good outcome in ocular conditions and to prevent vision loss.

f) Auditive problems

The animal auditory system is essential for survival and plays a key role in social communication, learning, and maintaining body postural balance. As one of the most developed senses in evolution, it depends on the proper function of all its components and the integration of the information these components receive (Fuchs & Tucker, 2015). Any disruption to the connections of the elements that make up the middle ear, or any loss of

[375] Open Vaers [Internet]. Data updated to September 29 2023. Searchable at: https://www.openvaers.com/vaersapp/reports.php

integrity of its tissues, can lead to signal loss and loss or alteration in sound conduction, potentially resulting in deafness.

There are many factors that can cause middle ear diseases, ranging from bacterial, viral, fungal, and helminthic infections to processes of inflammation and autoimmunity. The latter has been recognized for over 50 years when Leinhart (1984) reported that bilateral hearing loss could result from autoimmune processes in the middle ear. Since the late 1970s (McCabe 1970), reports of these cases have accumulated (revised in Zhai, 2015), as well as reports of treatments based on dexamethasone (a corticosteroid with a potent anti-inflammatory effect). Autoimmune middle ear disease is caused by autoantibodies mistakenly produced against self-antigens, triggering inflammatory and cytotoxic processes against tissues in this region of the ear (Zhai, 2015).

It is worth mentioning that the middle ear is considered a tissue with some immune privilege (Keithley, 2022), as it is protected by the blood-brain barrier. For example, the amount of IgG antibodies circulating in the lymph bathing the tissues of the middle ear is only a thousandth of its concentration in the blood. The only issue with this immune privilege is that problems of immunopathology and autoimmunity can more easily arise if middle ear cells undergo infection or damage that increases the expression of the pro-inflammatory cytokine interleukin 1b (IL-1b). This induces the migration of leukocytes into these tissues through the venous circulation of the ear (Keithley, 2022). In individuals predisposed to autoimmune diseases, whose lymphocytes exhibit reactivity to self-antigens, serious problems can be triggered in the inner ear (Agrup & Luxton, 2006).

In fact, several systemic autoimmune diseases such as lupus erythematosus, Sjögren's syndrome, Hashimoto's thyroiditis, antiphospholipid/anticardiolipin syndrome, Behcet's disease, Wegener's granulomatosis, etc., have been associated with hearing dysfunctions due to these autoimmune processes (Zhai, 2015).

Various clinical cases demonstrating hearing impairments that occurred after COVID vaccination have been published in the medical literature (e.g., Leong et al., 2023; Lin & Selleck, 2023; Kamogashira et al., 2022; Parrino et al., 2022; Tseng et al., 2021; Wichova et al., 2021). To highlight the potential severity of the problem, by September 2021, just nine months after the start of COVID vaccination in Europe, Eudravigilance reported 687 cases of ear and labyrinth disorders associated with Janssen's vaxgene, 3,769 cases associated with Moderna's vaxgene, 11,826 cases associated with AstraZeneca's vaxgene, and 14,027 cases associated with Pfizer's vaxgene[376]. The 30,309 cases mainly occurred in individuals aged 18 to 64, with full recovery rates ranging from 22 to 28% (almost three-quarters of the cases were unresolved at the time of the search). Collectively for the four vaxgenes, these disorders included 1,590 cases of deafness, 9,881 cases of tinnitus, and 11,741 cases of vertigo, with over 70% of cases unrecovered. The scenario is similar in the U.S. monitoring system (VAERS); an updated search shows 12,818 cases of deafness, tinnitus, and other hearing impairments in individuals who received vaxgenes[377].

In 2022, news reports indicated more than 10,000 cases of tinnitus in vaccinated individuals, occurring at a rate of 1 in every 21,000 vaccinated individuals[378]. The WHO acknowledged having knowledge of reports of tinnitus and other hearing impairments due to COVID vaccines[379]. Interestingly, while the CDC stated in an article that post-vaccination hearing problems did not exceed the incidence in the general population (Formeister et al., 2021), the FDA considered adverse events sufficient evidence to consider them a safety signal and suggested listing tinnitus as a side effect in Janssen's vectorized vaxgene. Unfortunately, there was no mention by the FDA, CDC, or WHO regarding other auditory serious adverse events (ESAVI), including sudden deafness and hearing loss.

In 2022, a scientific review on tinnitus cases associated with COVID vaxgenes was published (Ahmed et al., 2022). The article describes the occurrence of over 12,000 confirmed cases of tinnitus following

---

[376] Eudravigilance European Database of Suspected Adverse Drug Reaction Reports [Internet]. Search conducted September 8 2021. Database access at: https://www.adrreports.eu/en/search_subst.html#
[377] Open Vaers [Internet]. Data updated to September 29 2023. Searchable at: https://www.openvaers.com/vaersapp/reports.php
[378] https://www.youtube.com/watch?v=H6d0r0b9uCc (ABC news segment) Accessed September 16 2023.
[379] See page 6 of: https://apps.who.int/iris/bitstream/handle/10665/351326/9789240042452-eng.pdf Accessed September 20 2023.

vaccination reported in VAERS between December 2020 and September 2021. The authors also assessed clinical medical literature to identify case studies. They discuss mechanisms that could lead to tinnitus after vaccination and identify autoimmunity (provoked by the molecular similarity of parts of the Spike protein to human proteins) as a possibility. Other possibilities they considered include the potential ototoxicity of some vaccine components, stress, and genetic or physiological predisposition (Ahmed et al., 2022).

In the context of COVID vaccination, to understand the pathogenic mechanisms that could explain the causal association between tinnitus cases and other hearing impairments and COVID vaxgenes, it should be considered that: 1) Immunization will specifically focus on inducing immunity against the Spike protein of the virus through the transfection of the genetic material that encodes it, 2) Synthetic mRNA from COVID vaxgenes as well as the Spike protein cross the blood-brain barrier (Mörz et al., 2023), 3) Both vaccine mRNA and the Spike protein induce severe inflammation (Seneff et al., 2022), and 4) Similarities exist between Spike and some human proteins (Adiguzel et al., 2021; Obando-Pereda 2021; Vojdani et al., 2021; Kanduc and Shoenfeld, 2020; Marino Gammazza et al., 2020; Paladino et al., 2020).

6.6 Increased susceptibility to infections

The consequence of a state of lymphocyte depletion due to mono antigenic hyperstimulation (see section 5.8) or immune dysregulation (see section 5.3) would be an increased risk of various pathological processes, including a higher predisposition to infections and a greater likelihood of developing cancer. It is noteworthy that, to date, not a single experimental or observational study has been conducted to assess the possibility of lymphocyte depletion and immune dysregulation with repeated doses of mono antigenic vaccines.

Published studies have reported that some patients with severe COVID were characterized by having exhausted $CD8^+$ T lymphocytes (e.g., De Biasi et al., 2020; Zheng HY et al., 2020; Zheng M et al., 2020). However, other studies have failed to find evidence of lymphocyte depletion, even in severe cases. This probably reflects that the markers of lymphocyte exhaustion have some overlap with activation markers, at least for a time before they become exhausted. A study based on single-cell transcriptomic analysis (scRNA-seq)[380] reported that the expression pattern of $CD8^+$ T lymphocytes was not different in COVID patients compared to healthy individuals (Wilk et al., 2020). Another study that used a similar method along with Cellular Indexing of Transcriptomes and Epitopes[381] by Sequencing (CITE-seq) and T cell receptor sequencing showed that there were clusters of exhausted $CD8^+$ T lymphocytes, but these were not evidently associated with severe COVID (Liu C. et al., 2021).

It is possible that these results also indicate that most severe cases of COVID are due more to sustained inflammation than to sustained antigen production, as SARS-CoV-2, like all other coronaviruses, establishes acute infections, not latent or chronic ones and does not integrate into the host genome (Ravi et al., 2022). This means there is no active replication after a short period (typically less than 15 days; Hu et al., 2021). However, it has been demonstrated that various SARS-CoV-2 antigens can persist without viral replication in the intestines of patients with irritable bowel syndrome who had been infected, and the persistence of viral antigens could last for months (Zollner et al., 2022). The results of other studies have suggested that subgenomic RNA of SARS-CoV-2 can be found in immunosuppressed individuals for months, and in a fraction of samples, the cultivated virus could exert cytopathic effects, suggesting that the virus can remain competent for replication for months (Stein et al., 2022).

The discrepancy in the results of studies that have found evidence of antigen persistence and those that have not, and those that have detected lymphocyte exhaustion phenotypes, may be due to many factors, including differences in the immune senescence of patients according to their age

[380] Transcriptomics are those analyses that allow us to identify all the expressed genes in a biological sample at a given moment. It quantifies and identifies all mRNA molecules that the cells are transcribing.

[381] An epitope or antigenic determinant is a group of amino acids or other chemical groups that are exposed on the surface of a molecule (almost always a protein) that can cause an immune response, and are the ones that a specific antibody will bind to.

group, concomitant factors, and differences in the severity of COVID, among others (Rha and Shin, 2021).

There is some evidence that the immune function of some vaccinated individuals may have been impacted. For example, cases of herpesvirus activation (e.g., Mahendradas et al., 2023; Mishra et al., 2023; Sangoram et al., 2022) and even recurrence of retinoid toxoplasmosis have been reported in vaccinated individuals against COVID. It is worth noting that both the activation of latent herpesviruses and the reactivation of retinoid toxoplasmosis are associated with states of immune suppression (Lee et al., 2000).

Herpesviruses are large DNA viruses (Herpesviridae family)[382] that, depending on the genus, have an affinity for epithelial cells (skin and mucous membranes), immune cells (monocytes, dendritic cells, and lymphocytes, such as the herpesvirus that causes mononucleosis), or neurons (Adler et al., 2017). Once a herpesvirus successfully enters a susceptible and permissive cell, it can carry out its replication cycle, which, along with the responses and particular conditions of the susceptible host, can cause the characteristic signs of the associated disease. However, it can also enter latency by remaining episomal in the cell's cytoplasm without completing its replication cycle. Episomal herpesviruses can reactivate when there is a state of immune suppression (such as with AIDS, due to immunosuppressive drugs, or in cancer patients receiving chemotherapy or radiotherapy) or when a neuron is damaged.

Upon emerging from their dormant state, herpesviruses reactivate their replication cycle. This is why reactivation of herpesviruses is usually a sign of immune suppression. Although the phenomenon of herpesvirus reactivation is not completely understood, it is likely that when cytotoxic (CD8+) or helper ($CD4^+$) T lymphocytes are compromised, this reactivation occurs (Campbell et al., 2012). That is relevant in the context of COVID vaxgenes, because only considering VAERS, there are, to date, 15,878 reports of herpesvirus reactivations in vaccinated people[383]. This scenario

[382] Viralzone [Internet]. Available at: https://viralzone.expasy.org/176?outline=all_by_species
[383] Open Vaers [Internet]. Data updated to September 29 2023. Can be accessed at: https://www.openvaers.com/vaersapp/reports.php

suggests that the number of people who could be having poor immune competence due to the vaxgenes is not small.

Beyond the data from the adverse event monitoring systems (ESAVI), the reactivation of herpesviruses in individuals who received an COVID vaxgene has been epidemiologically analysed (Hertel et al., 2022). It was found that those who received the COVID vaxgene have a higher risk of reactivating herpesviruses if they had previously been infected by one. The objective of Hertel and colleagues' study (2022) was to determine if the frequency of herpes zoster (HZ) increases in vaccinated individuals compared to non-vaccinated individuals. They followed both cohorts, each consisting of over a million people, and compared the incidence of HZ over a 60-day period since receiving the vaccine at the medical centre (vaccinated cohort) or since visiting the medical centre for another reason (non-vaccinated cohort). They obtained data from the TriNetX database[384] in Germany and matched the data by age and gender to mitigate any potential bias that could confound the results. In the vaccinated cohort, 2,204 individuals had HZ within 60 days of receiving the COVID vaxgene. In contrast, in the non-vaccinated cohort, 1,223 people were diagnosed with HZ. This means that the risk of HZ reactivation is 0.20% for the vaccinated and 0.11% for the non-vaccinated, resulting in a statistically significant risk ratio of 1.8. In conclusion, being vaccinated against COVID carries almost twice the risk of reactivating a herpesvirus compared to those who are not vaccinated, strongly suggesting that COVID vaxgenes are the cause of the reactivation (Hertel et al., 2022). This can only be explained if COVID vaxgenes affect cellular immune function.

There is some evidence of this. A recent study showed that Pfizer's synthetic mRNA COVID vaxgene alters the immune responses of children. Specifically, it decreases cytokine production in response to heterologous stimuli, even one month after vaccination (Noé et al., 2023). This means that children who were vaccinated with Pfizer may not have the same ability to respond to challenges with other common microorganisms, such as *Staphylococcus aureus*, *Escherichia coli*, *Listeria monocytogenes*, *Haemophilus influenza*, *Candida albicans*, and the hepatitis B virus.

[384] TrinetX [Internet]. Available at: https://trinetx.com

Furthermore, the decreased response to viral challenges persisted over time, even six months after vaccination. Additionally, they found that the quantity of specific anti-Spike antibodies in vaccinated children did not explain the reduced ability to respond to other antigenic stimuli. The authors discussed that this could be due to Pfizer's synthetic mRNA affecting the signalling cascade of key elements for immune responses, as explained in section 4.3 and as detailed in (Acevedo-Whitehouse and Bruno, 2023; Seneff et al., 2022). They concluded that synthetic mRNA vaxgenes "*reprogram the innate and adaptive immune responses of children*", which could impact their ability to respond to other pathogens (Noé et al., 2023).

Finally, another mechanism through which immune suppression that increases susceptibility to infections could occur, as described in Chapter 2 for vectorized vaccines with adenovirus (AdV). Considering that AdVs are known to increase susceptibility to HIV in people at risk of infection (Gray et al., 2010; Gray et al., 2011; Duerr et al., 2012; Richie and Villasante, 2013), there is a possibility that at least some of the individuals who received COVID vaxgenes based on AdV5 (Janssen, CanSino, Sputnik) have a higher risk of contracting HIV/AIDS, as warned before the start of the vaccination campaign (Buchbinder et al., 2020).

6.7 V-ADE. Is it occurring?

In addition to herpesvirus reactivations suggesting impaired cellular immune function, it has also been reported that vaccinated individuals are at a higher risk of SARS-CoV-2 reinfection. This may seem counterintuitive but is not when considering lymphocytic exhaustion or anergy caused by monovalent antigenic overstimulation or direct immune suppression induced by vaxgenes, as described in section 6.6.

One of the effects associated with COVID vaxgenes is antibody-dependent enhancement (ADE). ADE is the worsening of a disease associated with an infection due to antibodies that are not adequately neutralizing. These antibodies fail to neutralize the virus, bacteria, or microorganism in question and, instead, increase the likelihood of infecting other cells, typically immune cells. When ADE occurs due to antibodies generated by vaccination, it is known as V-ADE or VDE.

It should be noted that COVID vaxgenes were designed based on the sequence of the *wild-type* SARS-CoV-2 virus, which, since mid-2020, is no longer the one currently circulating, particularly concerning the RBD N-terminal antigenic region of Spike (Ma et al., 2023). Therefore, antibodies generated in response to the mechanism of action of vaxgenes (see section 1.3) when people received one, two, or three doses of the 'original' vaccines are no longer efficient in neutralizing the Spike protein of the currently circulating variants. The same applies to bivalent vaxgenes: the variant of SARS-CoV-2 for which they were intended to provide protection is no longer prevalent. For instance, when vaccination began against the 'subvariants' BA.4 and BA.5 of the Omicron variant of SARS-CoV-2, these subvariants were no longer circulating significantly, but others like BQ.1, BQ.1.1, and BF.7 were (Shrestra et al., 2023).

Rather than conferring protection, non-neutralizing antibodies increase the virus's infectivity (Liu Y. et al., 2021). This has been known for at least three decades and has been reported for the Dengue virus and other coronaviruses, including the one causing Feline Infectious Peritonitis (Cloutier et al., 2020), a feline disease for which vaccination is not recommended as it increases infectivity through this mechanism (Venemma et al., 1990).

Before the onset of the COVID vaccination campaign, several scientists warned about the risk of Antibody-Dependent Enhancement (ADE) (Coish & MacNeil, 2020; Flanagan et al., 2020; Halstead & Katzelnick, 2020; Karthik et al., 2020), and some emphasized the necessity of disclosing this risk in the informed consent for those opting to be vaccinated against COVID (Cardozo & Veazey, 2021). These warnings were not unfounded; as mentioned in Chapter 2, vaccine safety expert committees, CEPI and SPEAC, concluded that they must "*evaluate vaccine candidates for any evidence of disease exacerbation*" (Lambert et al., 2020). However, the COVID vaccination strategy we know today was still implemented.

The challenge for public health is that if V-ADE is occurring due to the synthesis of non-neutralizing antibodies generated by COVID vaccination, it is clinically indistinguishable from a severe COVID case (Lee et al., 2020). Hence, it's not surprising that studies claiming no clinical evidence of V-ADE are published (e.g., Ikewaki et al., 2023; Yaugel-Novoa et al., 2023). However, what is complex to determine individually can be done at the population level. For instance, a prospective cohort epidemiological study conducted in Iceland between December 1, 2021, and February 13, 2022, found that the risk of SARS-CoV-2 reinfection increased 1.56 times at 18 months compared to the likelihood of initial infection, and the risk of reinfection was 1.42 times higher for individuals who had received two or more doses than those who had received one dose or none (Eythorsson et al., 2022). In line with these results, a more recent study showed that hospital admissions for people with COVID and admissions to the Intensive Care Unit increase significantly with the number of doses of COVID vaxgenes a person has received (Parry et al., 2023).

An epidemiological analysis investigating whether bivalent vaxgenes conferred protection against COVID found that out of the 51,011 people included in the study, 6,419 (13%) were unvaccinated. They found that the more doses of vaxgenes people had, the higher the incidence of COVID (Shrestha et al., 2023). In other words, the more doses you receive, the more likely you are to get infected with SARS-CoV-2. This could be due to V-ADE or direct or indirect immune suppression, or both phenomena, as they are not mutually exclusive. However, it completely contradicts the narrative of "the pandemic of the unvaccinated." The more people are vaccinated, the higher the chances of severe COVID. This pattern has also been observed at the population level. For example, a recent report showed that the Southern Hemisphere countries that vaccinated their population the most exhibited the highest COVID mortality (Rancourt et al., 2023).

6.8 Dysbiosis

COVID vaccines and vaxgenes have been found to be associated with alterations in the intestinal microbiota (Hazan et al., 2022b; Hazan et al., 2022c; Ng et al., 2022). Before describing these alterations, it's necessary to briefly explain what the intestinal microbiota is. It encompasses all bacteria, viruses, fungi, yeasts, and other microorganisms that are normally present in our intestines, particularly in the colon, and collaborate to maintain the health of this tissue. The most abundant and diverse component of the microbiota is bacterial, and bacteria are typically the focus of study when characterizing the microbiota.

There is a growing understanding that maintaining a stable microbiota in the intestine is important for human health. When the microbiota is disrupted, for example, after taking broad-spectrum antibiotics, alterations can occur that impact our metabolism and health.

"*Now, wait a minute*" – some might ask "*.What does the intestinal microbiota have to do with COVID vaccination?*". Well, it turns out that there is evidence that vaccines and vaxgenes can cause dysbiosis (Hazan et al., 2022b; Hazan et al., 2022c), similar to what has been reported in some individuals who were infected with SARS-CoV-2 (De and Dutta, 2022; Gang et al., 202; Hazan et al., 2022a).

The impact of vaccines and vaxgenes on the intestinal microbiota, as well as the impact of the intestinal microbiota on post-vaccination adverse events, is not something that should be ignored. Both the inactivated vaccine (Sinovac) and the synthetic mRNA vaxgene (Pfizer) induce a change in the bacterial diversity[385] of the intestine even a month after receiving the second dose (Ng et al., 2022). It's noteworthy that, despite being from different technological platforms, both the inactivated vaccine and the synthetic mRNA vaxgene caused a drastic decrease in bacteria from the phylum[386] Actinobacteria and the phylum Firmicutes. This could be explained by the intense systemic inflammation caused by these vaccines (Ciabattini et al., 2019), leading to alterations in the intestinal microbiota.

On the other hand, the presence of specific bacteria was associated with the magnitude of the vaccination response. Specifically, *Bifidobacterium adolescentis* was found to be more abundant in those with higher antibody levels after receiving the Sinovac vaccine, and they exhibited a bias in bacterial carbohydrate metabolism. In contrast, individuals with higher antibody levels who received Pfizer's vaxgene were associated with a greater abundance of flagellated bacteria such as *Roseburia faecis*. This is

---

[385] I am referring to alpha diversity (the measure of the diversity of microorganisms in an individual) and beta diversity (the measure of the similarity of diversity between two communities).
[386] Phylum (plural: phyla) is a taxonomic category that is situated between Kingdom and Class.

interesting for two reasons: firstly, it demonstrates that although both products induce antibody formation, the impact on other systems (in this case, the intestinal microbiota) is not the same for those who received an inactivated vaccine as for those who received a synthetic mRNA vaxgene; secondly, finding a high presence of the bacterium *Roseburia faecis* in the intestine of those who received the synthetic mRNA vaxgene implies a higher risk for the development of various diseases, including irritable bowel syndrome, obesity, type 2 diabetes, neurological diseases, and allergies (reviewed by Tamanai-Shacoori et al., 2017).

It was also reported that individuals who experienced fewer adverse events after genetic vaccination had a higher abundance of *Prevotella copri* as well as two species of the *Megamonas bacterium*. The study authors interpreted this as evidence that these bacteria play a crucial immunomodulatory and anti-inflammatory role (Ng et al., 2022). While their relevance in this context is acknowledged, it's essential to consider that the presence of *Prevotella copri* has also been associated with a higher risk of rheumatoid arthritis and Parkinson's disease (Abdelsalam and Hegazy, 2023).

Certainly, the impact on the microbiota is not a phenomenon specific to COVID vaccines, vaxgenes or SARS-CoV-2 infection. For example, the subcutaneous application of the *Bacillus* Calmette-Guérin (BCG) vaccine against tuberculosis is known to alter the intestinal and pulmonary microbiota, particularly affecting the relative abundance of two bacterial phyla: Firmicutes and Bacteroidetes. It modifies bacterial diversity, interpreted as a result of immune responses triggered by vaccination that have a systemic impact causing dysbiosis. This, in turn, may contribute to the immunopathogenesis of tuberculosis and influence susceptibility to other infections (Silva et al., 2022). This is because, in addition to inducing 'trained' lymphocytes against specific antigens in the bone marrow and peripheral blood, vaccination (as well as infections) induces memory in alveolar macrophages residing in the mucosa. This leads to an alteration of the intestinal and pulmonary microbiome affecting microbial metabolism. It's truly fascinating to think that there is a pathway mediated by commensal microorganisms in our mucosae that impacts the development of innate immune memory, even in distant areas from the anatomical site of vaccination or infection (Jeyanathan et al., 2022).

In the context of global mass vaccination with repeated booster doses, the potential impact of COVID vaxgenes on the microbiome is significant. Dysbiosis can have serious health consequences and may even be associated with a higher risk of developing chronic-degenerative diseases such as cancer (Helmink et al., 2017) and psychoneurological conditions like schizophrenia (Agorastos and Bozikas, 2019; Zuo and Ng, 2018). It is now known, for instance, that the severity of the condition known as COVID is associated with a delicate interaction between the intestinal microbiota, vitamin D levels, and the proper regulation of the renin-angiotensin axis (Shenoy, 2022). This could explain why the disease has been more severe in older individuals with comorbidities characterized by lower intestinal microbial diversity and vitamin D deficiency. In other words, the microbiota plays a role in maintaining homeostasis. Therefore, the relevance of caring for the microbiota to maintain health is increasingly appreciated (Harper et al., 2021). If COVID vaxgenes modify the abundance and diversity of the intestinal, respiratory, and potentially skin, genital mucosa, and conjunctival mucosa microbiota, it is not unreasonable to suggest that this could increase the risk of opportunistic infections in these tissues. The stability of the microbiota helps prevent the colonization of other potentially harmful microorganisms (Wu et al., 2022). There is some evidence that this might be happening. For example, a search in the U.S. adverse event monitoring system shows, at the time of writing this book, 496 reports of candidiasis in individuals who received at least one dose of COVID vaxgene[387], which is associated with both immune suppression and dysbiosis (Černáková and Rodrigues, 2020).

Dysbiosis can also be associated with a higher risk of developing Crohn's disease, ulcerative colitis, and other inflammatory diseases, as well as colorectal cancer, allergies, type 1 diabetes, autism, and obesity (DeGruttola et al., 2016). Considering the action of the active compounds and excipients of COVID vaxgenes, as well as the persistence of synthetic mRNA in the cell cytoplasm (see section 5.3) and the potential for immune

[387] OpenVaers [Internet]. Data updated to September 23 2023. Available at: https://openvaers.com

dysregulation caused by multiple mono antigenic stimulations (see section 5.8), these conditions are already a risk. To this risk, the effect of possible dysbiosis due to the action of vaxgenes must be added.

6.9 Rapid onset and hyper progression of cancer

Around six months after the start of mass COVID vaccinations, following emergency authorization, there were reports from doctors claiming to observe many more cancer cases than usual in their practices. In fact, the term 'turbo cancer' was coined to explain the sudden appearance and rapid development of cancer in some vaccinated individuals. The term 'turbo cancer' is not a medical term. However, the excessively rapid development of a cancerous tumour does have an accepted medical term: it's called "hyper progression" and reflects a phenomenon that has been known for several years. During therapeutic immune stimulation, such as in cancer immunotherapy, sometimes tumours being treated, instead of decreasing in size, grow and spread rapidly.

It is valid and pertinent to ask whether vaxgenes based on synthetic mRNA, such as those from Pfizer, Moderna, or vectorized vaxgenes, can increase the risk of cancer and tumour hyperproliferation. In section 5.3 and section 5.5, I described various mechanisms by which synthetic mRNA can interact with molecules and cells, causing damage and altering biochemical pathways, as well as lead to the sustained production of Spike. This antigenic overstimulation leads to states of immune dysregulation, either sustained immune suppression or hyperactivity. Both scenarios may be related to an increased risk of malignant cellular transformation that goes undetected and uncontrolled by the immune system. As early as 2022, a warning had been issued that the use of these vaxgenes could increase the risk of cancer, especially causing rapid progression in individuals already having cancer (Brest et al., 2022). The authors emphasized that administering COVID vaxgenes to individuals receiving oncologic immunotherapy, especially 'checkpoint inhibitor therapy' (CPI), might be counterproductive. According to Brest and colleagues, tumour hyperproliferation would occur due to the expansion of T and B cell populations in response to sustained antigenic stimulation induced by these vaxgenes.

On the other hand, the fact that synthetic mRNA vaxgenes contain DNA from the bacterial plasmids used in the manufacturing process (see section 5.6) further increases the risk of insertional mutagenesis. This risk is even higher for individuals who received Pfizer's vaxgene, as the plasmid used to manufacture them contains the eukaryotic promoter of SV40 along with a nuclear insertion-enhancing region (McKernan et al., 2023; Speicher et al., 2023). Additionally, as explained in section 5.3, synthetic mRNA impacts the structure and function of ribosomes, alters the expression of microRNAs, and can activate the LINE-1 transposable element, leading to more chromosomal instability and promoting a cancerous state. Adding to this, the Spike protein produced based on the genetic information of the vaxgenes interacts with the tumour suppressor protein p53 (see section 5.5), resulting in an increased risk of cancer and rapid cancer progression. This risk is even more significant with an increasing number of doses received (see section 5.8).

The matter becomes even more complex since it is now known that modified synthetic mRNA COVID vaxgenes (like those of Pfizer and Moderna) are associated with a change in the abundance and diversity of intestinal bacteria, known as dysbiosis, a phenomenon that can also increase the risk of hyper progression of tumour cells, as described in some individuals who were infected with SARS-CoV-2 (Hazan et al., 2022a). The following graphic summarizes these mechanisms that may explain the occurrence of hyper progressive cancer (Fig. 25).

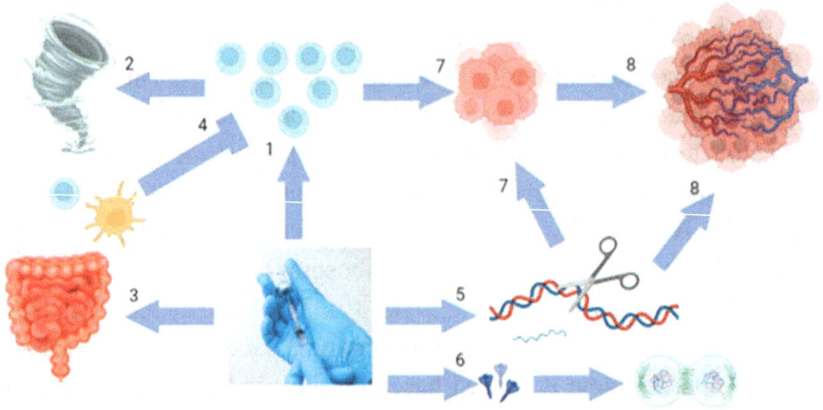

Figure 25. *Mechanisms by which the COVID vaxgenes can be related to cancer hyper progression. 1) The vaxgene induces a clonal expansion of lymphocytes. 2) A cytokine storm can occur (Au et al., 2021). 3) The intestinal microbiota can become altered, leading to dysbiosis, which reduces the activation of T-cells and dendritic cells. 4) This can lead to the inhibition of lymphocyte activity. 5) The synthetic mRNA can activate LINE-1 and deregulate the expression of microRNAs. 6) The vaxgene leads to the production of Spike protein, that binds to P53, with the possibility of uncontrolled cell division occurring. 7) The described events can lead to cancerous tumours. 8) These can progress quickly.*

The risk of hyperproliferative cancer due to COVID vaxgenes is not limited to oncology patients undergoing immunotherapy. Cellular transformation processes frequently occur and are counteracted by a functional immune system (Ikeda and Togashi, 2022). When any factor dysregulates immune function, the anti-tumour response is impacted, increasing the chances of promoting cancer. As explained in sections 5.8, 6.6, and 6.7, this is precisely what vaxgenes do: deregulate immune function.

Several clinical cases have been published describing the onset of various types of cancer following COVID vaccination, including malignant lymphomas (Tachita et al., 2023; Sekizawa et al., 2022; Gamblicher et al., 2021; Goldman et al., 2021), carcinomas (Kyriakopoulos et al., 2023; Ooi et al., 2022), lymphangioma (Sasa et al., 2022), and neuroendocrine tumours (Yildiz Tasci et al., 2022), as well as cases of cancer reactivation or worsening following COVID vaccination (e.g., Adin et al., 2022; Panou et al., 2022; Tripathy et al., 2022; Brumfiel et al., 2021; Sumi et al., 2021). Among the cancer cases recorded in adverse event monitoring systems, breast cancer associated with COVID vaxgenes appears to have a disproportionately high number of reports. For example, in the adverse event monitoring system of the United States, between December 2020 and the end of September 2023, 3,849 cases of breast cancer were registered, occurring after the receipt of COVID vaxgenes[388]. If we apply the underreporting factor, we would be talking about 119,319 possible cases of breast cancer associated with COVID vaxgenes in the United States.

There is evidence, both official and testimonial, suggesting an increase in cases of certain types of cancer following the widespread administration of COVID vaxgenes. For example, based on information provided in April 2022 in response to a request made to Mexico's National Institute of Transparency, Access to Information, and Protection of Personal Data (INAI), it is known that the incidence of breast cancer cases increased in 2021 compared to the five-year average (2016 to 2020) (Fig. 26).

The increase observed in Figure 26 for the year 2021 is not trivial. For instance, in girls aged 10 to 14, there was an increase of 518%, in adolescents aged 15 to 19, it was 348%, and the age group where the increase was most evident was young women aged 20 to 24, with an increase of 3,249%. Additionally, there was a shift in the age group with the highest number of cases, previously in women aged 50 to 59 and in 2021, it was in the 45 to 49 age group.

It's worth mentioning that the increase in breast cancer incidence may not necessarily imply a causal association with COVID vaxgenes but instead could be a non-causal correlation reflecting some as yet unknown phenomenon. Nevertheless, it undoubtedly represents a relevant epidemiological change that urgently requires further study.

[388] OpenVaers [Internet]. Data updated to September 23 2023. Available at: https://openvaers.com

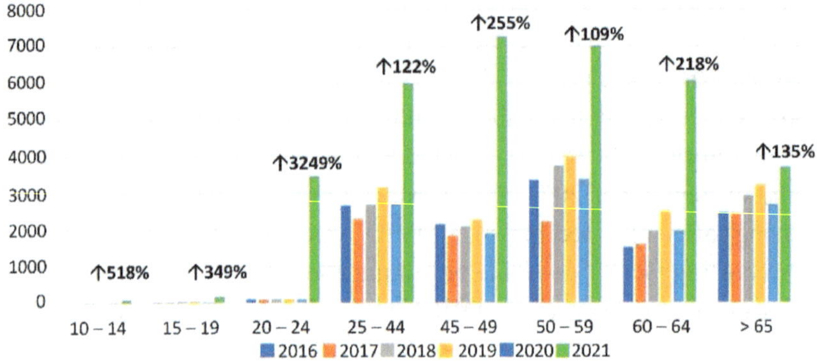

Figure 26. *Annual incidence of breast cancer in women in Mexico, between 2016 and 2021. Data from the Health Ministry in response to the Freedom of Information Request INAI 330026922006519.*

The data align with observations in other countries. For instance, Dr. Üte Kruger, a German pathologist specializing in breast cancer histopathology for 19 years, reported during a 2023 Pathology conference that since the fall of 2021, she had been receiving more breast biopsy samples from younger patients than expected for breast cancer. The tumours were growing faster and more aggressively, larger than expected (over 4 cm and up to 16 cm), and there was an increased frequency of multifocal tumour growth and bilateral malignancies compared to before 2021[389].

Undoubtedly, the vaxgenes induces changes in breast tissue and the immune tissue associated with the mammary gland. There is a growing number of publications reporting cases of mammary lymphadenopathies[390] (e.g., Mema et al., 2023; Raj et al., 2022; Wolfson et al., 2022; Edmonds et al., 2021) or changes in breast tissue (e.g., Adam et al., 2022; Kim & Reig, 2022; Soeder et al., 2022) following the receipt of the COVID vaxgene. This should not be surprising; the vaxgene is distributed to virtually all organs of the body (see section 5.2), and we know that synthetic mRNA from the COVID vaxgene can be found in breast milk of vaccinated

[389] DailyClout. Report 61: Histopathology Series Part 3 – Ute Krüger, MD, Breast Cancer Specialist, Reveals Increase in Cancers and Occurrences of "Turbo Cancers" Following Genetic Therapy "Vaccines" [Internet]. Available at: https://dailyclout.io/report-61-ute-kruger-md-breast-cancer-specialist-reveals-increase-in-cancers-and-occurrences-of-turbo-cancers-following-genetic-therapy-vaccines/

[390] Inflammation of lymphatic nodes.

mothers (Hanna et al., 2022). However, even if this broad distribution did not occur, the lymph nodes closest to the site of application of the vaxgene in the deltoid muscle are the axillary nodes. Due to the mechanism of action of the synthetic mRNA, dendritic cells in which the synthetic mRNA has entered will migrate to these lymph nodes. If the processes described above occur in the lymph nodes or in the epithelium of the mammary ducts, the probability of tumorigenesis is not low. On the other hand, the risk may be exacerbated with each additional dose of the vaxgene received. There is experimental evidence for this: a study in mice demonstrated that malignant lymphoma could occur as little as two days after receiving a booster of Pfizer's vaxgene (Eens et al., 2023). Therefore, it is crucial for oncologists and women to recognize that this process can occur and understand that the risk increases with each additional dose received.

In this chapter, I have described and explained the most common adverse events occurring in individuals who received one or more doses of vaxgenes. It is important to emphasize that these described events are not exhaustive; many other infrequent events have also been associated with COVID vaxgenes (Afshar et al., 2022), and it is possible that there are still undiscovered conditions related to this technology.

Chapter 7. What can be done to mitigate the effects of vaxgenes?

If the answer is simple, God is speaking.

Albert Einstein

After reading Chapter 6 of this book, you may have identified clinical conditions in yourselves or your family and friends who received one or more doses of COVID vaxgenes, and these conditions may have seemed to occur without a deeper explanation than 'bad luck'. If you read Chapter 5, you now know the mechanisms that explain these clinical conditions, and if you read Chapter 4, you can now identify which causality criteria are met to have more certainty that COVID vaxgenes may have been the cause of these ailments. The next logical and obvious question is, "*What can be done?*"

It is not the goal of this book to offer medical advice or indicate protocols that may help counteract the adverse effects of vaxgenes. However, if the pathophysiology of the components of vaxgenes is understood, it should not be complicated for doctors to envision possible avenues for treating their patients, and it would be less complex for them to propose, based on that knowledge, their own protocols to help their patients suffering from the adverse effects of COVID vaxgenes.

As I mentioned at the beginning of Chapter 6, the various clinical conditions that are occurring in people who received one or more vaxgenes are grouped into inflammatory, autoimmune, degenerative, and uncontrolled cell proliferation disorders. I also explained why these effects can be seen in all types of tissues, from capillary endothelia to neurons and in all organs. Once the pathophysiology is understood, a constant headache and general malaise in a patient who received one or more doses of vaxgenes, who has no history of migraines, has not been exposed to heparin, has no infectious condition, and has not had any traumatic events explaining the pain, will no longer be simply an 'idiopathic headache' but a possible sign of vaccine-induced thrombotic thrombocytopenia (VITT; see Section

6.2), or even the onset of Bell's palsy (Hsiao et al., 2023). If, in addition to persistent headaches, the patient has petechiae[391], it is even more justified to propose VITT as a presumptive diagnosis. Therefore, requesting blood tests to count the number of circulating platelets, to search for antibodies against platelet factor 4 (PF4), and to quantify D-dimers in the blood would be important to confirm the diagnosis of VITT and propose treatment. Of course, if brain and cerebral blood vessel imaging studies can also be performed, more elements will be available to identify this clinical picture. This simple action: using the knowledge learned to open one's eyes to the possibility that vaxgenes caused a coagulopathy, could save the patient's life. The fact that a doctor does not understand the pathophysiology of COVID vaxgenes and, because of that ignorance, dismisses headaches and general malaise as “normal”, could lead to a very different outcome for the patient.

This same criterion, based on scientific evidence about the pathophysiology of vaxgenes, can be used for any of the clinical conditions that many doctors are seeing in their practice, at rates higher than observed during decades. These conditions range from hyper progressive cancer, recurrence of cancer in patients who have been in remission for years, and atypical cancers in young people, to autoimmune diseases, severe inflammatory disorders, coagulopathies, reactivation of herpetic conditions, clinical immune suppression, blindness or decreased vision, deafness or hearing impairments, menstrual disturbances, infertility, etc. (see Chapter 6). The main thing, after understanding that it is possible and plausible that a COVID vaxgene is the cause of the patient's clinical condition (or one's own), is to carry out the necessary laboratory tests to help understand which associated mechanisms are causing the clinical signs and symptoms and initiate the corresponding treatment. For this, it is also essential to understand that adverse events do not only occur days after receiving vaxgenes but can occur long after (Finsterer & Scorza, 2022) and can affect many areas of the affected individuals' lives (Krumholz et al., 2023).

[391] Small red dots, like pinpricks, on the skin, that appear in different parts of the body with no discharge and without having been caused by an insect.

There are clinical analyses that provide valuable information, are not very expensive, and only require a blood sample, such as measuring troponin, creatine kinase, and lactate dehydrogenase if there is suspicion that the COVID vaxgenes caused cardiac damage (Basit & Huecker, 2023; Federspiel et al., 2023; Jeet Kaur et al., 2021), measuring D-dimers, blood-clotting times (prothrombin time and partial thromboplastin time), tissue factor, and antibodies against PF4 if there is suspicion that COVID vaxgenes caused endothelial damage and thrombotic thrombocytopenia (Müller & Griesmacher, 2000). Furthermore, measuring C-reactive protein, ferritin, serum amyloid A, and pro-inflammatory cytokines (such as IL-1, IFN-I, TNF-α, IL-6, and IL-8) can be very useful if there is suspicion that COVID vaxgenes caused an autoinflammatory state (Chuamanochan et al., 2019). Depending on their country, individuals can undergo these tests in a clinical analysis laboratory without a prescription or medical recommendation and then bring the results to a doctor who has already understood the pathophysiology of the components of COVID vaxgenes. However, beyond laboratory tests, the most important aspect to consider is the patient's full medical history. It is essential to have information about the number of doses of COVID vaxgenes received, the brand, the batch number (if possible), and the date of vaccination. It is not justified to say, "*It was three, six, or nine months ago, so it cannot be related*". If you still think that way, I recommend revisiting Chapter 3, Chapter 4, and Chapter 5.

Once the clinical picture and its cause are understood, treatment should necessarily include measures to limit and stop further damage. This means, first and foremost, avoiding any new dose of COVID vaxgenes. Additionally, it makes sense to use blockers of the Spike protein, which, as explained, can continue to be produced for months in those who received COVID vaxgenes (see section 5.5) and, potentially, in those who are exposed to vaccinated individuals who are shedding the Spike protein or the active compounds of the vaxgenes (see section 5.9). Once further exposure to damage is stopped, efforts can be made to repair the damage already caused (Halma et al., 2023b).

I have invested a lot of time and effort in explaining the *what*, *how*, *where*, and *when* (and, between the lines, the *why*) of the adverse events associated with COVID vaxgenes. From now on, the effort will have to be yours, as healthcare professionals, of course, but also, regardless of your profession, as individuals who have understood the importance of taking charge of your health and the health of your dependents based on sound knowledge. There are things that can be done to reduce, mitigate, and treat adverse events. There are several ways to do this, using generic compounds with broad nonspecific effects. If we understand that the vaxgenes can cause immune dysregulation, then it becomes logical that immune modulators can be used; if we understand that they can affect the vascular endothelium, then it becomes logical that endothelial protectors can be used; if we understand that they can cause dysbiosis, then it becomes logical that helping to regulate and restore the intestinal microbiota will be beneficial. How to do this will depend on each person's preference: from using healthy food, nutraceuticals, probiotics, prebiotics, micronutrients, to using specific compounds and drugs to achieve these goals (see Table 1 in Halma et al., 2023b).

The good news is that there are many protocols that have been developed by physicians and are available to everyone. For example, the World Council for Health (WCH)[392] has proposed a Spike protein detox protocol based on the recommendation of physicians from different countries who have been successfully treating patients who suffered adverse events. If you wish, you can consult it at: https://worldcouncilforhealth.org/resources/spike-protein-detox-guide/.

This is not the only protocol that exists; I mention it here precisely because it is a compilation of many protocols and because it is accessible to many people, being available in different languages. You can even look for protocols that were published since 2020 with the intention of minimizing or counteracting the effects of the SARS-CoV-2 Spike protein (e.g., Dhasmana et al., 2020), as vaxgenes lead to the endogenous production of this same protein (McCullough et al., 2023). Of course, at the

[392] The World Council for Health is a not for profit organization that was founded in 2021 with the goal of increasing knowledge on public health and help take decisions based on common sense. It is not financed by any agency and is informed and funded by the people. Their global coalition of health-focused initiatives and civil society groups seeks to broaden public health knowledge and sense-making through science and shared wisdom.

time of writing this book, there is no medical protocol that can truthfully claim to counteract each and every possible harmful effect caused by COVID vaxgenes because we still do not know them all; however, as I have said before, if the pathophysiology of their components is understood, it is at least possible to aspire to counteract or treat the effects described to date. My recommendation is that if what you have read and understood in this book seems important to consider, take the time to search for and compare protocols and make your own decisions. No one is more responsible for their health and life than oneself.

Regardless of the available medical protocols, it seems pertinent to make it clear that no protocol, no matter how good it is, will overlook an unhealthy lifestyle. Part of being responsible for our health involves striving to live a healthier life. Unfortunately, there are no magic formulas. If we are accustomed to living in an unhealthy way, sleeping less than we should, consuming food of poor nutritional value, leading sedentary lifestyles, constantly exposing ourselves to sources of electromagnetic radiation and chemical pollutants, and engaging in practices or seeking relationships that harm us emotionally, there will be no pill, tablet, or liquid that can restore our health. The decision and the responsibility for the decision lie entirely with us, as will be its consequence on our body and our life.

Chapter 8. Looking towards the future

Hope is being able to see that there is light despite the darkness.

Desmond Tutu

You have almost reached the end of the book, which means that, if you did not skip sections, you have already read 292 pages. I sense that, at times, these pages were difficult to read, not so much due to technicality but because of their emotional impact. I know this because it was tough for me to write many of these pages. Despite being familiar with all the information shared here, revisiting each reference to articulate the information and to present the evidence in black and white, in a sequential and logical manner, was very painful. Each section I finished writing allowed me to see more clearly the magnitude of the assault on humanity that has been the pandemic and has allowed me to understand that it has not yet shown all its facets.

I have been questioned many times, especially over the past 12 months, about why I continue to make efforts to share and explain scientific information about the adverse effects if '*what happened is already done*' and '*this has already ended*'. Sometimes, I have perceived some discomfort, annoyance, or outright anger underlying those questions. Part of me understands it: when one has received one (or more) of these vaxgenes, or when their family and loved ones did so, learning about everything that vaxgenes can do in the body and discovering the often murky history surrounding their clinical trials must not be pleasant. Some may even think it is an act of cruelty on my part to write about this. I assure you it is not. I have been trying for over three years to communicate responsibly the scientific information that the media did not, and that most doctors were not aware of, with the hope that people would have at least some elements to decide responsibly whether to accept these vaxgenes.

I continue to do what I do because this—not the pandemic, but everything that has moved because of it—has not ended. I continue to do what I do because due to the components and nature of these vaxgenes, their consequences could manifest later. I continue to do what I do because people whose health or that of their loved ones was affected need to know what happened to aspire to treat themselves, mitigate the effects, or prevent them from worsening. I continue to do what I do to honour the memory of those who died because of having received vaxgenes, by acknowledging what happened. I continue to do what I do because the implications of what I have presented in the previous chapters go far beyond anti-COVID vaxgenes and far beyond the COVID pandemic.

I continue to do what I do because we need to ensure that what has happened never happens again. That is why and for what I do it. You can be sure that vaxgenes will not stop being developed and used when the public loses fear of COVID. Their rapid manufacturing, low manufacturing cost, and the very lubricated path to regulatory approvals mean that this genetic technology, specifically synthetic mRNA technology, is intended to replace traditional childhood vaccines as well as those that many adults receive every year. This is not the product of a wild imagination; these are concrete facts. Currently, 165 clinical trials are underway with synthetic mRNA vaxgenes against HIV, influenza virus, Nipah virus, zika virus, rabies virus, cytomegalovirus, respiratory syncytial virus, metapneumovirus, parainfluenza, Epstein-Barr virus, herpes zoster virus, Ebola virus, hepatitis B virus, Marburg virus, as well as vaxgenes against typhoid fever, tuberculosis, and various types of cancer[393]. 165 clinical trials! The fact that vaxgenes against wrinkles (You et al., 2023) are also being promoted shows how trivially the safety risks of this technology are being considered. On the other hand, synthetic mRNA vaxgenes are being developed and used to immunize livestock and other consumption animals (Kitikoon et al., 2023; Le et al., 2022), without a single study having evaluated the risks it would pose to humans that consume meat, milk, or eggs from these animals and without a single study having examined the potential bioaccumulation of these products. If no studies have been conducted on the risk of synthetic mRNA shedding or the resulting protein among humans, even less is known about this potential risk for humans who consume animals that received vaxgenes.

[393] Clinical Trials. Search terms: [(mRNA AND vaccine) NOT COVID]

If that seems concerning to you, I must tell you that the situation is worse. This is because synthetic self-replicating mRNA vaxgenes are also being developed. I didn't mention them in previous chapters because these have not been authorized against COVID to date; however, clinical trials are being conducted with them, and if the consequences of synthetic mRNA are persistent and severe, imagine what they will be if a technology is used that allows the generation of more copies of synthetic mRNA than those injected into a person. To give you an idea of what this technology means, if you already understood what I explained in Chapter 1, imagine a scenario where synthetic mRNA does not degrade within the cell but produces more and more and more; hence the term 'self-replicating'.

It is important to note that the self-replicating synthetic mRNA technology did not arise in the context of the pandemic. It was proposed since 1989 to increase the duration of gene therapy drugs without the need for continuous application (Xiong et al., 1989). However, it was only recently that clinical trials of vaxgenes based on self-replicating synthetic mRNA began. Precisely, the COVID pandemic seems to have been fertile ground for the growing interest in this vaccine technology.

The central idea of self-replicating synthetic mRNA technology is to administer, in addition to the gene of interest (such as the Spike gene in the case of synthetic mRNA-based COVID vaccines), a specific fragment of the genome of another virus, usually an alphavirus (Togaviridae Family), which has a single-stranded RNA genome of just under 12,000 nucleotides (that is, almost three times smaller than SARS-CoV-2) and can be easily read by ribosomes by simply entering the cytoplasm (see Introduction and Chapter 1). The fragment of the alphavirus genome included is the one that contains the instructions to produce the polymerase enzyme, whose function is to make more copies of the RNA genetic material. That is precisely what is sought: to produce an enzyme that copies and copies and copies the sequence of the alphavirus enzyme and the target gene. This is very concerning because everything I explained about the biological mechanisms by which synthetic mRNA vaxgenes can cause problems (see section 5.3) would likely occur, although potentially worse, since the foreign genetic material within cells would last even longer than what has been seen so far.

At the time of writing this book, there are eight clinical trials of anticancer therapy based on self-replicating synthetic mRNA, and 11 phase 1, 2, and 3 clinical trials with vaxgenes based on these products against various viruses, from HIV to rabies (Aliahmad et al., 2023). Among them is one against COVID by Pfizer, which started clinical trials in 2020 (the product is registered as BNT162c2[394]). Almost nothing has been said about it, but I am forced to ask: *how many people who participated in the trial may have received this self-replicating technology?* The information presented on the clinical trial page is so brief that we cannot know, and to date, there is not a single scientific study published on the results of the clinical trials of BNT162c2.

Of course, Pfizer is not the only one interested in this technology. In Japan, the pharmaceutical company VLP Therapeutics is evaluating a self-replicating synthetic mRNA vaxgene against COVID (jRCT2051210164)[395]. To date, only one study reporting the findings of the phase 1 clinical trial of VLP Therapeutics has been published, where it was reported that 70 to 80% of the volunteers who received the highest dose of the self-replicating synthetic mRNA vaxgenes had local and systemic adverse events (Akahata et al., 2023). On the other hand, the pharmaceutical company Glaxo-Smith Kline developed three vaxgenes based on this technology[396], one against herpesvirus, one against COVID, and one against rabies, but so far, they do not seem to have published any results.

In that sense, looking to the future, I find it indispensable that you know about these technologies, especially because the trend is that this will be the one used to make vaccines and gene therapies in the near future, unless, from knowledge and with a cool head, we demand safety assurances for its use, in the short, medium, and long term in humans and even in domestic animals (Kitikoon et al., 2023). Any politician, doctor, health personnel,

---

[394] National Library of Medicine. National Center for Biotechnology Information. A Trial Investigating the Safety and Effects of Four BNT162 Vaccines Against COVID-2019 in Healthy and Immunocompromised Adults [Internet]. Available at: https://clinicaltrials.gov/ct2/show/NCT04380701

[395] JPRN Search Portal. A phase 1 study of VLPCOV-01 in COVID vaccinated healthy subjects. VLP Therapeutics. [Internet]. Available at: https://rctportal.niph.go.jp/en/detail?trial_id=jRCT2051210164

[396] National Library of Medicine. National Center for Biotechnology Information [Internet]. Available at: https://clinicaltrials.gov/ct2/show/NCT04762511, https://clinicaltrials.gov/ct2/show/NCT04758962, https://clinicaltrials.gov/ct2/show/NCT04062669

and even influencers can articulate words to say 'they are safe products'. But those words have no foundation. Why? Because there is not a single study that has evaluated, in humans, the safety, nor has a single study evaluated interactions with the genome, genotoxicity, mutagenicity, stimulation of autoinflammatory states, in any animal used as a model (see Chapter 2). To give you an idea, the few studies that have been published about the safety of self-replicating synthetic mRNA were done using rodents as models (Donahue et al., 2023; Maruggi et al., 2022; McCafferty et al., 2022), and only one was done using a primate (Bogers et al., 2015). These studies found evidence of liver impact in vaccinated animals (Donahue et al., 2023; Bogers et al., 2015), that lipid nanoparticles are distributed to all organs and tissues examined and are detectable even 60 days after vaccination (Maruggi et al., 2022). The only honest thing that could be said is that to date, we do not know, remotely, the range of consequences that could occur, although we can infer it from what we already know is associated with synthetic mRNA (see section 5.3).

If we say nothing, it is likely that soon synthetic mRNA technology (or even self-replicating synthetic mRNA) will be the basis for the immunizations they ask, demand, or order us to apply in the next epidemic outbreak, or simply as part of the annual vaccinations that some rush to apply. After all, the official narrative boasts synthetic mRNA technology as a 'panacea,' and the fact that the Nobel Prize in Physiology and Medicine was awarded to Katalin Karikó and Drew Weissman in 2023 for proposing the use of modified nucleosides for synthetic mRNA vaxgenes[397] would appear to confer validity to this technology. What an honour! But before applauding, perhaps it would be good to understand that the awards granted do not nullify the evidence of the harms of synthetic mRNA, that prestigious recognitions do not replace irregularities in the manufacturing, purification, and authorization process. Just as an appeal to authority is not an argument, a prize is not evidence of safety.

It would be advisable for scientists and doctors who applauded the award to remember their principles of scientific ethics and medical

[397] Nobel Prize. Press release 2/10/2023 [Internet]. Available at: https://www.nobelprize.org/prizes/medicine/2023/press-release/

deontology, but it seems that we still have a long way to go. Examples of this are the responses given by Professors Rickard Sandberg and Olle Kampe to a reporter's question on the day the Nobel Committee of the Karolinska Institute announced the winners at a press conference[398]. The question was valid: "*with synthetic mRNA, we have no data on long-term safety, so do you have any concerns about it?*" The answers given were not. On the part of Prof. Rickard Sandberg: "*Yes, synthetic mRNA vaccines have only been given for a certain time, but the mRNA administered is transient. 13,000,000,000 people have received the viral, sorry, vaccine virus* [sic], *and the amount of adverse effects noticed to date is extremely low*". On the part of Prof. Olle Kampe: "*It cannot be integrated into the nucleus; that was a safety check... the adverse effects are really only myocarditis and mild myocarditis, mainly in young men, and it usually resolves without long-term effects*". If you have read this book, you already know the hundreds of scientific studies published that show that these responses reflect two scenarios that are not mutually exclusive; they arise from either ignorance or malice. Now that the WHO is serious about combating what they call *misinformation* (false information transmitted without harmful intent) and *disinformation* (false or misleading information transmitted with harmful intent), and now that they have included strategies to combat such misinformation and disinformation in the proposal for the 2024 Pandemic Treaty[399], we should demand, for the sake of consistency, that they file a complaint against the Nobel Committee of the Karolinska Institute[400].

Now, after reading this book, you may understand why it is not correct to consider Pfizer's, Moderna's, AstraZeneca's, Janssen's, Sputnik's, and CanSino's COVID products as if they were traditional vaccines. They must be understood as vaxgenes or vaxgenes because they are a type of gene therapy technology. That is precisely their mechanism of action: to

---

[398] Press Conference of the announcement of the winners of the Nobel Prize 2023 in Physiology or Medicine with Thomas Perlmann, Secretary of the Nobel Committee of the Karolinska Institute in Stockholm. Transmitted live on October 2 2023 [Internet]. Available at: https://www.youtube.com/watch?v=5DM3F376t48 From minute 33:10 onwards you can find the question made by the reporter and the answers she was given.

[399] Seventh meeting of the Intergovernmental Negotiating body to draft and negotiate a WHO Convention, Agreement or other International instrument on pandemic Prevention, preparedness and response. A/INB/7/3 30/10/2023 [Document]. Available at: https://apps.who.int/gb/inb/pdf_files/inb7/A_INB7_3-en.pdf

[400] Much subtlety is lost in paper. My tone was sarcastic when writing that sentence.

introduce genetic information into a cell to produce a desired protein. I also hope that you now know that the manufacturing process of these vaxgenes for the vials used in clinical trials was different from the one used (and continue to be used) to manufacture the vials that would be used for the general public. I hope you can infer the serious legal implications of these disparities yourselves[401].

I wish it is clear to you that the components of vaxgenes interact at various levels within cells and the body, and in some people, they may have much more serious consequences than pain at the injection site, fever, and muscle pain. Some of you who have read this book may now question cases of aggressive cancers, thromboembolisms, myocarditis, sudden heart attacks, and autoimmune and autoinflammatory diseases that may have occurred in your loved ones unexpectedly. If so, I also hope you have understood that determining causality between exposure to something (in this case, vaxgenes) and a particular outcome (in this case, adverse events) goes far beyond simply saying 'I *feel* it was because of the vaxgene' If you read Chapter 4, you will recall that the causality criteria are met for most of the unprecedented adverse events that are occurring.

If this book has helped you in that understanding, then it has achieved its goal. I know that in some way, I have opened Pandora's box for the readers, and I know that once you know, you cannot go back to ignorance. But I also know that, just as it happened in Greek mythology, hope is also contained in these pages. That hope is very powerful. I am not referring to the stale, superficial hope that is often used in conversations without meaning anything. I am not referring to hope that serves as an excuse to continue being victims while clinging to it. No. I am referring to living hope, the one that is real and goes deep within us to remind us that it is possible to help change things, that no one is so small that their actions are insignificant when born from that living hope. Certainly, we cannot reverse what has happened, at the level of humanity or individually, but we can prevent it from continuing; I have hope and certainty of that.

---

[401] With all my heart, I hope that at least one lawyer that has written this book decides to consider these inconsistencies and use them in a necessary mission to protect humanity.

As humanity, we stand at a crossroads. The responsibility to choose which path to take is entirely ours. On one side, there is a short and straight path, where 'security' and 'protection' against any health threat are promised if we do as we are told. Whatever we are told; whether it's one dose or two or six, or annual doses. Anything! We simply must go and let ourselves be injected, without murmuring, without questioning, without investigating, without thinking. If we follow that path, there will be no space for any thought that differs from the official one, and the official one will be dictated by pharmaceutical conglomerates, those business entities linked economically to media, prestigious universities, medical and scientific journals, various non-profit organizations, drug regulatory agencies, and the World Health Organization.

On the other side, a long and winding path awaits us, where we will have to assume responsibilities, be willing to question and learn (and relearn), let go of beliefs and certainties that are not supported by truths, even if doing so is painful. It is a path that requires courage and strength, but it is the only path through which we will prevent further erosion of individual freedoms and guarantees, where we can demand respect for our freedom to choose whether to consent to the application or non-application of a product and make that decision for our minor children. This is not an easy path, but it is the one I choose. Which path do you choose?

You have reached the end of this book, and that already tells me that perhaps you have a clearer idea of which of these two paths you will consciously choose. I look towards the future and can see a world that is not bleak. Although sometimes more pessimistic thoughts may sneak into my visualization of what I desire and consider possible, I refuse to accept as the only possible future one where absolutism and dogmatism prevail, and free and independent thinking is considered undesirable and even dangerous.

That's why I have dedicated so much time and energy to this book; that's why I am glad to know that you have read this far. Your persistence helps me remember that we can indeed shape and inhabit another future.

Thank you for your trust. Thank you for reading what I could share with you in this book

Karina AW

Glossary

Acrosome: Structure covering the anterior part of the sperm cell head. It contains hydrolytic and proteolytic enzymes that the sperm uses to penetrate the ovule.

Active Compound: In a drug, refers to the main ingredient responsible for the desired effect.

Adenovirus: Virus of the Adenoviridae family. Characterized by a large double-stranded DNA genome and lacking an envelope. Has a broad host range, including humans. Often associated with asymptomatic or mild infections. Used as vectors in gene therapy.

Allergen: Chemical or biological substance that triggers an allergic response.

Amenorrhea: Absence of menstruation.

Amyotrophic lateral sclerosis (ALS): A disease affecting motor neurons responsible for movement, characterized by progressive and fatal degeneration. Also known as Lou Gehrig's disease.

Anaphylaxis: Acute allergic reaction that, if not promptly treated, can be fatal.

Antibody: Protein (Immunoglobulin) secreted by B lymphocytes that binds to antigens on the surface of viruses or bacteria, activating various immune responses to resolve associated disease processes.

Antigen Presentation: The process by which immune phagocytic cells (macrophages and dendritic cells) display foreign antigens to lymphocytes through proteins on their membrane, known as the major histocompatibility complex (MHC). This process is essential for initiating adaptive immune responses, including antibody production and the activation of T lymphocytes.

Antigen: Fragment of a molecule that the immune system can recognize and generate a response against. Antigens are usually protein fragments but can also be lipid, carbohydrate, or nucleic acid fragments.

Apoptosis: Programmed cell death. A biological process essential for preventing cancer and limiting viral infections.

Area postrema: An anatomical region located outside the blood-brain barrier on each side of the fourth cerebral ventricle which receives neurons from the brain, spinal cord and medulla oblongata. Functions as a receptor for chemical signals that activate the vomiting reflex.

Astrocytes: Nervous system cells with a star-like shape, supporting the development and proper functioning of neurons.

Avidity: In immunology, the sum of interaction strength at all binding sites between an antibody and an antigen. Higher avidity indicates a stronger bond.

Base pairs (bp): Two complementary bases (nucleotides) that pair up to form part of a DNA chain. Since the DNA in cells is double-stranded, the concept of bp is used to refer to its size. If it is a single strand of DNA or RNA, the term "bases" (b) would be used to refer to its size.

Biological significance: Biological significance is the rational and supported interpretation of biological processes that explains the detected statistical significance.

Cap: Methylated guanine nucleotide linked to mRNA via a triphosphate bond at the 5' end; specifically, a 7-methylguanosine cap.

Carcinogen: Physical, chemical, or biological agent capable of inducing cancer in a healthy organism.

Cholinergic nervous system: Includes neurons from the anterior basal forebrain, cerebral cortex, and hippocampus. Cognition depends on the functioning of this cholinergic system.

Chromosomal instability: Occurs when there is an abnormally high rate of improper chromosome segregation during mitosis due to defective cell cycle quality control mechanisms. It can result in a higher number of chromosome copies than the 46 that somatic cells in humans should have.

Codon: Three nucleotides read in ribosomes as one amino acid. Genes are written as sequences of codons.

Competent Cells: In virology, cells that have all the elements required for a specific virus to complete its replication cycle.

Complement Cascade: A series of sequential steps that enhance the activity of antibodies and immune cells to eliminate microorganisms and damaged cells, promoting inflammation.

Covariance: Statistical measure of the relationship between two random variables.

Crystallizable fraction of antibodies: The part of an antibody's 'tail' that interacts with Fc receptors on various immune cells. It is the region of antibodies that activates the complement system and other immune processes.

Cytokines: Molecules playing a crucial role in various actions, such as inducing or preventing inflammation, regulating immune responses, directing lymphocyte responses, inducing programmed cell death (apoptosis), and preventing tumour formation.

Dalton (Da): Unit of the atomic mass of a protein. One kilodalton (kDa) is equal to 1,000 Da.

Diversity: Referring to alpha diversity (a measure of microbial diversity within an individual) and beta diversity (a measure of the similarity of diversity between two communities).

Efficacy: Refers to the reduction in relative risk between the group receiving the product and the group receiving a placebo.

Eicosanoids: Lipid molecules resulting from the oxidation of fatty acids, with activities related to inflammation.

Electrophoresis: Technique used to separate DNA, RNA, or protein molecules in a matrix (usually a gel) based on their size and electric charge. An electric current is applied, causing the molecules to move through the matrix.

Embryogenesis: The process of embryo formation.

Energy-dispersive X-ray spectroscopy (EDX): Analytical technique allowing the chemical characterization of materials.

Erythema: Reddening of the skin due to inflammation.

Esterification: The process of combining an organic acid with an alcohol to form an ester and water.

Eukaryote: Cells with a nucleus and membrane-bound organelles. All multicellular organisms (plants, animals, and many fungi) have these cells, as do many unicellular organisms such as amoebas, yeasts, zooplankton, etc. Also known as eukaryotic cells.

Excipients: Inactive substance in a drug that serves as a vehicle or stabilizer for the active compound.

Gene therapy: Refers to the use of genetic information to treat or correct a disease caused by an altered or non-functional version of a specific gene. It also refers to the use of genetic information to make cells produce a specific protein to treat a disease or for immunization. Gene therapy can be carried out using DNA plasmids, viral vectors, bacterial vectors, or synthetic mRNA (the latter is also known as RNA therapy).

Genotoxicity: Processes that alter the structure, information, or segregation of DNA, not necessarily resulting from mutations.

Germ cells: Ovules and sperm.

Glia: The set of different cells that assist neurons, either by providing nutrients, insulating them, or defending them.

Glycosylation: Process by which a protein is attached to a carbohydrate (typically a sugar molecule).

Haematuria: Presence of blood in the urine.

Histone: Histone proteins bind to DNA, helping chromosomes maintain their proper shape and control gene expression.

Hypersensitivity: Reaction that occurs after contact with a chemical, physical, or biological agent that triggers a danger signal in the body, excessively activating the immune response, causing tissue damage. Allergy is a type of hypersensitivity reaction, attributable to the effects of excess immunoglobulin E (IgE).

Iatrogenesis: Refers to a medical error that causes harm to health.

Idiopathic: A process or syndrome with several probable causes, but the specific cause is unknown.

Immune complexes: Molecules formed by the binding of several antigens with several antibodies.

Immunoglobulins: Also called antibodies. Glycoproteins composed of two heavy chains and two light chains. Produced and secreted by B lymphocytes, immunoglobulins can be found in blood, mucous membranes, and other tissues.

Immunopathology: Damage caused by exacerbated immune responses.

In silico: Study conducted on a computer to understand or simulate a biological process.

In vitro: Biological study conducted outside an organism. Typically involves the use of cell cultures.

Incidence: The number of new cases in a specific population during a specified time. Usually expressed as cases per 100,000 people per year.

Inductively coupled plasma analysis (ICP): Analytical technique for determining and quantifying most elements of the periodic table in a sample, even at trace levels.

Insertional mutagenesis: Generation of mutations in a cell's DNA due to the addition of one or more nucleotides in the sequence.

Intussusception: A condition in which one part of the intestine slides into another. It is a medical emergency as it can be fatal if not treated promptly.

Ischemia: Refers to what happens when blood does not reach a tissue or organ adequately. One cause is the presence of a clot blocking the flow in a blood vessel.

Lymphocytes: Immune system cells produced, like all blood cells, in the bone marrow of long bones. There are two major groups: B lymphocytes and T lymphocytes, and T lymphocytes further characterize into different populations, such as CD4+ T lymphocytes and CD8+ T lymphocytes. Lymphocytes are the only cells in the body that undergo a process in which their genome undergoes changes and rearrangements, allowing the generation of a lot of diversity in their cellular receptors. This process enables the generation of billions of different lymphocytes in each individual. Once activated, they also differentiate into effector cells and memory cells.

Macrophages: Immune cells specialized in detecting, phagocytizing, and destroying bacteria and other microorganisms. After phagocytosis, they present fragments of the bacteria and other microorganisms they 'ate' (phagocytized) to T lymphocytes, activating inflammation and ultimately leading to the generation of antibodies and cytotoxic responses.

Mass spectroscopy (MS): Quantitative analytical technique used to identify unknown compounds in a sample, determine the structure and chemical properties of molecules, and quantify known compounds.

Mesothelioma: A type of cancer that originates in the layer of cells lining the lungs, known as the pleura.

Mitosis: The process of cell division used by all cells in the body to make copies of themselves. During mitosis, cells copy their chromosomes and then segregate them, producing two identical nuclei.

Modified synthetic mRNA: Chain of RNA molecules generated in vitro or in a cellular system, containing modified bases.

mRNA (Messenger RNA): RNA molecule corresponding to the genetic sequence of a specific gene, readable by ribosomes to produce a specific protein.

Myelin: A layer of lipids, water, and associated proteins that covers neurons in the central and peripheral nervous systems.

Myelitis: A type of myelopathy characterized by unregulated inflammation of the spinal cord.

Myelopathy: Refers to diseases of the spinal cord.

Nanolipids: Very small particles composed of various types of lipids used as a drug or genetic material delivery system.

Neutrophil extracellular trap (NET): A network formed by DNA strands from neutrophils (one of the types of white blood cells) when they die. Its function is to trap bacteria, although it also promotes clotting.

Neutrophils: Immune system cells that are the first to arrive when there is a damage signal or a molecule associated with a considered pathogenic microorganism. They are the most abundant immune cells in the blood.

NF-κB Transcription Factor: Functions to allow the expression of genes involved in innate and adaptive immune responses. Its activation induces, among other things, sustained inflammation.

Oligodendrocytes: Cells that produce myelin for neurons in the central nervous system.

Oncogenic: Indicating that it promotes the generation of malignant tumours.

Paracrine: Inducing changes in nearby cells.

Paresis: Muscle weakness ranging from mild to moderate.

Pericytes: Cells found on the inner wall of capillaries.

Pharmacodynamics: Study of the biochemical and physiological effects of a drug in the receiving organism.

Pharmacokinetics: Study of the absorption, distribution, metabolism, and excretion of a drug.

Placebo: Substance with no therapeutic effect used as a control in clinical trials of a new drug or vaccine.

Plasmid: Circular, double-stranded DNA that naturally exchanges between bacteria but can be synthesized in the laboratory to contain desired information. By introducing it into bacteria, they can produce more copies of the plasmid or produce the desired protein.

Polymerase chain reaction (PCR): A technique involving the *in vitro* amplification of millions of copies of a fragment of a known sequence in a sample.

Polymerase: Cellular enzyme whose function is to copy nucleic acids. There are RNA polymerases, which perform transcription (the process of copying DNA into RNA), DNA polymerases that copy DNA, and some viruses have a reverse transcriptase that generates DNA from RNA.

Prokaryote: Cells with a cell wall, lacking a nucleus and membrane-bound organelles. All bacteria and archaea are prokaryotic cells. Also known as prokaryotic cells.

Promoter: Refers to a genetic sequence of 100 to 1000 base pairs containing a site to which the enzyme RNA polymerase (RNApol II) binds. It is located before a gene and allows the gene to be transcribed, meaning a copy of the information is produced but written in RNA instead of DNA. The promoter sequence controls the transcription of a gene and determines in which tissues the protein will be expressed.

Proto-oncogenes: A group of genes that, when expressed, induces continuous cell division. They can cause cancer when mutated (in this case, they become known as oncogenes) or when turned on out of schedule due to a dysregulation in gene expression.

Raman spectroscopy coupled microscopy: Non-quantitative analytical technique based on light diffraction to measure the vibrational energy of the elements comprising a sample.

Recombinant: Term used to denote an organism, cell, or genetic material containing parts of genetic material from another organism.

Reverse Transcription: Conversion of an RNA sequence into DNA using an enzyme called reverse transcriptase.

Ribosome: Cellular organelle where protein translation occurs. They are found in the cytoplasm, usually attached to the endoplasmic reticulum.

SDS Page: A protein identification technique. In this method, proteins are extracted from a sample and placed in an acrylamide gel for electrophoresis with detergents and heat. As proteins have a negative charge, applying electricity causes them to move towards the positive electrode. Proteins have different molecular weights, so we can observe 'bands' of a specific molecular weight for each different protein.

Solvent: A chemical substance that dissolves a solid, liquid, or gas solute.

Somatic cells: Any nucleated cell in the body except ovules and sperm.

Statistical power: Refers to the probability that the hypothesis being challenged in a study is accepted as true. It depends on various factors, including the sample size. If the sample size is insufficient, there may be low statistical power in the analysis, making it difficult to detect a real difference.

Statistical significance: The result of a statistical test that indicates there is a relationship that numerically is not due to chance. Statistical significance does not necessarily imply a real variation or a real effect in a biological system.

Stillbirths: Refers to babies born dead. In contrast, foetal death occurs within the uterus before childbirth.

Surfactant: A chemical compound that reduces the surface tension between two liquids, between a liquid and a solid, and between a liquid and a gas. They can function as emulsifiers, detergents, or dispersants.

Teratogenic: The ability of a chemical, physical, or biological agent to cause deformities or anomalies in the foetus.

Thrombocytopenia: Decrease in the number of platelets in the blood.

Thrombotic thrombocytopenia: A clinical condition characterized by a low number of platelets coinciding with the formation of many blood clots.

Toll-Like receptors: Proteins expressed on the cell membrane that play a significant role in regulating the inflammatory process.

Transcription: In Biology, it refers to the process by which a gene (written as DNA) is copied into mRNA within the nucleus (in eukaryotic cells) or in the cytoplasm (in bacteria and archaea). It is the step before translation, and in eukaryotic cells, it occurs in the nucleus, while in prokaryotic cells, it occurs in the cytoplasm.

Transcriptomics: Transcriptomic analyses identify all the genes being expressed in a sample at a given moment, quantifying and identifying all the mRNA molecules that cells are producing.

Transfect: The process of introducing foreign genetic material into a cell.

Transgenerational effects: Refers to adverse effects on the offspring of an individual exposed to a chemical, physical, or biological agent.

Translation: In Biology, it refers to the process by which mRNA is read in ribosomes to produce the protein according to the specific instructions contained in the mRNA.

Tumour suppressor genes: Genes that, when expressed, inhibit cell proliferation and the development of cancerous tumours.

Vaccine: A product that, when administered intramuscularly, orally, intranasally, or dermally, induces a specific immune response in the organism without causing the disease it aims to prevent with vaccination. Vaccines can be made from the complete but attenuated microorganism (live attenuated vaccines), from the complete inactivated microorganism (inactivated vaccines), or from proteins of the microorganism (protein subunit vaccines).

Vaccinology: The science and engineering that deal with the development of vaccines to immunize someone against a specific antigen or a particular disease.

Vector: In molecular biology, it refers to a genetic element that can be carried into the nucleus of a cell to be inserted or to undergo transcription and translation of genetic material. In vaccinology, it mainly refers to the use of a recombinant virus that serves as a method of delivering genetic material to the cells of a person or animal.

Virion: The individual unit of a specific virus. The analogy that seems most useful to understand it is that if a virus is to a human, a virion is to a person.

References

Abara, W. E., Gee, J., Marquez, P., Woo, J., Myers, T. R., DeSantis, A., Baumblatt, J. A. G., Woo, E. J., Thompson, D., Nair, N., Su, J. R., Shimabukuro, T. T., & Shay, D. K. (2023). Reports of Guillain-Barré Syndrome After COVID-19 Vaccination in the United States. *JAMA Network Open*, *6*(2), e2253845. https://doi.org/10.1001/jamanetworkopen.2022.53845

Abbate, A., Gavin, J., Madanchi, N., Kim, C., Shah, P. R., Klein, K., Boatman, J., Roberts, C., Patel, S., & Danielides, S. (2021). Fulminant myocarditis and systemic hyperinflammation temporally associated with BNT162b2 mRNA COVID-19 vaccination in two patients. *International Journal of Cardiology*, *340*, 119–121. https://doi.org/10.1016/j.ijcard.2021.08.018

Abdelhady, M., Husain, M. A., Hawas, Y., Elazb, M. A., Mansour, L. S., Mohamed, M., Abdelwahab, M. M., Aljabali, A., & Negida, A. (2023). Encephalitis following COVID-19 Vaccination: A Systematic Review. *Vaccines*, *11*(3), 576. https://doi.org/10.3390/vaccines11030576

Abdelsalam, N. A., Hegazy, S. M., & Aziz, R. K. (2023). The curious case of Prevotella copri. *Gut Microbes*, *15*(2). https://doi.org/10.1080/19490976.2023.2249152

Abdillah, D. A., Kereilwe, O., Ferdousy, R. N., Saito, R., & Kadokawa, H. (2022). Spike protein of SARS-CoV-2 suppresses gonadotrophin secretion from bovine anterior pituitaries. *Journal of Reproduction and Development*, *68*(2), 2021–2126. https://doi.org/10.1262/jrd.2021-126

Abdullah, L., Awada, B., Kurban, M., & Abbas, O. (2022). Comment on 'Vitiligo in a COVID-19-vaccinated patient with ulcerative colitis: coincidence?': Type I interferons as possible link between COVID-19 vaccine and vitiligo. *Clinical and Experimental Dermatology*, *47*(2), 436–437. https://doi.org/10.1111/ced.14932

Abu Mouch, S., Roguin, A., Hellou, E., Ishai, A., Shoshan, U., Mahamid, L., Zoabi, M., Aisman, M., Goldschmid, N., & Berar Yanay, N. (2021). Myocarditis following COVID-19 mRNA vaccination. *Vaccine*, *39*(29), 3790–3793. https://doi.org/10.1016/j.vaccine.2021.05.087

Abu-Rumeileh, S., Abdelhak, A., Foschi, M., Tumani, H., & Otto, M. (2021). Guillain–Barré syndrome spectrum associated with COVID-19: an up-to-date systematic review of 73 cases. *Journal of Neurology*, *268*(4), 1133–1170. https://doi.org/10.1007/s00415-020-10124-x

Acevedo-Whitehouse, K., & Bruno, R. (2023). Potential health risks of mRNA-based vaccine therapy: A hypothesis. *Medical Hypotheses*, *171*, 111015. https://doi.org/10.1016/j.mehy.2023.111015

Acharya, B., KC, S., Karki, S., Thapa, P., & KC, P. (2023). Guillain-Barré syndrome following the second dose of COVID AstraZeneca vaccine in a 78-year-old male: a case report from Nepal. *Annals of Medicine & Surgery*, *85*(3), 498–501. https://doi.org/10.1097/MS9.0000000000000193

Actis, G. C., Ribaldone, D. G., & Pellicano, R. (2022). COVID vaccine's hot problems: erratic serious blood clotting, ill-defined prion-like reactogenicity of the spike, unclear roles of other factors. *Minerva Medica*, *112*(6). https://doi.org/10.23736/S0026-4806.21.07769-7

Adam, R., Duong, T., Hodges, L., Staeger-Hirsch, C., & Maldjian, T. (2022). Mammographic findings of diffuse axillary tail trabecular thickening following immunization with mRNA COVID-19 vaccines: Case series study. *Radiology Case Reports*, *17*(8), 2841–2849. https://doi.org/10.1016/j.radcr.2022.04.028

Adiguzel, Y. (2021). Molecular mimicry between SARS-CoV-2 and human proteins. *Autoimmunity Reviews*, *20*(4), 102791. https://doi.org/10.1016/j.autrev.2021.102791

Adin, M. E., Wu, J., Isufi, E., Tsui, E., & Pucar, D. (2022). Ipsilateral Malignant Axillary Lymphadenopathy and Contralateral Reactive Lymph Nodes in a COVID-19 Vaccine Recipient With Breast Cancer. *Journal of Breast Cancer*, *25*(2), 140. https://doi.org/10.4048/jbc.2022.25.e12

Adler, B., Sattler, C., & Adler, H. (2017). Herpesviruses and Their Host Cells: A Successful Liaison. *Trends in Microbiology*, *25*(3), 229–241. https://doi.org/10.1016/j.tim.2016.11.009

Afshar, Z. M., Pirzaman A. T., Liang, J. J., Sharma, A., Pirzadeh, M., Babazadeh, A., Hashemi, E., Deravi, N., Abdi, S., Allahgholipour, A., Hosseinzadeh, R., Vaziri, Z., Sio, T. T., Sullman, M. J. M., Barary, M., Ebrahimpour, S. (2022). Do we miss rare adverse events induced by COVID-19 vaccination? *Frontiers in Medicine (Lausanne), 9*, 933914. https://doi.org/10.3389/fmed.2022.933914

Agorastos, A., & Bozikas, V. P. (2019). Gut microbiome and adaptive immunity in schizophrenia. *Psychiatriki*, *30*(3), 189–192. https://doi.org/10.22365/jpsych.2019.303.189

Ågrup, C., & Luxon, L. M. (2006). Immune-mediated inner-ear disorders in neuro-otology. *Current Opinion in Neurology*, *19*(1), 26–32. https://doi.org/10.1097/01.wco.0000194143.02171.46

Ahmadian, E., Hosseiniyan Khatibi, S. M., Razi Soofiyani, S., Abediazar, S., Shoja, M. M., Ardalan, M., & Zununi Vahed, S. (2021). Covid-19 and kidney injury: Pathophysiology and molecular mechanisms. *Reviews in Medical Virology*, *31*(3). https://doi.org/10.1002/rmv.2176

Ahmed, S. H., Waseem, S., Shaikh, T. G., Qadir, N. A., Siddiqui, S. A., Ullah, I., Waris, A., & Yousaf, Z. (2022). SARS-CoV-2 vaccine-associated-tinnitus: A review. *Annals of Medicine & Surgery*, *75*. https://doi.org/10.1016/j.amsu.2022.103293

Akahata, W., Sekida, T., Nogimori, T., Ode, H., Tamura, T., Kono, K., Kazami, Y., Washizaki, A., Masuta, Y., Suzuki, R., Matsuda, K., Komori, M., Morey, A. L., Ishimoto, K., Nakata, M., Hasunuma, T., Fukuhara, T., Iwatani, Y., Yamamoto, T., … Sato, N. (2023). Safety and immunogenicity of SARS-CoV-2 self-amplifying RNA vaccine expressing an anchored RBD: A randomized, observer-blind phase 1 study. *Cell Reports Medicine*, *4*(8), 101134. https://doi.org/10.1016/j.xcrm.2023.101134

Aksenova, A. Y., Likhachev, I. V., Grishin, S. Y., & Galzitskaya, O. V. (2022). The Increased Amyloidogenicity of Spike RBD and pH-Dependent Binding to ACE2 May Contribute to the Transmissibility and Pathogenic Properties of SARS-CoV-2 Omicron as Suggested by In Silico Study. *International Journal of Molecular Sciences*, *23*(21), 13502. https://doi.org/10.3390/ijms232113502

Aktas, H., & Ertuğrul, G. (2022). Vitiligo in a COVID-19-vaccinated patient with ulcerative colitis: coincidence? *Clinical and Experimental Dermatology*, *47*(1), 143–144. https://doi.org/10.1111/ced.14842

Al Kadri, H. M., Al Sudairy, A. A., Alangari, A. S., Al Khateeb, B. F., & El-Metwally, A. A. (2023). COVID-19 vaccination and menstrual disorders among women: Findings from a meta-analysis study. *Journal of Infection and Public Health, 16*(5), 697–704. https://doi.org/10.1016/j.jiph.2023.02.019

Albert, E., Aurigemma, G., Saucedo, J., & Gerson, D. S. (2021). Myocarditis following COVID-19 vaccination. *Radiology Case Reports, 16*(8), 2142–2145. https://doi.org/10.1016/j.radcr.2021.05.033

Aldén, M., Olofsson Falla, F., Yang, D., Barghouth, M., Luan, C., Rasmussen, M., & De Marinis, Y. (2022). Intracellular Reverse Transcription of Pfizer BioNTech COVID-19 mRNA Vaccine BNT162b2 In Vitro in Human Liver Cell Line. *Current Issues in Molecular Biology, 44*(3), 1115–1126. https://doi.org/10.3390/cimb44030073

Alderson, P. (2004). Absence of evidence is not evidence of absence. *BMJ, 328*(7438), 476–477. https://doi.org/10.1136/bmj.328.7438.476

Alexander, N. J. (1989). Natural and induced immunological infertility. *Current Opinion in Immunology, 1*(6), 1125–1130. https://doi.org/10.1016/0952-7915(89)90003-4

Algahtani, H. A., Shirah, B. H., Albeladi, Y. K., & Albeladi, R. K. (2023). Guillain-Barré Syndrome Following the BNT162b2 mRNA COVID-19 Vaccine. *Acta Neurologica Taiwanica, 32*(2), 82–85.

Alhashim, A., Hadhiah, K., Al khalifah, Z., Alhaddad, F. M., Al ARhain, S. A., Bin Saif, F. H., Abid, A., Al Gamdi, O., Alsulaiman, F., & AlQarni, M. (2022). Extensive Cerebral Venous Sinus Thrombosis (CVST) After the First Dose of Pfizer-BioNTech BNT162b2 mRNA COVID-19 Vaccine without Thrombotic Thrombocytopenia Syndrome (TTS) in a Healthy Woman. *American Journal of Case Reports, 23*. https://doi.org/10.12659/AJCR.934744

Aliahmad, P., Miyake-Stoner, S. J., Geall, A. J., & Wang, N. S. (2023). Next generation self-replicating RNA vectors for vaccines and immunotherapies. *Cancer Gene Therapy, 30*(6), 785–793. https://doi.org/10.1038/s41417-022-00435-8

Alipon, S. B., Takashima, Y., Avagyan, T., Grabovac, V., Aslam, S. K., Bayutas, B., Logronio, J., Wang, X., Shrestha, A., Neupane, S., Roces, M. C., Apostol, L. N., & Sucaldito, N. (2022). Emergence of vaccine-derived poliovirus type 2 after using monovalent type 2 oral poliovirus vaccine in an outbreak response, Philippines. *Western Pacific Surveillance Response Journal, 13*(2), 1–7. https://doi.org/10.5365/wpsar.2022.13.2.904.

Aljeshi, A. A., Abdelrahim, A. S. I., & Aljeshi, M. A. (2022). Psychosis Associated With COVID-19 Vaccination. *The Primary Care Companion For CNS Disorders, 24*(1). https://doi.org/10.4088/PCC.21cr03160

Al-kuraishy, H. M., Al-Gareeb, A. I., Kaushik, A., Kujawska, M., & Batiha, G. E.-S. (2022). Hemolytic anemia in COVID-19. *Annals of Hematology, 101*(9), 1887–1895. https://doi.org/10.1007/s00277-022-04907-7

Alleman, M. M., Jorba, J., Henderson, E., Diop, O. M., Shaukat, S., Traoré, M. A., Wiesen, E., Wassilak, S. G. F., & Burns, C. C. (2021). Update on Vaccine-Derived Poliovirus Outbreaks - Worldwide, January 2020-June 2021. *MMWR Morbidity and Mortality Weekly Report, 70*(49), 1691–1699. https://doi.org/10.15585/mmwr.mm7049a1.

Allen, A. J., & Kudenchak, L. N. (2023). Acute Recurrent Pancreatitis in a Pediatric Patient in the Setting of Viral Infection and COVID-19 Vaccination. *Cureus*. https://doi.org/10.7759/cureus.40564

Allen, C. M., Ramsamy, S., Tarr, A. W., Tighe, P. J., Irving, W. L., Tanasescu, R., & Evans, J. R. (2021). Guillain–Barré Syndrome Variant Occurring after SARS-CoV-2 Vaccination. *Annals of Neurology*, *90*(2), 315–318. https://doi.org/10.1002/ana.26144

Alloush, T. K., Alloush, A. T., Abdelazeem, Y., Shokri, H. M., Abdulghani, K. O., & Elzoghby, A. (2023). Creutzfeldt–Jakob disease in a post-COVID-19 patient: did SARS-CoV-2 accelerate the neurodegeneration? *The Egyptian Journal of Neurology, Psychiatry and Neurosurgery*, *59*(1), 69. https://doi.org/10.1186/s41983-023-00666-y

Al-Maqbali, J. S., Al Rasbi, S., Kashoub, M. S., Al Hinaai, A. M., Farhan, H., Al Rawahi, B., & Al Alawi, A. M. (2021). A 59-Year-Old Woman with Extensive Deep Vein Thrombosis and Pulmonary Thromboembolism 7 Days Following a First Dose of the Pfizer-BioNTech BNT162b2 mRNA COVID-19 Vaccine. *American Journal of Case Reports*, *22*. https://doi.org/10.12659/AJCR.932946

Almuqrin, A., Davidson, A. D., Williamson, M. K., Lewis, P. A., Heesom, K. J., Morris, S., Gilbert, S. C., & Matthews, D. A. (2021). SARS-CoV-2 vaccine ChAdOx1 nCoV-19 infection of human cell lines reveals low levels of viral backbone gene transcription alongside very high levels of SARS-CoV-2 S glycoprotein gene transcription. *Genome Medicine*, *13*(1), 43. https://doi.org/10.1186/s13073-021-00859-1

Alphonso, H., DeMoss, D., Hurd, C., Oliphant, N., Davis, J. K., & Rush, A. J. (2022). Vaccine-Induced Psychosis as an Etiology to Consider in the Age of COVID-19. *The Primary Care Companion For CNS Disorders*, *24*(6). https://doi.org/10.4088/PCC.22cr03324

Altamirano, J., Sarnquist, C., Behl, R., García-García, L., Ferreyra-Reyes, L., Leary, S., & Maldonado, Y. (2018). OPV Vaccination and Shedding Patterns in Mexican and US Children. *Clinical Infectious Diseases, 67*(suppl_1), S85–S89. https://doi.org/10.1093/cid/ciy636.

Altman, D. G., & Bland, J. M. (1995). Statistics notes: Absence of evidence is not evidence of absence. *BMJ*, *311*(7003), 485–485. https://doi.org/10.1136/bmj.311.7003.485

Anamnart, C., Tisavipat, N., Owattanapanich, W., Apiwattanakul, M., Savangned, P., Prayoonwiwat, N., Siritho, S., Rattanathamsakul, N., & Jitprapaikulsan, J. (2022). Newly diagnosed neuromyelitis optica spectrum disorders following vaccination: Case report and systematic review. *Multiple Sclerosis and Related Disorders*, *58*, 103414. https://doi.org/10.1016/j.msard.2021.103414

Anand, R., Biswal, S., Bhatt, R., & Tiwary, B. N. (2020). Computational perspectives revealed prospective vaccine candidates from five structural proteins of novel SARS corona virus 2019 (SARS-CoV-2). *PeerJ*, *8*, e9855. https://doi.org/10.7717/peerj.9855

Ando, H., Ukena, K., & Nagata, S. (2021). Gonadal hormones. In *Handbook of Hormones* (Second Edition, pp. 553–554). Academic Press . https://doi.org/10.1016/B978-0-12-820649-2.00140-6

Anjum, Z., Iyer, C., Naz, S., Jaiswal, V., Nepal, G., Laguio-vila, M., Anandaram, S., & Thapaliya, S. (2022). Guillain-Barré syndrome after mRNA-1273 (Moderna)

COVID-19 vaccination: A case report. *Clinical Case Reports*, *10*(4). https://doi.org/10.1002/ccr3.5733

Aochi, S., Uehara, M., & Yamamoto, M. (2023). IgG4-related Disease Emerging after COVID-19 mRNA Vaccination. *Internal Medicine*, *62*(10), 1125–22. https://doi.org/10.2169/internalmedicine.1125-22

Aomar-Millán, I. F., Martínez de Victoria-Carazo, J., Peregrina-Rivas, J. A., & Villegas-Rodríguez, I. (2021). COVID-19, Guillain-Barré y vacuna. Una mezcla peligrosa. *Revista Clínica Española*, *221*(9), 555–557. https://doi.org/10.1016/j.rce.2021.05.005

Appelbaum, J., Arnold, D. M., Kelton, J. G., Gernsheimer, T., Jevtic, S. D., Ivetic, N., Smith, J. W., & Nazy, I. (2022). SARS-CoV-2 spike-dependent platelet activation in COVID-19 vaccine-induced thrombocytopenia. *Blood Advances*, *6*(7), 2250–2253. https://doi.org/10.1182/bloodadvances.2021005050

Arand, M. (2021). Opinion: A serious issue with the standardization of the adenovirus-based COVID-19 vaccines? *Archives of Toxicology*, *95*(9), 3137–3139. https://doi.org/10.1007/s00204-021-03126-9

Arepally, G. M., & Padmanabhan, A. (2020). Heparin-Induced Thrombocytopenia. *Arteriosclerosis, Thrombosis, and Vascular Biology*. https://doi.org/10.1161/ATVBAHA.120.315445

Artamonova, I. N., Petrova, N. A., Lyubimova, N. A., Kolbina, N. Y., Bryzzhin, A. V., Borodin, A. V., Levko, T. A., Mamaeva, E. A., Pervunina, T. M., Vasichkina, E. S., Nikitina, I. L., Zlotina, A. M., Efimtsev, A. Yu., & Kostik, M. M. (2022). Case Report: COVID-19-Associated ROHHAD-Like Syndrome. *Frontiers in Pediatrics*, *10*. https://doi.org/10.3389/fped.2022.854367

Atassi, M. Z., Casali, P., Atassi, M. Z., & Casali, P. (2008). Molecular mechanisms of autoimmunity. *Autoimmunity*, *41*(2), 123–132. https://doi.org/10.1080/08916930801929021

Attia, A., Badr, B., Albalaihad, R., Alharshan, R., & Almukhhaitah, A. (2023). Creutzfeldt-Jakob disease after the second dosage of the novel Pfizer-BioNtech messenger ribonucleic acid (mRNA) COVID-19 vaccination: a case report. *HIV Nursing*, *23*(1), 743–747.

Au, L., Fendler, A., Shepherd, S. T. C., Rzeniewicz, K., Cerrone, M., Byrne, F., Carlyle, E., Edmonds, K., Del Rosario, L., Shon, J., Haynes, W. A., Ward, B., Shum, B., Gordon, W., Gerard, C. L., Xie, W., Joharatnam-Hogan, N., Young, K., Pickering, L., … Turajlic, S. (2021). Cytokine release syndrome in a patient with colorectal cancer after vaccination with BNT162b2. *Nature Medicine*, *27*(8), 1362–1366. https://doi.org/10.1038/s41591-021-01387-6

Avolio, E., Carrabba, M., Milligan, R., Kavanagh Williamson, M., Beltrami, A. P., Gupta, K., Elvers, K. T., Gamez, M., Foster, R. R., Gillespie, K., Hamilton, F., Arnold, D., Berger, I., Davidson, A. D., Hill, D., Caputo, M., & Madeddu, P. (2021). The SARS-CoV-2 Spike protein disrupts human cardiac pericytes function through CD147 receptor-mediated signalling: a potential non-infective mechanism of COVID-19 microvascular disease. *Clinical Science*, *135*(24), 2667–2689. https://doi.org/10.1042/CS20210735

Azlan, A., Salamonsen, L. A., Hutchison, J., & Evans, J. (2020). Endometrial inflammasome activation accompanies menstruation and may have implications for systemic inflammatory events of the menstrual cycle. *Human Reproduction*, *35*(6), 1363–1376. https://doi.org/10.1093/humrep/deaa065

Azzaz, F., Yahi, N., Di Scala, C., Chahinian, H., & Fantini, J. (2022). *Ganglioside binding domains in proteins: Physiological and pathological mechanisms* (pp. 289–324). https://doi.org/10.1016/bs.apcsb.2021.08.003

Baden, L. R., El Sahly, H. M., Essink, B., Kotloff, K., Frey, S., Novak, R., Diemert, D., Spector, S. A., Rouphael, N., Creech, C. B., McGettigan, J., Khetan, S., Segall, N., Solis, J., Brosz, A., Fierro, C., Schwartz, H., Neuzil, K., Corey, L., … Zaks, T. (2021). Efficacy and Safety of the mRNA-1273 SARS-CoV-2 Vaccine. *New England Journal of Medicine*, *384*(5), 403–416. https://doi.org/10.1056/NEJMoa2035389

Badoiu, A., Moranne, O., Coudray, S., & Ion, I. M. (2021). Clinical Variant of Guillain–Barre Syndrome With Prominent Facial Diplegia After AstraZeneca Coronavirus Disease 2019 Vaccine. *Journal of Clinical Neuromuscular Disease*, *23*(2), 115–116. https://doi.org/10.1097/CND.0000000000000383

Badrawi, N., Kumar, N., & Albastaki, U. (2021). Post COVID-19 vaccination neuromyelitis optica spectrum disorder: Case report & MRI findings. *Radiology Case Reports*, *16*(12), 3864–3867. https://doi.org/10.1016/j.radcr.2021.09.033

Baena-García, L., Aparicio, V. A., Molina-López, A., Aranda, P., Cámara-Roca, L., & Ocón-Hernández, O. (2022). Premenstrual and menstrual changes reported after COVID-19 vaccination: The EVA project. *Women's Health*, *18*, 174550572211122. https://doi.org/10.1177/17455057221112237

Bahl, K., Senn, J. J., Yuzhakov, O., Bulychev, A., Brito, L. A., Hassett, K. J., Laska, M. E., Smith, M., Almarsson, Ö., Thompson, J., Ribeiro, A. (Mick), Watson, M., Zaks, T., & Ciaramella, G. (2017). Preclinical and Clinical Demonstration of Immunogenicity by mRNA Vaccines against H10N8 and H7N9 Influenza Viruses. *Molecular Therapy*, *25*(6), 1316–1327. https://doi.org/10.1016/j.ymthe.2017.03.035

Bai, H., Lester, G. M. S., Petishnok, L. C., & Dean, D. A. (2017). Cytoplasmic transport and nuclear import of plasmid DNA. *Bioscience Reports*, *37*(6). https://doi.org/10.1042/BSR20160616

Baiersdörfer, M., Boros, G., Muramatsu, H., Mahiny, A., Vlatkovic, I., Sahin, U., & Karikó, K. (2019). A Facile Method for the Removal of dsRNA Contaminant from In Vitro-Transcribed mRNA. *Molecular Therapy - Nucleic Acids*, *15*, 26–35. https://doi.org/10.1016/j.omtn.2019.02.018

Balasubramanian, I., Faheem, A., Padhy, S. K., & Menon, V. (2022). Psychiatric adverse reactions to COVID-19 vaccines: A rapid review of published case reports. *Asian Journal of Psychiatry*, *71*, 103129. https://doi.org/10.1016/j.ajp.2022.103129

Baldo, A., Leunda, A., Willemarck, N., & Pauwels, K. (2021). Environmental Risk Assessment of Recombinant Viral Vector Vaccines against SARS-Cov-2. *Vaccines*, *9*(5), 453. https://doi.org/10.3390/vaccines9050453

Ball-Burack, M. R., & Kosowsky, J. M. (2022). A Case of Leukocytoclastic Vasculitis Following SARS-COV-2 Vaccination. *The Journal of Emergency Medicine*, *63*(2), e62–e65. https://doi.org/10.1016/j.jemermed.2021.10.005

Banerji, A., Wickner, P. G., Saff, R., Stone, C. A., Robinson, L. B., Long, A. A., Wolfson, A. R., Williams, P., Khan, D. A., Phillips, E., & Blumenthal, K. G. (2021). mRNA Vaccines to Prevent COVID-19 Disease and Reported Allergic Reactions: Current Evidence and Suggested Approach. *The Journal of Allergy and*

Clinical Immunology: In Practice, *9*(4), 1423–1437. https://doi.org/10.1016/j.jaip.2020.12.047

Bangolo, A., Cherian, J., Ahmed, M., Atoot, A., Gupta, B., & Atoot, A. (2022). A Case Report of DVT following the Johnson and Johnson Vaccine against the Novel SARS-CoV-2. *Case Reports in Infectious Diseases*, 1–3. https://doi.org/10.1155/2022/1292754

Bangolo, A. I., Akhter, M., Auda, A., Akram, R., Nagesh, V. K., Athem, D., Thomas, R., Tibalan, L., Trivedi, M., Mushtaq, S., Singh, N., Bagale, P., Arana, G. V., Khan, T., Sharma, S., Mynedi, S., Patel, D. D., Saini, M., Chinthakuntla, M. R., … Weissman, S. (2023). A Case Report of Acute Severe Necrotizing Pancreatitis following the Johnson & Johnson Vaccine against the Novel SARS-CoV-2. *Case Reports in Infectious Diseases*, 1–4. https://doi.org/10.1155/2023/9965435

Banoun, H. (2023). mRNA: Vaccine or Gene Therapy? The Safety Regulatory Issues. *International Journal of Molecular Sciences*, *24*(13), 10514. https://doi.org/10.3390/ijms241310514

Banoun, H (2022). Current state of knowledge on the excretion of mRNA and spike produced by anti-COVID-19 mRNA vaccines; possibility of contamination of the entourage of those vaccinated by these products. *Infectious Disease Research*, *3*(4). https://doi.org/10.53388/IDR20221125022.

Bansal, S., Perincheri, S., Fleming, T., Poulson, C., Tiffany, B., Bremner, R. M., & Mohanakumar, T. (2021). Cutting Edge: Circulating Exosomes with COVID Spike Protein Are Induced by BNT162b2 (Pfizer–BioNTech) Vaccination prior to Development of Antibodies: A Novel Mechanism for Immune Activation by mRNA Vaccines. *The Journal of Immunology*, *207*(10), 2405–2410. https://doi.org/10.4049/jimmunol.2100637

Barale, C., Melchionda, E., Morotti, A., & Russo, I. (2021). Prothrombotic Phenotype in COVID-19: Focus on Platelets. *International Journal of Molecular Sciences*, *22*(24), 13638. https://doi.org/10.3390/ijms222413638

Barrios, Y., Alava-Cruz, C., Franco, A., & Matheu, V. (2022). Long Term Cell Immune Response to COVID-19 Vaccines Assessment Using a Delayed-Type Hypersensitivity (DTH) Cutaneous Test. *Diagnostics*, *12*(6), 1421. https://doi.org/10.3390/diagnostics12061421

Barry, M. (2018). Single-cycle adenovirus vectors in the current vaccine landscape. *Expert Review of Vaccines*, 1–11. https://doi.org/10.1080/14760584.2018.1419067

Bartoszek, K., & Okrój, M. (2022). Controversies around the statistical presentation of data on mRNA-COVID 19 vaccine safety in pregnant women. *Journal of Reproductive Immunology*, *151*, 103503. https://doi.org/10.1016/j.jri.2022.103503

Basit, H., & Huecker, M. R. (2023). Myocardial Infarction Serum Markers. [Updated 2023 Aug 14]. *In*: StatPearls [Internet]. Treasure Island (FL): StatPearls Publishing; 2023 Jan-. Available from: https://www.ncbi.nlm.nih.gov/books/NBK532966/

Bassi, A., Mazzatenta, C., Sechi, A., Cutrone, M., & Piccolo, V. (2022). Not only toes and fingers: COVID vaccine-induced chilblain-like lesions of the knees. *Journal of the European Academy of Dermatology and Venereology*, *36*(7). https://doi.org/10.1111/jdv.18025

Batot, C., Chea, M., Zeidan, S., Mongin, M., Pop, G., Mazoyer, J., & Degos, B. (2022). Clinical and Radiological Follow-Up of a Pfizer-BioNTech COVID-19

Vaccine-Induced Hemichorea-Hemiballismus. *Tremor and Other Hyperkinetic Movements*, *12*(1). https://doi.org/10.5334/tohm.688
Batova, I. N., Richardson, R. T., Widgren, E. E., & O'Rand, M. G. (2000). Analysis of the autoimmune epitopes on human testicular NASP using recombinant and synthetic peptides. *Clinical and Experimental Immunology*, *121*(2), 201–209. https://doi.org/10.1046/j.1365-2249.2000.01303.x
Baugh, R. F., Basura, G. J., Ishii, L. E., Schwartz, S. R., Drumheller, C. M., Burkholder, R., Deckard, N. A., Dawson, C., Driscoll, C., Gillespie, M. B., Gurgel, R. K., Halperin, J., Khalid, A. N., Kumar, K. A., Micco, A., Munsell, D., Rosenbaum, S., & Vaughan, W. (2013). Clinical Practice Guideline: Bell's Palsy. *Otolaryngology–Head and Neck Surgery*, *149*(S3). https://doi.org/10.1177/0194599813505967
Baumeier, C., Aleshcheva, G., Harms, D., Gross, U., Hamm, C., Assmus, B., Westenfeld, R., Kelm, M., Rammos, S., Wenzel, P., Münzel, T., Elsässer, A., Gailani, M., Perings, C., Bourakkadi, A., Flesch, M., Kempf, T., Bauersachs, J., Escher, F., & Schultheiss, H.-P. (2022). Intramyocardial Inflammation after COVID-19 Vaccination: An Endomyocardial Biopsy-Proven Case Series. *International Journal of Molecular Sciences*, *23*(13), 6940. https://doi.org/10.3390/ijms23136940
Bautista García, J., Peña Ortega, P., Bonilla Fernández, J. A., Cárdenes León, A., Ramírez Burgos, L., & Caballero Dorta, E. (2021). Acute myocarditis after administration of the BNT162b2 vaccine against COVID-19. *Revista Española de Cardiología (English Edition)*, *74*(9), 812–814. https://doi.org/10.1016/j.rec.2021.04.005
Bazrafshan, H., Sadat Mohamadi Jahromi, L., Parvin, R., & Ashraf, A. (2022). A case of Guillain-Barre syndrome after the second dose of AstraZeneca COVID-19 vaccination. *Turkish Journal of Physical Medicine and Rehabilitation*, *68*(2), 295–299. https://doi.org/10.5606/tftrd.2022.9984
Beatty, A. L., Peyser, N. D., Butcher, X. E., Cocohoba, J. M., Lin, F., Olgin, J. E., Pletcher, M. J., & Marcus, G. M. (2021). Analysis of COVID-19 Vaccine Type and Adverse Effects Following Vaccination. *JAMA Network Open*, *4*(12), e2140364. https://doi.org/10.1001/jamanetworkopen.2021.40364
Beaudoin, C. A., Jamasb, A. R., Alsulami, A. F., Copoiu, L., van Tonder, A. J., Hala, S., Bannerman, B. P., Thomas, S. E., Vedithi, S. C., Torres, P. H. M., & Blundell, T. L. (2021). Predicted structural mimicry of spike receptor-binding motifs from highly pathogenic human coronaviruses. *Computational and Structural Biotechnology Journal*, *19*, 3938–3953. https://doi.org/10.1016/j.csbj.2021.06.041.
Becker, E. C., Siddique, O., Kapur, D., Patel, K., & Mehendiratta, V. (2023). Type 1 Autoimmune Pancreatitis Unmasked by COVID-19 Vaccine. *ACG Case Reports Journal*, *10*(1), e00950. https://doi.org/10.14309/crj.0000000000000950
Bedrosian, T. A., Quayle, C., Novaresi, N., & Gage, Fred. H. (2018). Early life experience drives structural variation of neural genomes in mice. *Science*, *359*(6382), 1395–1399. https://doi.org/10.1126/science.aah3378
Beh, S. C., Greenberg, B. M., Frohman, T., & Frohman, E. M. (2013). Transverse Myelitis. *Neurologic Clinics*, *31*(1), 79–138. https://doi.org/10.1016/j.ncl.2012.09.008

Bellucci, M., Germano, F., Grisanti, S., Castellano, C., Tazza, F., Mobilia, E. M., Visigalli, D., Novi, G., Massa, F., Rossi, S., Durando, P., Cabona, C., Schenone, A., Franciotta, D., & Benedetti, L. (2022). Case Report: Post-COVID-19 Vaccine Recurrence of Guillain–Barré Syndrome Following an Antecedent Parainfectious COVID-19–Related GBS. *Frontiers in Immunology*, *13*. https://doi.org/10.3389/fimmu.2022.894872

Belyi, V. A., Levine, A. J., & Skalka, A. M. (2010). Unexpected Inheritance: Multiple Integrations of Ancient Bornavirus and Ebolavirus/Marburgvirus Sequences in Vertebrate Genomes. *PLoS Pathogens*, *6*(7), e1001030. https://doi.org/10.1371/journal.ppat.1001030

Ben-Yosef, T. (2022). Inherited Retinal Diseases. *International Journal of Molecular Science*, *23*(21),13467. https://doi.org/10.3390/ijms232113467.

Berbic, M., & Fraser, I. S. (2013). Immunology of Normal and Abnormal Menstruation. *Women's Health*, *9*(4), 387–395. https://doi.org/10.2217/WHE.13.32

Berga, S. L., Mortolo, J. F., Girton, L., Suh, B., Lauglin, G., Pham, P., & Yen, S. S. C. (1989). Neuroendocrine Aberrations in Women With Functional Hypothalamic Amenorrhea*. *The Journal of Clinical Endocrinology & Metabolism*, *68*(2), 301–308. https://doi.org/10.1210/jcem-68-2-301

Bernardini, A., Gigli, G. L., Janes, F., Pellitteri, G., Ciardi, C., Fabris, M., & Valente, M. (2022). Creutzfeldt-Jakob disease after COVID-19: infection-induced prion protein misfolding? A case report. *Prion*, *16*(1), 78–83. https://doi.org/10.1080/19336896.2022.2095185

Berrim, K., Lakhoua, G., Zaiem, A., Charfi, O., Aouinti, I., Kastalli, S., Daghfous, R., & El Aidli, S. (2023). Guillain-Barré syndrome after COVID-19 vaccines: A Tunisian case series. *British Journal of Clinical Pharmacology*, *89*(2), 574–578. https://doi.org/10.1111/bcp.15601

Bert, F., Scaioli, G., Vola, L., Accortanzo, D., Lo Moro, G., & Siliquini, R. (2022). Booster Doses of Anti COVID-19 Vaccines: An Overview of Implementation Policies among OECD and EU Countries. *International Journal of Environmental Research and Public Health*, *19*(12), 7233. https://doi.org/10.3390/ijerph19127233

Beyaz, Ş., Öksüzer Çimşir, D., Çelebi Sözener, Z., Soyyiğit, Ş., & Öner Erkekol, F. (2022). Delayed-type hypersensitivity reactions to Pfizer BioNTech SARS-CoV-2 vaccine. *Postgraduate Medical Journal*, *98*(1163), 658–659. https://doi.org/10.1136/postgradmedj-2021-141420

Bhardwaj, T., Gadhave, K., Kapuganti, S. K., Kumar, P., Brotzakis, Z. F., Saumya, K. U., Nayak, N., Kumar, A., Joshi, R., Mukherjee, B., Bhardwaj, A., Thakur, K. G., Garg, N., Vendruscolo, M., & Giri, R. (2023). Amyloidogenic proteins in the SARS-CoV and SARS-CoV-2 proteomes. *Nature Communications*, *14*(1), 945. https://doi.org/10.1038/s41467-023-36234-4

Biswas, A., & Pandey, S. (2022). Guillain–Barre syndrome after the first dose of Anti-SARS-CoV-2 vaccination is a rare side effect and the second jab is controversial in these cases. *Indian Journal of Public Health*, *66*(4), 535. https://doi.org/10.4103/ijph.ijph_1360_22

Blumenthal, K. G., Ahola, C., Anvari, S., Samarakoon, U., & Freeman, E. E. (2022). Delayed large local reactions to Moderna COVID-19 vaccine: A follow-up report after booster vaccination. *JAAD International*, *8*, 3–6. https://doi.org/10.1016/j.jdin.2022.03.017

Boczkowski, D., Nair, S. K., Snyder, D., & Gilboa, E. (1996). Dendritic cells pulsed with RNA are potent antigen-presenting cells *in vitro* and *in vivo*. *Journal of Experimental Medicine*, *184*(2), 465-72. https://doi.org/ 10.1084/jem.184.2.465.

Bogers, W. M., Oostermeijer, H., Mooij, P., Koopman, G., Verschoor, E. J., Davis, D., Ulmer, J. B., Brito, L. A., Cu, Y., Banerjee, K., Otten, G. R., Burke, B., Dey, A., Heeney, J. L., Shen, X., Tomaras, G. D., Labranche, C., Montefiori, D. C., Liao, H.-X., … Barnett, S. W. (2015). Potent Immune Responses in Rhesus Macaques Induced by Nonviral Delivery of a Self-amplifying RNA Vaccine Expressing HIV Type 1 Envelope With a Cationic Nanoemulsion. *Journal of Infectious Diseases*, *211*(6), 947–955. https://doi.org/10.1093/infdis/jiu522

Boissinot, S., & Sookdeo, A. (2016). The Evolution of Line-1 in Vertebrates. *Genome Biology and Evolution*, evw247. https://doi.org/10.1093/gbe/evw247

Bok, K., Sitar, S., Graham, B. S., & Mascola, J. R. (2021). Accelerated COVID-19 vaccine development: milestones, lessons, and prospects. *Immunity*, *54*(8), 1636–1651. https://doi.org/10.1016/j.immuni.2021.07.017

Bollenbach, L., Buske, J., Mäder, K., & Garidel, P. (2022). Poloxamer 188 as surfactant in biological formulations – An alternative for polysorbate 20/80? *International Journal of Pharmaceutics*, *620*, 121706. https://doi.org/10.1016/j.ijpharm.2022.121706

Bolletta, E., Iannetta, D., Mastrofilippo, V., De Simone, L., Gozzi, F., Croci, S., Bonacini, M., Belloni, L., Zerbini, A., Adani, C., Fontana, L., Salvarani, C., & Cimino, L. (2021). Uveitis and Other Ocular Complications Following COVID-19 Vaccination. *Journal of Clinical Medicine*, *10*(24), 5960. https://doi.org/10.3390/jcm10245960

Bonifacio, G. B., Patel, D., Cook, S., Purcaru, E., Couzins, M., Domjan, J., Ryan, S., Alareed, A., Tuohy, O., Slaght, S., Furby, J., Allen, D., Katifi, H. A., & Kinton, L. (2022). Bilateral facial weakness with paraesthesia variant of Guillain-Barré syndrome following Vaxzevria COVID-19 vaccine. *Journal of Neurology, Neurosurgery & Psychiatry*, *93*(3), 341–342. https://doi.org/10.1136/jnnp-2021-327027

Borchers, A. T., & Gershwin, M. E. (2012). Transverse myelitis. *Autoimmunity Reviews*, *11*(3), 231–248. https://doi.org/10.1016/j.autrev.2011.05.018

Boskabadi, S. J., Ala, S., Heydari, F., Ebrahimi, M., & Jamnani, A. N. (2023). Acute pancreatitis following COVID-19 vaccine: A case report and brief literature review. *Heliyon*, *9*(1), e12914. https://doi.org/10.1016/j.heliyon.2023.e12914

Bouattour, N., Hdiji, O., Sakka, S., Fakhfakh, E., Moalla, K., Daoud, S., Farhat, N., Damak, M., & Mhiri, C. (2022). Guillain-Barré syndrome following the first dose of Pfizer-BioNTech COVID-19 vaccine: case report and review of reported cases. *Neurological Sciences*, *43*(2), 755–761. https://doi.org/10.1007/s10072-021-05733-x

Bozkurt, B., Kamat, I., & Hotez, P. J. (2021). Myocarditis With COVID-19 mRNA Vaccines. *Circulation*, *144*(6), 471–484. https://doi.org/10.1161/CIRCULATIONAHA.121.056135

Bravo Vázquez, L. A., Moreno Becerril, M. Y., Mora Hernández, E. O., León Carmona, G. G. de, Aguirre Padilla, M. E., Chakraborty, S., Bandyopadhyay, A., & Paul, S. (2021). The Emerging Role of MicroRNAs in Bone Diseases and Their

Therapeutic Potential. *Molecules*, *27*(1), 211. https://doi.org/10.3390/molecules27010211

Brest, P., Mograbi, B., Hofman, P., & Milano, G. (2022). COVID-19 vaccination and cancer immunotherapy: should they stick together? *British Journal of Cancer*, *126*(1), 1–3. https://doi.org/10.1038/s41416-021-01618-0

Brisse, M., & Ly, H. (2019). Comparative Structure and Function Analysis of the RIG-I-Like Receptors: RIG-I and MDA5. *Frontiers in Immunology*, *10*. https://doi.org/10.3389/fimmu.2019.01586

Brock, A. R., & Thornley, S. (2021). Spontaneous Abortions and Policies on COVID-19 mRNA Vaccine Use During Pregnancy. *Science, Public Health Policy, and the Law*, *4*, 130–143. chrome-extension://efaidnbmnnnibpcajpcglclefindmkaj/https://cf5e727d-d02d-4d71-89ff-9fe2d3ad957f.filesusr.com/ugd/adf864_2bd97450072f4364a65e5cf1d7384dd4.pdf

Brogna, C., Cristoni, S., Marino, G., Montano, L., Viduto, V., Fabrowski, M., Lettieri, G., & Piscopo, M. (2023). Detection of recombinant Spike protein in the blood of individuals vaccinated against SARS-CoV-2: Possible molecular mechanisms. *PROTEOMICS – Clinical Applications*. https://doi.org/10.1002/prca.202300048

Brook, B., Sodhi, N., & Bradshaw, C. (2008). Synergies among extinction drivers under global change. *Trends in Ecology & Evolution*, *23*(8), 453–460. https://doi.org/10.1016/j.tree.2008.03.011

Brouha, B., Schustak, J., Badge, R. M., Lutz-Prigge, S., Farley, A. H., Moran, J. V., & Kazazian, H. H. (2003). Hot L1s account for the bulk of retrotransposition in the human population. *Proceedings of the National Academy of Sciences*, *100*(9), 5280–5285. https://doi.org/10.1073/pnas.0831042100

Bruce Yu, Y., Taraban, M. B., & Briggs, K. T. (2021). All vials are not the same: Potential role of vaccine quality in vaccine adverse reactions. *Vaccine*, *39*(45), 6565–6569. https://doi.org/10.1016/j.vaccine.2021.09.065

Brumfiel, C. M., Patel, M. H., DiCaudo, D. J., Rosenthal, A. C., Pittelkow, M. R., & Mangold, A. R. (2021). Recurrence of primary cutaneous CD30-positive lymphoproliferative disorder following COVID-19 vaccination. *Leukemia & Lymphoma*, *62*(10), 2554–2555. https://doi.org/10.1080/10428194.2021.1924371

Buchbinder, S. P., McElrath, M. J., Dieffenbach, C., & Corey, L. (2020). Use of adenovirus type-5 vectored vaccines: a cautionary tale. *The Lancet*, *396*(10260), e68–e69. https://doi.org/10.1016/S0140-6736(20)32156-5

Buergin, N., Lopez-Ayala, P., Hirsiger, J. R., Mueller, P., Median, D., Glarner, N., Rumora, K., Herrmann, T., Koechlin, L., Haaf, P., Rentsch, K., Battegay, M., Banderet, F., Berger, C. T., & Mueller, C. (2023). Sex-specific differences in myocardial injury incidence after COVID-19 mRNA-1273 booster vaccination. *European Journal of Heart Failure*. https://doi.org/10.1002/ejhf.2978

Bukhari, A. E. (2022). New-onset of vitiligo in a child following COVID-19 vaccination. *JAAD Case Reports*, *22*, 68–69. https://doi.org/10.1016/j.jdcr.2022.02.021

Bularca, E., Monte-Serrano, J., Villagrasa-Boli, P., Lapeña-Casado, A., & de-la-Fuente, S. (2022). Reply to "COVID vaccine–induced lichen planus on areas previously affected by vitiligo." *Journal of the European Academy of Dermatology and Venereology*, *36*(6). https://doi.org/10.1111/jdv.18001

Burbelo, P. D., Riedo, F. X., Morishima, C., Rawlings, S., Smith, D., Das, S., Strich, J. R., Chertow, D. S., Davey, R. T., & Cohen, J. I. (2020). Sensitivity in Detection of Antibodies to Nucleocapsid and Spike Proteins of Severe Acute Respiratory Syndrome Coronavirus 2 in Patients With Coronavirus Disease 2019. *The Journal of Infectious Diseases*, *222*(2), 206–213. https://doi.org/10.1093/infdis/jiaa273

Burnap, S. A., Ortega-Prieto, A. M., Jimenez-Guardeño, J. M., Ali, H., Takov, K., Fish, M., Shankar-Hari, M., Giacca, M., Malim, M. H., & Mayr, M. (2023). Cross-Linking Mass Spectrometry Uncovers Interactions Between High-Density Lipoproteins and the SARS-CoV-2 Spike Glycoprotein. *Molecular & Cellular Proteomics*, *22*(8), 100600. https://doi.org/10.1016/j.mcpro.2023.100600

Burns, C. C., Diop, O. M., Sutter, R. W., & Kew, O. M. (2014).Vaccine-derived polioviruses. *Journal of Infection and Disease,* 210(Suppl 1), S283–S293. https://doi.org/10.1093/infdis/jiu295.

Butler, D. L., Imberti, L., Quaresima, V., Fiorini, C., Barnett, J., Chauvin, S., Cheng, X., Danielson, J., Dobbs, K., Garabedian, E., Kuram, V., Lau, W., Li, Z., Magliocco, M., Matthews, H., Nambiar, M., Samuel, S., Shaw, E., Stack, M., … Gildersleeve, J. C. (2022). Abnormal antibodies to self-carbohydrates in SARS-CoV-2-infected patients. *PNAS Nexus*, *1*(3). https://doi.org/10.1093/pnasnexus/pgac062

Buzhdygan, T. P., DeOre, B. J., Baldwin-Leclair, A., Bullock, T. A., McGary, H. M., Khan, J. A., Razmpour, R., Hale, J. F., Galie, P. A., Potula, R., Andrews, A. M., & Ramirez, S. H. (2020). The SARS-CoV-2 spike protein alters barrier function in 2D static and 3D microfluidic in-vitro models of the human blood–brain barrier. *Neurobiology of Disease*, *146*, 105131. https://doi.org/10.1016/j.nbd.2020.105131

Cabanillas, B., & Novak, N. (2021). Allergy to COVID-19 vaccines: A current update. *Allergology International*, *70*(3), 313–318. https://doi.org/10.1016/j.alit.2021.04.003

Cacdac, R., Jamali, A., Jamali, R., Nemovi, K., Vosoughi, K., & Bayraktutar, Z. (2022). Acute pancreatitis as an adverse effect of COVID-19 vaccination. *SAGE Open Medical Case Reports*, *10*, 2050313X2211311. https://doi.org/10.1177/2050313X221131169

Cai, H., Zhou, R., Jiang, F., Zeng, Q., & Yang, H. (2022). Vaccination in neuromyelitis optica spectrum disorders: Friend or enemy? *Multiple Sclerosis and Related Disorders*, *58*, 103394. https://doi.org/10.1016/j.msard.2021.103394

Campbell, J., Trgovcich, J., Kincaid, M., Zimmerman, P. D., Klenerman, P., Sims, S., & Cook, C. H. (2012). Transient CD8-memory contraction: a potential contributor to latent cytomegalovirus reactivation. *Journal of Leukocyte Biology*, *92*(5), 933–937. https://doi.org/10.1189/jlb.1211635

Campra-Madrid, P. (2021). *Detección de grafeno en vacunas COVID19 por espectroscopia micro-RAMAN*. chrome-extension://efaidnbmnnnibpcajpcglclefindmkaj/https://joaomfjorge.files.wordpress.com/2021/06/informetecnicofinaldeteccindegrafenoenvacunascovidconanexoresultados-1.pdf

Cao, S., Song, Z., Rong, J., Andrikopoulos, N., Liang, X., Wang, Y., Peng, G., Ding, F., & Ke, P. C. (2023). Spike Protein Fragments Promote Alzheimer's Amyloidogenesis. *ACS Applied Materials & Interfaces*, *15*(34), 40317–40329. https://doi.org/10.1021/acsami.3c09815

Cao, W., He, L., Cao, W., Huang, X., Jia, K., & Dai, J. (2020). Recent progress of graphene oxide as a potential vaccine carrier and adjuvant. *Acta Biomaterialia*, *112*, 14–28. https://doi.org/10.1016/j.actbio.2020.06.009

Carabelli, A. M., Peacock, T. P., Thorne, L. G., Harvey, W. T., Hughes, J., de Silva, T. I., Peacock, S. J., Barclay, W. S., de Silva, T. I., Towers, G. J., & Robertson, D. L. (2023). SARS-CoV-2 variant biology: immune escape, transmission and fitness. *Nature Reviews Microbiology*. https://doi.org/10.1038/s41579-022-00841-7

Carbone, M. L., Madonna, G., Capone, A., Bove, M., Mastroeni, S., Levati, L., Capone, M., Ascierto, P. A., De Galitiis, F., D'Atri, S., Fortes, C., Volpe, E., & Failla, C. M. (2022). Vitiligo-specific soluble biomarkers as early indicators of response to immune checkpoint inhibitors in metastatic melanoma patients. *Scientific Reports*, *12*(1), 5448. https://doi.org/10.1038/s41598-022-09373-9

Cardozo, T., & Veazey, R. (2021). Informed consent disclosure to vaccine trial subjects of risk of COVID-19 vaccines worsening clinical disease. *International Journal of Clinical Practice*, *75*(3). https://doi.org/10.1111/ijcp.13795

Caroppo, F., Deotto, M. L., Tartaglia, J., & Belloni Fortina, A. (2022). Vitiligo worsened following the second dose of mRNA SARS-CoV-2 vaccine. *Dermatologic Therapy*, *35*(6). https://doi.org/10.1111/dth.15434

Carrillo-Garcia, P., Sánchez-Osorio, L., & Gómez-Pavón, J. (2022). Leukocytoclastic vasculitis in possible relation to the BNT162b2 mRNA COVID-19 vaccine. *Journal of the American Geriatrics Society*, *70*(4), 971–973. https://doi.org/10.1111/jgs.17675

Casati, L., Ciceri, S., Maggi, R., & Bottai, D. (2023). Physiological and pharmacological overview of the gonadotropin releasing hormone. *Biochemical Pharmacology*, *212*, 115553. https://doi.org/10.1016/j.bcp.2023.115553

Casavant, CH., & Youmans, GP. (1975). The induction of delayed hypersensitivity in guinea pigs to poly U and poly A:U. *J Immunol*, *114*(5).

Català, A., Muñoz-Santos, C., Galván-Casas, C., Roncero Riesco, M., Revilla Nebreda, D., Solá-Truyols, A., Giavedoni, P., Llamas-Velasco, M., González-Cruz, C., Cubiró, X., Ruíz-Villaverde, R., Gómez-Armayones, S., Gil Mateo, M. P., Pesqué, D., Marcantonio, O., Fernández-Nieto, D., Romaní, J., Iglesias Pena, N., Carnero Gonzalez, L., … Guilabert, A. (2022). Cutaneous reactions after SARS-CoV-2 vaccination: a cross-sectional Spanish nationwide study of 405 cases. *British Journal of Dermatology*, *186*(1), 142–152. https://doi.org/10.1111/bjd.20639

Čenščák, D., Ungermann, L., Štětkářová, I., & Ehler, E. (2021). Guillan-Barré Syndrome after First Vaccination Dose against COVID-19: Case Report. *Acta Medica (Hradec Kralove, Czech Republic)*, *64*(3), 183–186. https://doi.org/10.14712/18059694.2021.31

Centers for Disease Control and Prevention, CDC. (2004). Suspension of rotavirus vaccine after reports of intussusception--United States, 1999. *MMWR Morbidity and Mortality Weekly Report*, 53(34), 786–789.

Černáková, L., & Rodrigues, C. F. (2020). Microbial interactions and immunity response in oral Candida species. *Future Microbiology*, *15*(17), 1653–1677. https://doi.org/10.2217/fmb-2020-0113

Ceschia, N., Scheggi, V., Gori, A. M., Rogolino, A. A., Cesari, F., Giusti, B., Cipollini, F., Marchionni, N., Alterini, B., & Marcucci, R. (2021). Diffuse prothrombotic syndrome after ChAdOx1 nCoV-19 vaccine administration: a case report. *Journal of Medical Case Reports*, *15*(1), 496. https://doi.org/10.1186/s13256-021-03083-y

Chahed, F., Ben Fadhel, N., Maamri, K., Abdelali, M., Ben Romdhane, H., Chadli, Z., Ben Fredj, N., Zrig, A., Aouam, K., & Chaabane, A. (2023). An unusual occurrence of autoimmune pancreatitis after gam-Covid-Vac (Sputnik V): A case report and literature review. *British Journal of Clinical Pharmacology*, *89*(9), 2915–2919. https://doi.org/10.1111/bcp.15817

Chakrabarti, S. S., Tiwari, A., Jaiswal, S., Kaur, U., Kumar, I., Mittal, A., Singh, A., Jin, K., & Chakrabarti, S. (2022). Rapidly Progressive Dementia with Asymmetric Rigidity Following ChAdOx1 nCoV-19 Vaccination. *Aging and Disease*, *13*(3), 633. https://doi.org/10.14336/AD.2021.1102

Chalela, J. A., Andrews, C., Bashmakov, A., Kapoor, N., & Snelgrove, D. (2023). Reports of Guillain–Barre Syndrome Following COVID-19 Vaccination in the USA: An Analysis of the VAERS Database. *Journal of Clinical Neurology*, *19*(2), 179. https://doi.org/10.3988/jcn.2022.0237

Chamling, B., Vehof, V., Drakos, S., Weil, M., Stalling, P., Vahlhaus, C., Mueller, P., Bietenbeck, M., Reinecke, H., Meier, C., & Yilmaz, A. (2021). Occurrence of acute infarct-like myocarditis following COVID-19 vaccination: just an accidental co-incidence or rather vaccination-associated autoimmune myocarditis? *Clinical Research in Cardiology*, *110*(11), 1850–1854. https://doi.org/10.1007/s00392-021-01916-w

Chang, Y.-L., & Chang, S.-T. (2022). The effects of intravascular photobiomodulation on sleep disturbance caused by Guillain-Barré syndrome after Astrazeneca vaccine inoculation. *Medicine*, *101*(6), e28758. https://doi.org/10.1097/MD.0000000000028758

Changeux, J.-P., Amoura, Z., Rey, F. A., & Miyara, M. (2020). A nicotinic hypothesis for Covid-19 with preventive and therapeutic implications. *Comptes Rendus. Biologies*, *343*(1), 33–39. https://doi.org/10.5802/crbiol.8

Chaudhuri, T. K., & Paul, S. (2006). Protein-misfolding diseases and chaperone-based therapeutic approaches. *The FEBS Journal*, *273*(7), 1331–1349. https://doi.org/10.1111/j.1742-4658.2006.05181.x

Chavda, V., Bezbaruah, R., Valu, D., Patel, B., Kumar, A., Prasad, S., Kakoti, B., Kaushik, A., & Jesawadawala, M. (2023). Adenoviral Vector-Based Vaccine Platform for COVID-19: Current Status. *Vaccines*, *11*(2), 432. https://doi.org/10.3390/vaccines11020432

Checkoway, H., Lundin, J., & Kelada, S. (2011). Neurodegenerative diseases. *IARC Scientific Publications*, *163*, 407–419.

Chen, Q.-T., Liu, Y., Chen, Y.-C., Chou, C.-H., Lin, Y.-P., Lin, Y.-Q., Tsai, M.-C., Chang, B.-K., Ho, T.-H., Lu, C.-C., & Sung, Y.-F. (2022). Case report: Vaccine-induced immune thrombotic thrombocytopenia complicated by acute cerebral venous thrombosis and hemorrhage after AstraZeneca vaccines followed by Moderna COVID-19 vaccine booster and surgery. *Frontiers in Neurology*, *13*. https://doi.org/10.3389/fneur.2022.989730

Chen, Y.-C., Smith, T., Hicks, R. H., Doekhie, A., Koumanov, F., Wells, S. A., Edler, K. J., van den Elsen, J., Holman, G. D., Marchbank, K. J., & Sartbaeva, A. (2017). Thermal stability, storage and release of proteins with tailored fit in silica. *Scientific Reports*, *7*(1), 46568. https://doi.org/10.1038/srep46568

Chereshnev, V., Pichugova, S., Beikin, Y., Chereshneva, M., Iukhta, A., Stroev, Y., & Churilov, L. (2021). Pathogenesis of Autoimmune Male Infertility: Juxtacrine, Paracrine, and Endocrine Dysregulation. *Pathophysiology*, *28*(4), 471–488. https://doi.org/10.3390/pathophysiology28040030

Chesney, A. D., Maiti, B., & Hansmann, U. H. E. (2023). SARS-COV-2 spike protein fragment eases amyloidogenesis of α-synuclein. *The Journal of Chemical Physics*, *159*(1). https://doi.org/10.1063/5.0157331

Chew, M. C., Wiryasaputra, S., Wu, M., Khor, W. B., & Chan, A. S. Y. (2022). Incidence of COVID-19 Vaccination-Related Uveitis and Effects of Booster Dose in a Tertiary Uveitis Referral Center. *Frontiers in Medicine*, *9*. https://doi.org/10.3389/fmed.2022.925683

Cho, J. Y., Kim, K. H., Lee, N., Cho, S. H., Kim, S. Y., Kim, E. K., Park, J.-H., Choi, E.-Y., Choi, J.-O., Park, H., Kim, H. Y., Yoon, H. J., Ahn, Y., Jeong, M. H., & Cho, J. G. (2023). COVID-19 vaccination-related myocarditis: a Korean nationwide study. *European Heart Journal*, *44*(24), 2234–2243. https://doi.org/10.1093/eurheartj/ehad339

Choi, S., Lee, S., Seo, J.-W., Kim, M., Jeon, Y. H., Park, J. H., Lee, J. K., & Yeo, N. S. (2021). Myocarditis-induced Sudden Death after BNT162b2 mRNA COVID-19 Vaccination in Korea: Case Report Focusing on Histopathological Findings. *Journal of Korean Medical Science*, *36*(40). https://doi.org/10.3346/jkms.2021.36.e286

Choong, W.-K., & Sung, T.-Y. (2022). Multiaspect Examinations of Possible Alternative Mappings of Identified Variant Peptides: A Case Study on the HEK293 Cell Line. *ACS Omega*, *7*(19), 16454–16467. https://doi.org/10.1021/acsomega.2c00466

Chorin, O., Markovich, M. P., Avramovich, E., Rahmani, S., Sofer, D., Weil, M., Shohat, T., Chorin, E., Tasher, D., & Somekh, E. (2023). Oral and fecal polio vaccine excretion following bOPV vaccination among Israeli infants. *Vaccine*, *41*(28), 4144–4150. https://doi.org/10.1016/j.vaccine.2023.05.036.

Christensen, S., Ballegaard, M., & Boesen MS. (2021). Guillian Barré syndromeafter mRNA-1273 vaccination against COVID-19. *Ugeskr Laeger*, *183*(35).

Chuamanochan, M., Weller, K., Feist, E., Kallinich, T., Maurer, M., Kümmerle-Deschner, J., & Krause, K. (2019). State of care for patients with systemic autoinflammatory diseases - Results of a tertiary care survey. *World Allergy Organization Journal, 12*(3), 100019. https://doi.org/10.1016/j.waojou.2019.100019.

Chue, K. M., Tok, N. W. K., & Gao, Y. (2022). Spontaneous rare visceral pseudoaneurysm presenting with rupture after COVID -19 vaccination. *ANZ Journal of Surgery*, *92*(4), 915–917. https://doi.org/10.1111/ans.17199

Chuong, E. B., Elde, N. C., & Feschotte, C. (2016). Regulatory evolution of innate immunity through co-option of endogenous retroviruses. *Science*, *351*(6277), 1083–1087. https://doi.org/10.1126/science.aad5497

Ciabattini, A., Olivieri, R., Lazzeri, E., & Medaglini, D. (2019). Role of the Microbiota in the Modulation of Vaccine Immune Responses. *Frontiers in Microbiology*, *10*. https://doi.org/10.3389/fmicb.2019.01305

Ciccarese, G., Drago, F., Boldrin, S., Pattaro, M., & Parodi, A. (2022). Sudden onset of vitiligo after COVID-19 vaccine. *Dermatologic Therapy*, *35*(1). https://doi.org/10.1111/dth.15196

Cieślewicz, A., Dudek, M., Krela-Kaźmierczak, I., Jabłecka, A., Lesiak, M., & Korzeniowska, K. (2021). Pancreatic Injury after COVID-19 Vaccine—A Case Report. *Vaccines*, *9*(6), 576. https://doi.org/10.3390/vaccines9060576

Cimaglia, P., Tolomeo, P., & Rapezzi, C. (2022). Acute myocarditis after SARS-CoV-2 vaccination in a 24-year-old man. *Revista Portuguesa de Cardiologia, 41*(1), 71–72. https://doi.org/10.1016/j.repc.2021.07.005

Cincotta, M., & Walker, R. H. (2022). Clinical and Radiological Follow-Up of a Pfizer-BioNTech COVID-19 Vaccine-Induced Hemichorea-Hemiballismus; Insights Into Mechanisms of Basal Ganglia Dysfunction. *Tremor and Other Hyperkinetic Movements, 12*(1). https://doi.org/10.5334/tohm.697

Clarke, K. E. N., Jones, J. M., Deng, Y., Nycz, E., Lee, A., Iachan, R., Gundlapalli, A. V., Hall, A. J., & MacNeil, A. (2022). Seroprevalence of Infection-Induced SARS-CoV-2 Antibodies — United States, September 2021–February 2022. *MMWR. Morbidity and Mortality Weekly Report, 71*(17), 606–608. https://doi.org/10.15585/mmwr.mm7117e3

Classen, J. B. (2021a). COVID-19 RNA Based Vaccines and the Risk of Prion Disease. *Microbiology & Infectious Diseases, 5*(1), 1–3.

Classen, J. B. (2021b). Review of COVID-19 Vaccines and the Risk of Chronic Adverse Events Including Neurological Degeneration. *Journal of Medical - Clinical Research & Reviews, 5*(3), 1–7.

Cloutier, M., Nandi, M., Ihsan, A. U., Chamard, H. A., Ilangumaran, S., & Ramanathan, S. (2020). ADE and hyperinflammation in SARS-CoV2 infection-comparison with dengue hemorrhagic fever and feline infectious peritonitis. *Cytokine, 136*, 155256. https://doi.org/10.1016/j.cyto.2020.155256

Coish, J. M., & MacNeil, A. J. (2020). Out of the frying pan and into the fire? Due diligence warranted for ADE in COVID-19. *Microbes and Infection, 22*(9), 405–406. https://doi.org/10.1016/j.micinf.2020.06.006

Cole, J., Evans, E., Mwangi, M., & Mar, S. (2019). Acute Disseminated Encephalomyelitis in Children: An Updated Review Based on Current Diagnostic Criteria. *Pediatric Neurology, 100*, 26–34. https://doi.org/10.1016/j.pediatrneurol.2019.06.017

Consolini, R., Costagliola, G., Spada, E., Colombatto, P., Orsini, A., Bonuccelli, A., Brunetto, M. R., & Peroni, D. G. (2022). Case Report: MIS-C With Prominent Hepatic and Pancreatic Involvement in a Vaccinated Adolescent – A Critical Reasoning. *Frontiers in Pediatrics, 10*. https://doi.org/10.3389/fped.2022.896903

Corbett, K. S., Edwards, D. K., Leist, S. R., Abiona, O. M., Boyoglu-Barnum, S., Gillespie, R. A., Himansu, S., Schäfer, A., Ziwawo, C. T., DiPiazza, A. T., Dinnon, K. H., Elbashir, S. M., Shaw, C. A., Woods, A., Fritch, E. J., Martinez, D. R., Bock, K. W., Minai, M., Nagata, B. M., … Graham, B. S. (2020). SARS-CoV-2 mRNA vaccine design enabled by prototype pathogen preparedness. *Nature, 586*(7830), 567–571. https://doi.org/10.1038/s41586-020-2622-0

Cortés, H., Hernández-Parra, H., Bernal-Chávez, S. A., Prado-Audelo, M. L. Del, Caballero-Florán, I. H., Borbolla-Jiménez, F. V., González-Torres, M., Magaña, J. J., & Leyva-Gómez, G. (2021). Non-Ionic Surfactants for Stabilization of Polymeric Nanoparticles for Biomedical Uses. *Materials, 14*(12), 3197. https://doi.org/10.3390/ma14123197

Cosentino, C., Torres, L., Vélez, M., Nuñez, Y., Sánchez, D., Armas, C., & Alvarado, M. (2022). SARS-CoV-2 Vaccines and Motor Symptoms in Parkinson's Disease. *Movement Disorders, 37*(1), 233–233. https://doi.org/10.1002/mds.28851

Coudrey, L. (1998). The Troponins. *Archives of Internal Medicine, 158*(11), 1173. https://doi.org/10.1001/archinte.158.11.1173

Crisafulli, S., Sultana, J., Fontana, A., Salvo, F., Messina, S., & Trifirò, G. (2020). Global epidemiology of Duchenne muscular dystrophy: an updated systematic review and meta-analysis. *Orphanet Journal of Rare Diseases*, *15*(1),141. https://doi.org/10.1186/s13023-020-01430-8.

Crommelin, D. J. A., Anchordoquy, T. J., Volkin, D. B., Jiskoot, W., & Mastrobattista, E. (2021). Addressing the Cold Reality of mRNA Vaccine Stability. *Journal of Pharmaceutical Sciences*, *110*(3), 997–1001. https://doi.org/10.1016/j.xphs.2020.12.006

Crystal, R. G. (2014). Adenovirus: The First Effective In Vivo Gene Delivery Vector. *Human Gene Therapy*, *25*(1), 3–11. https://doi.org/10.1089/hum.2013.2527

Cueva-Recalde, J. F., Ibáñez-Muñoz, D., Meseguer-González, D., Sola-Moreno, T., Yanguas-Barea, N., & Ruiz-Arroyo, J. R. (2023). Acute myocarditis after administration of BNT162b2 vaccine against COVID-19. *Archivos de Cardiología de México*, *93*(2). https://doi.org/10.24875/ACM.21000270

Cuspoca, F. A., Estrada, I. P., & Velez-van-Meerbeke, A. (2022). Molecular Mimicry of SARS-CoV-2 Spike Protein in the Nervous System: A Bioinformatics Approach. *Computational and Structural Biotechnology Journal*, *20*, 6041–6054. https://doi.org/10.1016/j.csbj.2022.10.022

Cutillo, G., Saariaho, A.-H., & Meri, S. (2020). Physiology of gangliosides and the role of antiganglioside antibodies in human diseases. *Cellular & Molecular Immunology*, *17*(4), 313–322. https://doi.org/10.1038/s41423-020-0388-9

Czakó, C., Sándor, G., Ecsedy, M., Récsán, Z., Horváth, H., Szepessy, Z., Nagy, Z. Z., & Kovács, I. (2019). Decreased retinal capillary density is associated with a higher risk of diabetic retinopathy in patients with diabetes. *Retina*, *39*(9), 1710–1719. https://doi.org/10.1097/IAE.0000000000002232

Czekay, D. P., & Kothe, U. (2021). H/ACA Small Ribonucleoproteins: Structural and Functional Comparison Between Archaea and Eukaryotes. *Frontiers in Microbiology*, *12*, 654370. https://doi.org/ 10.3389/fmicb.2021.654370.

Dabbousi, A. A., El Masri, J., El Ayoubi, L. M., Ismail, O., Zreika, B., & Salameh, P. (2023). Menstrual abnormalities post-COVID vaccination: a cross-sectional study on adult Lebanese women. *Irish Journal of Medical Science (1971 -)*, *192*(3), 1163–1170. https://doi.org/10.1007/s11845-022-03089-5

D'Agati, V. D., Kudose, S., Bomback, A. S., Adamidis, A., & Tartini, A. (2021). Minimal change disease and acute kidney injury following the Pfizer-BioNTech COVID vaccine. *Kidney International*, *100*(2), 461–463. https://doi.org/10.1016/j.kint.2021.04.035.

Dalmau, J., Gleichman, A. J., Hughes, E. G., Rossi, J. E., Peng, X., Lai, M., Dessain, S. K., Rosenfeld, M. R., Balice-Gordon, R., & Lynch, D. R. (2008). Anti-NMDA-receptor encephalitis: case series and analysis of the effects of antibodies. *The Lancet Neurology*, *7*(12), 1091–1098. https://doi.org/10.1016/S1474-4422(08)70224-2

Dalmau, J., Lancaster, E., Martinez-Hernandez, E., Rosenfeld, M. R., & Balice-Gordon, R. (2011). Clinical experience and laboratory investigations in patients with anti-NMDAR encephalitis. *The Lancet Neurology*, *10*(1), 63–74. https://doi.org/10.1016/S1474-4422(10)70253-2

Dalwadi, V., Hancock, D., Ballout, A. A., & Geraci, A. (2021). Axonal-Variant Guillian-Barre Syndrome Temporally Associated With mRNA-Based Moderna SARS-CoV-2 Vaccine. *Cureus*. https://doi.org/10.7759/cureus.18291

Damase, T. R., Sukhovershin, R., Boada, C., Taraballi, F., Pettigrew, R. I., & Cooke, J. P. (2021). The Limitless Future of RNA Therapeutics. *Frontiers in Bioengetics Biotechnology*, *9*,628137. https://doi.org/10.3389/fbioe.2021.628137.

Dang, Y. L., & Bryson, A. (2021). Miller-Fisher Syndrome and Guillain-Barre Syndrome overlap syndrome in a patient post Oxford-AstraZeneca SARS-CoV-2 vaccination. *BMJ Case Reports*, *14*(11), e246701. https://doi.org/10.1136/bcr-2021-246701

D'Angelo, T., Cattafi, A., Carerj, M. L., Booz, C., Ascenti, G., Cicero, G., Blandino, A., & Mazziotti, S. (2021). Myocarditis After SARS-CoV-2 Vaccination: A Vaccine-Induced Reaction? *Canadian Journal of Cardiology*, *37*(10), 1665–1667. https://doi.org/10.1016/j.cjca.2021.05.010

Darrow, J. J., Avorn, J., & Kesselheim, A. S. (2020). FDA Approval and Regulation of Pharmaceuticals, 1983-2018. *JAMA*, *323*(2), 164. https://doi.org/10.1001/jama.2019.20288

Dash, S., Pai, A. R., Kamath, U., & Rao, P. (2015). Pathophysiology and diagnosis of Guillain–Barré syndrome – challenges and needs. *International Journal of Neuroscience*, *125*(4), 235–240. https://doi.org/10.3109/00207454.2014.913588

Dash, S., Sirka, C. S., Mishra, S., & Viswan, P. (2021). COVID-19 vaccine-induced Stevens–Johnson syndrome. *Clinical and Experimental Dermatology*, *46*(8), 1615–1617. https://doi.org/10.1111/ced.14784

Dassanayaka, W., Liyanaarachchi, K. S., Ala, A., & Bagwan, I. N. (2023). IgG4-related disease: an analysis of the clinicopathological spectrum: UK centre experience. *Journal of Clinical Pathology*, *76*(1), 53–58. https://doi.org/10.1136/jclinpath-2021-207748

Datta, P., Zhang, F., Dordick, J. S., Linhardt, R. J. (2021). Platelet factor 4 polyanion immune complexes: heparin induced thrombocytopenia and vaccine-induced immune thrombotic thrombocytopenia. *Thrombosis Journal, 19*(1), 66. https://doi.org/10.1186/s12959-021-00318-2.

De Biasi, S., Meschiari, M., Gibellini, L., Bellinazzi, C., Borella, R., Fidanza, L., Gozzi, L., Iannone, A., Lo Tartaro, D., Mattioli, M., Paolini, A., Menozzi, M., Milić, J., Franceschi, G., Fantini, R., Tonelli, R., Sita, M., Sarti, M., Trenti, T., … Cossarizza, A. (2020). Marked T cell activation, senescence, exhaustion and skewing towards TH17 in patients with COVID-19 pneumonia. *Nature Communications*, *11*(1), 3434. https://doi.org/10.1038/s41467-020-17292-4

De Domingo, B., López, M., Lopez-Valladares, M., Ortegon-Aguilar, E., Sopeña-Perez-Argüelles, B., & Gonzalez, F. (2022). Vogt-Koyanagi-Harada Disease Exacerbation Associated with COVID-19 Vaccine. *Cells*, *11*(6), 1012. https://doi.org/10.3390/cells11061012

De, R., & Dutta, S. (2022). Role of the Microbiome in the Pathogenesis of COVID-19. *Frontiers in Cellular and Infection Microbiology*, *12*. https://doi.org/10.3389/fcimb.2022.736397

de Vrieze, J. (2020, December 21). Suspicions grow that nanoparticles in Pfizer's COVID-19 vaccine trigger rare allergic reactions. *Science.*

Dean, D. A., Dean, B. S., Muller, S., & Smith, L. C. (1999). Sequence Requirements for Plasmid Nuclear Import. *Experimental Cell Research*, *253*(2), 713–722. https://doi.org/10.1006/excr.1999.4716

Deb, A., Abdelmalek, J., Iwuji, K., & Nugent, K. (2021). Acute Myocardial Injury Following COVID-19 Vaccination: A Case Report and Review of Current

Evidence from Vaccine Adverse Events Reporting System Database. *Journal of Primary Care & Community Health*, *12*, 215013272110292. https://doi.org/10.1177/21501327211029230

DeGruttola, A. K., Low, D., Mizoguchi, A., & Mizoguchi, E. (2016). Current Understanding of Dysbiosis in Disease in Human and Animal Models. *Inflammatory Bowel Diseases*, *22*(5), 1137–1150. https://doi.org/10.1097/MIB.0000000000000750

Deligeoroglou, E., & Karountzos, V. (2018). Abnormal Uterine Bleeding including coagulopathies and other menstrual disorders. *Best Practice & Research Clinical Obstetrics & Gynaecology*, *48*, 51–61. https://doi.org/10.1016/j.bpobgyn.2017.08.016

Deniz, C., Dltunan, B., & Unal, A. (2023). Anti-GAD Encephalitis Following Covid-19 Vaccination: A Case Report. *Archives of Neuropsychiatry*, *60*(3), 283–287. https://doi.org/10.29399/npa.28251

Deshayes, S., Aouba, A., Grateau, G., & Georgin-Lavialle, S. (2021). Infections and AA amyloidosis: An overview. *International Journal of Clinical Practice*, *75*(6). https://doi.org/10.1111/ijcp.13966

Detels, R., Kim, K. S., Gale, J. L, Grayston, J. T. (1971). Viral shedding in Chinese children following vaccination with HPV-77 and Cendehill-51 live attenuated rubella vaccines. *American Journal of Epidemiology*, *94*(5),473–478. https://doi.org/10.1093/oxfordjournals.aje.a121344.

Dettlaff-Pokora, A., & Swierczynski, J. (2021). Dysregulation of the Renin-Angiotensin-Aldosterone System (RAA) in Patients Infected with SARS-CoV-2-Possible Clinical Consequences. *International Journal of Molecular Sciences*, *22*(9), 4503. https://doi.org/10.3390/ijms22094503

Devarbhavi, H., Asrani, S. K., Arab, J. P., Nartey, Y. A., Pose, E., & Kamath, P. S. (2023). Global burden of liver disease: 2023 update. *Journal of Hepatology*, *79*(2), 516–537. https://doi.org/10.1016/j.jhep.2023.03.017

deVeber, G. A., Kirton, A., Booth, F. A., Yager, J. Y., Wirrell, E. C., Wood, E., Shevell, M., Surmava, A.-M., McCusker, P., Massicotte, M. P., MacGregor, D., MacDonald, E. A., Meaney, B., Levin, S., Lemieux, B. G., Jardine, L., Humphreys, P., David, M., Chan, A. K. C., … Bjornson, B. H. (2017). Epidemiology and Outcomes of Arterial Ischemic Stroke in Children: The Canadian Pediatric Ischemic Stroke Registry. *Pediatric Neurology*, *69*, 58–70. https://doi.org/10.1016/j.pediatrneurol.2017.01.016

Dewailly, D., Andersen, C. Y., Balen, A., Broekmans, F., Dilaver, N., Fanchin, R., Griesinger, G., Kelsey, T. W., La Marca, A., Lambalk, C., Mason, H., Nelson, S. M., Visser, J. A., Wallace, W. H., & Anderson, R. A. (2014). The physiology and clinical utility of anti-Müllerian hormone in women. *Human Reproduction Update*, *20*(3), 370–385. https://doi.org/10.1093/humupd/dmt062

Dey, R. K., Ilango, H., Bhatta, S., Shaheed, A., Dole, S., Zooshan, A., Faisham, M., & Murad, M. (2022). Acute pancreatitis in pregnancy following COVID-19 vaccine: a case report. *Journal of Medical Case Reports*, *16*(1), 354. https://doi.org/10.1186/s13256-022-03607-0

Dhasmana, A., Kashyap, V. K., Dhasmana, S., Kotnala, S., Haque, S., Ashraf, G. M., Jaggi, M., Yallapu, M. M., & Chauhan, S. C. (2020). Neutralization of SARS-CoV-2 Spike Protein via Natural Compounds: A Multilayered High Throughput

Virtual Screening Approach. *Current Pharmaceutical Design, 26*(41), 5300–5309. https://doi.org/10.2174/1381612826999200820162937.

Diaz, G. A., Parsons, G. T., Gering, S. K., Meier, A. R., Hutchinson, I. V., & Robicsek, A. (2021). Myocarditis and Pericarditis After Vaccination for COVID-19. *JAMA*, *326*(12), 1210. https://doi.org/10.1001/jama.2021.13443

Dicks, M. D. J., Spencer, A. J., Edwards, N. J., Wadell, G., Bojang, K., Gilbert, S. C., Hill, A. V. S., & Cottingham, M. G. (2012). A Novel Chimpanzee Adenovirus Vector with Low Human Seroprevalence: Improved Systems for Vector Derivation and Comparative Immunogenicity. *PLoS ONE*, *7*(7), e40385. https://doi.org/10.1371/journal.pone.0040385

Dingledine, R., Borges, K., Bowie, D., & Traynelis, S. F. (1999). The glutamate receptor ion channels. *Pharmacological Reviews*, *51*(1), 7–61.

Dinoto, A., Sechi, E., Ferrari, S., Gajofatto, A., Orlandi, R., Solla, P., Maccabeo, A., Maniscalco, G. T., Andreone, V., Sartori, A., Manganotti, P., Rasia, S., Capra, R., Mancinelli, C. R., & Mariotto, S. (2022). Risk of disease relapse following COVID-19 vaccination in patients with AQP4-IgG-positive NMOSD and MOGAD. *Multiple Sclerosis and Related Disorders*, *58*, 103424. https://doi.org/10.1016/j.msard.2021.103424

Dionne, A., Sperotto, F., Chamberlain, S., Baker, A. L., Powell, A. J., Prakash, A., Castellanos, D. A., Saleeb, S. F., de Ferranti, S. D., Newburger, J. W., & Friedman, K. G. (2021). Association of Myocarditis With BNT162b2 Messenger RNA COVID-19 Vaccine in a Case Series of Children. *JAMA Cardiology*, *6*(12), 1446. https://doi.org/10.1001/jamacardio.2021.3471

DiPiazza, A. T., Leist, S. R., Abiona, O. M., Moliva, J. I., Werner, A., Minai, M., Nagata, B. M., Bock, K. W., Phung, E., Schäfer, A., Dinnon, K. H., Chang, L. A., Loomis, R. J., Boyoglu-Barnum, S., Alvarado, G. S., Sullivan, N. J., Edwards, D. K., Morabito, K. M., Mascola, J. R., … Ruckwardt, T. J. (2021). COVID-19 vaccine mRNA-1273 elicits a protective immune profile in mice that is not associated with vaccine-enhanced disease upon SARS-CoV-2 challenge. *Immunity*, *54*(8), 1869-1882.e6. https://doi.org/10.1016/j.immuni.2021.06.018

Do, K., Kawana, E., Do, J., & Diaz, L. (2023). Onset of Guillain-Barre Syndrome and Transverse Myelitis Following COVID-19 Vaccination. *Cureus*. https://doi.org/10.7759/cureus.41009

Doğru, Y., & Kehaya, S. (2022). Do Severe Acute Respiratory Syndrome Coronavirus 2 Vaccines Change Creutzfeldt-Jakob Disease Prognosis? *Balkan Medical Journal*, *39*(5), 381–382. https://doi.org/10.4274/balkanmedj.galenos.2022.2022-6-83

Domazet-Lošo, T. (2022). mRNA Vaccines: Why Is the Biology of Retroposition Ignored? *Genes*, *13*(5), 719. https://doi.org/10.3390/genes13050719

Domińska, K. (2020). Involvement of ACE2/Ang-(1-7)/MAS1 Axis in the Regulation of Ovarian Function in Mammals. *International Journal of Molecular Sciences*, *21*(13), 4572. https://doi.org/10.3390/ijms21134572

Donahue, D. A., Ballesteros, C., Maruggi, G., Glover, C., Ringenberg, M. A., Marquis, M., Ben Abdeljelil, N., Ashraf, A., Rodriguez, L.-A., & Stokes, A. H. (2023). Nonclinical Safety Assessment of Lipid Nanoparticle-and Emulsion-Based Self-Amplifying mRNA Vaccines in Rats. *International Journal of Toxicology*, *42*(1), 37–49. https://doi.org/10.1177/10915818221138781

Donaldson, K., Murphy, F. A., Duffin, R., & Poland, C. A. (2010). Asbestos, carbon nanotubes and the pleural mesothelium: a review and the hypothesis regarding the role of long fibre retention in the parietal pleura, inflammation and mesothelioma. *Particle and Fibre Toxicology*, *7*(1), 5. https://doi.org/10.1186/1743-8977-7-5

Donaldson, L., & Margolin, E. (2023). Variant Guillain–Barre Syndrome Following SARS-CoV-2 Vaccination: Case Report and Review of the Literature. *Canadian Journal of Neurological Sciences / Journal Canadien Des Sciences Neurologiques*, *50*(1), 138–140. https://doi.org/10.1017/cjn.2021.492

Donnelly, J. J., Ulmer, J. B., Shiver, J. W., & Liu, M. A. (1997). DNA VACCINES. *Annual Review of Immunology*, *15*(1), 617–648. https://doi.org/10.1146/annurev.immunol.15.1.617

Dotan, A., & Shoenfeld, Y. (2021). Perspectives on vaccine induced thrombotic thrombocytopenia. *Journal of Autoimmunity*, *121*, 102663. https://doi.org/10.1016/j.jaut.2021.102663

Duerr, A., Huang, Y., Buchbinder, S., Coombs, R. W., Sanchez, J., del Rio, C., Casapia, M., Santiago, S., Gilbert, P., Corey, L., & Robertson, M. N. (2012). Extended Follow-up Confirms Early Vaccine-Enhanced Risk of HIV Acquisition and Demonstrates Waning Effect Over Time Among Participants in a Randomized Trial of Recombinant Adenovirus HIV Vaccine (Step Study). *Journal of Infectious Diseases*, *206*(2), 258–266. https://doi.org/10.1093/infdis/jis342

Dufour, C., Co, T.-K., & Liu, A. (2021). GM1 ganglioside antibody and COVID-19 related Guillain Barre Syndrome – A case report, systemic review and implication for vaccine development. *Brain, Behavior, & Immunity - Health*, *12*, 100203. https://doi.org/10.1016/j.bbih.2021.100203

Dugger, B. N., & Dickson, D. W. (2017). Pathology of Neurodegenerative Diseases. *Cold Spring Harbor Perspectives in Biology*, *9*(7), a028035. https://doi.org/10.1101/cshperspect.a028035

Dumont, C. A., Monserrat, L., Soler, R., Rodríguez, E., Fernández, X., Peteiro, J., Bouzas, B., Piñón, P., & Castro-Beiras, A. (2007). Significado clínico del realce tardío de gadolinio con resonancia magnética en pacientes con miocardiopatía hipertrófica. *Revista Española de Cardiología*, *60*(1), 15–23. https://doi.org/10.1157/13097921

Dumont, J., Euwart, D., Mei, B., Estes, S., & Kshirsagar, R. (2016). Human cell lines for biopharmaceutical manufacturing: history, status, and future perspectives. *Critical Reviews in Biotechnology*, *36*(6), 1110–1122. https://doi.org/10.3109/07388551.2015.1084266

Dunbar, C. E., & Larochelle, A. (2010). Gene therapy activates EVI1, destabilizes chromosomes. *Nature Medicine*, *16*(2), 163–165. https://doi.org/10.1038/nm0210-163

Dupont, J., Reverchon, M., Bertoldo, M. J., & Froment, P. (2014). Nutritional signals and reproduction. *Molecular and Cellular Endocrinology*, *382*(1), 527–537. https://doi.org/10.1016/j.mce.2013.09.028

Dutta, D., Nagappa, M., Sreekumaran Nair, B. V., Das, S. K., Wahatule, R., Sinha, S., Vasanthapuram, R., Taly, A. B., & Debnath, M. (2022). Variations within Toll-like receptor (TLR) and TLR signaling pathway-related genes and their synergistic effects on the risk of Guillain-Barré syndrome. *Journal of the Peripheral Nervous System*, *27*(2), 131–143. https://doi.org/10.1111/jns.12484

Dutta Majumder, P., Sadhu, S., González-López, J. J., & Mochizuki, M. (2023). A COVID-19 perspective of Vogt–Koyanagi–Harada disease. *Indian Journal of Ophthalmology, 71*(6), 2587–2591. https://doi.org/10.4103/IJO.IJO_172_23

Eder, P. S., DeVine, R. J., Dagle, J. M., & Walder, J. A. (1991). Substrate Specificity and Kinetics of Degradation of Antisense Oligonucleotides by a 3′ Exonuclease in Plasma. *Antisense Research and Development, 1*(2), 141–151. https://doi.org/10.1089/ard.1991.1.141

Edmonds, C. E., Zuckerman, S. P., & Conant, E. F. (2021). Management of Unilateral Axillary Lymphadenopathy Detected on Breast MRI in the Era of COVID-19 Vaccination. *American Journal of Roentgenology, 217*(4), 831–834. https://doi.org/10.2214/AJR.21.25604

Eens, S., Van Hecke, M., Favere, K., Tousseyn, T., Guns, P.-J., Roskams, T., & Heidbuchel, H. (2023). B-cell lymphoblastic lymphoma following intravenous BNT162b2 mRNA booster in a BALB/c mouse: A case report. *Frontiers in Oncology, 13*. https://doi.org/10.3389/fonc.2023.1158124

Eren, F., Aygul, R., Tenekeci, S., & Ozturk, S. (2022). Multifocal motor neuropathy after SARS-CoV-2 vaccination: a causal or coincidental association? *Journal of International Medical Research, 50*(7), 030006052211107. https://doi.org/10.1177/03000605221110709

Erro, R., Buonomo, A. R., Barone, P., & Pellecchia, M. T. (2021). Severe Dyskinesia After Administration of SARS-CoV2 mRNA Vaccine in Parkinson's Disease. *Movement Disorders, 36*(10), 2219–2219. https://doi.org/10.1002/mds.28772

Eslait-Olaciregui, S., Llinás-Caballero, K., Patiño-Manjarrés, D., Urbina-Ariza, T., Cediel-Becerra, J. F., & Domínguez-Domínguez, C. A. (2023). Serious neurological adverse events following immunization against SARS-CoV-2: a narrative review of the literature. *Therapeutic Advances in Drug Safety, 14*, 204209862311656. https://doi.org/10.1177/20420986231165674

Etemadifar, M., Nouri, H., Salari, M., & Sedaghat, N. (2022). Detection of anti-NMDA receptor antibodies following BBIBP-CorV COVID-19 vaccination in a rituximab-treated person with multiple sclerosis presenting with manifestations of an acute relapse. *Human Vaccines & Immunotherapeutics, 18*(1). https://doi.org/10.1080/21645515.2022.2033540

Evans, J., & Salamonsen, L. A. (2012). Inflammation, leukocytes and menstruation. *Reviews in Endocrine and Metabolic Disorders, 13*(4), 277–288. https://doi.org/10.1007/s11154-012-9223-7

Eythorsson, E., Runolfsdottir, H. L., Ingvarsson, R. F., Sigurdsson, M. I., & Palsson, R. (2022). Rate of SARS-CoV-2 Reinfection During an Omicron Wave in Iceland. *JAMA Network Open, 5*(8), e2225320. https://doi.org/10.1001/jamanetworkopen.2022.25320

Ezzat, K., & Espay, A. J. (2023). *The allure and pitfalls of the prion-like aggregation in neurodegeneration* (pp. 17–22). https://doi.org/10.1016/B978-0-323-85555-6.00004-7

Fakhari, M. S., Poorsaadat, L., & Mahmoodiyeh, B. (2022). Guillain-Barré syndrome following COVID-19 vaccine: A case report. *Clinical Case Reports, 10*(10). https://doi.org/10.1002/ccr3.6451

Falk, R. H., Alexander, K. M., Liao, R., & Dorbala, S. (2016). AL (Light-Chain) Cardiac Amyloidosis. *Journal of the American College of Cardiology, 68*(12), 1323–1341. https://doi.org/10.1016/j.jacc.2016.06.053

Fallaux, F. J., Bout, A., van der Velde, I., van den Wollenberg, D. J. M., Hehir, K. M., Keegan, J., Auger, C., Cramer, S. J., van Ormondt, H., van der Eb, A. J., Valerio, D., & Hoeben, R. C. (1998). New Helper Cells and Matched Early Region 1-Deleted Adenovirus Vectors Prevent Generation of Replication-Competent Adenoviruses. *Human Gene Therapy*, *9*(13), 1909–1917. https://doi.org/10.1089/hum.1998.9.13-1909

Falsey, A. R., Sobieszczyk, M. E., Hirsch, I., Sproule, S., Robb, M. L., Corey, L., Neuzil, K. M., Hahn, W., Hunt, J., Mulligan, M. J., McEvoy, C., DeJesus, E., Hassman, M., Little, S. J., Pahud, B. A., Durbin, A., Pickrell, P., Daar, E. S., Bush, L., … Gonzalez-Lopez, A. (2021). Phase 3 Safety and Efficacy of AZD1222 (ChAdOx1 nCoV-19) Covid-19 Vaccine. *New England Journal of Medicine*, *385*(25), 2348–2360. https://doi.org/10.1056/NEJMoa2105290

Farland, L. V., Khan, S. M., Shilen, A., Heslin, K. M., Ishimwe, P., Allen, A. M., Herbst-Kralovetz, M. M., Mahnert, N. D., Pogreba-Brown, K., Ernst, K. C., & Jacobs, E. T. (2023). COVID-19 vaccination and changes in the menstrual cycle among vaccinated persons. *Fertility and Sterility*, *119*(3), 392–400. https://doi.org/10.1016/j.fertnstert.2022.12.023

Farsalinos, K., Niaura, R., Le Houezec, J., Barbouni, A., Tsatsakis, A., Kouretas, D., Vantarakis, A., & Poulas, K. (2020). Editorial: Nicotine and SARS-CoV-2: COVID-19 may be a disease of the nicotinic cholinergic system. *Toxicology Reports*, *7*, 658–663. https://doi.org/10.1016/j.toxrep.2020.04.012

Fasano, G., Bennardo, L., Ruffolo, S., Passante, M., Ambrosio, A. G., Napolitano, M., Provenzano, E., Nisticò, S. P., & Patruno, C. (2022). Erythema Migrans-like COVID Vaccine Arm: A Literature Review. *Journal of Clinical Medicine*, *11*(3), 797. https://doi.org/10.3390/jcm11030797

Faulkner, G. J., & Garcia-Perez, J. L. (2017). L1 Mosaicism in Mammals: Extent, Effects, and Evolution. *Trends in Genetics*, *33*(11), 802–816. https://doi.org/10.1016/j.tig.2017.07.004

Fedak, K. M., Bernal, A., Capshaw, Z. A., & Gross, S. (2015). Applying the Bradford Hill criteria in the 21st century: how data integration has changed causal inference in molecular epidemiology. *Emerging Themes in Epidemiology*, *12*(1), 14. https://doi.org/10.1186/s12982-015-0037-4

Federspiel, J. M., Ramsthaler, F., Kettner, M., & Mall, G. (2023). Diagnostics of messenger ribonucleic acid (mRNA) severe acute respiratory syndrome-corona virus-2 (SARS-CoV-2) vaccination-associated myocarditis-A systematic review. *Rechtsmedizin* (Berl). 33(2), 125–131. https://doi.org/10.1007/s00194-022-00587-9.

Feghali, E. junior, Challa, A., Mahdi, M., Acosta, E., & Jackson, J. (2023). New-Onset Amyotrophic Lateral Sclerosis in a Patient who Received the J&J/Janssen COVID-19 Vaccine. *Kansas Journal of Medicine*, *16*(1), 69–70. https://doi.org/10.17161/kjm.vol16.18969

Fei, P., Feng, H., Li, J., Liu, M., Luo, J., Ye, H., & Zhao, P. (2022). Inflammatory ocular events after inactivated COVID-19 vaccination. *Human Vaccines & Immunotherapeutics*, *18*(6). https://doi.org/10.1080/21645515.2022.2138051

Feldman, E. L., Goutman, S. A., Petri, S., Mazzini, L., Savelieff, M. G., Shaw, P. J., & Sobue, G. (2022). Amyotrophic lateral sclerosis. *The Lancet*, *400*(10360), 1363–1380. https://doi.org/10.1016/S0140-6736(22)01272-7

Ferin, M. (1999). Stress and the Reproductive Cycle. *The Journal of Clinical Endocrinology & Metabolism*, *84*(6), 1768–1774. https://doi.org/10.1210/jcem.84.6.5367

Fernández, P., Alaye, M. L., Chiple, M. E. G., Arteaga, J. De, Douthat, W., Fuente, J. D. La, & Chiurchiu, C. (2023). Glomerulopathies after vaccination against COVID-19. Four cases with three different vaccines in Argentina. *Nefrología*, *43*(5), 655–657. https://doi.org/10.1016/j.nefro.2021.09.003

Ferris, R. L., Lu, B., & Kane, L. P. (2014). Too Much of a Good Thing? Tim-3 and TCR Signaling in T Cell Exhaustion. *The Journal of Immunology*, *193*(4), 1525–1530. https://doi.org/10.4049/jimmunol.1400557

Fertig, T. E., Chitoiu, L., Marta, D. S., Ionescu, V.-S., Cismasiu, V. B., Radu, E., Angheluta, G., Dobre, M., Serbanescu, A., Hinescu, M. E., & Gherghiceanu, M. (2022). Vaccine mRNA Can Be Detected in Blood at 15 Days Post-Vaccination. *Biomedicines*, *10*(7), 1538. https://doi.org/10.3390/biomedicines10071538

Fijak, M., & Meinhardt, A. (2006). The testis in immune privilege. *Immunological Reviews*, *213*(1), 66–81. https://doi.org/10.1111/j.1600-065X.2006.00438.x

Filicori, M., Cognigni, G., Dellai, P., Arnone, R., Sambataro, M., Falbo, A., Pecorari, R., Carbone, F., & Meriggiola, M. C. (1993). Role of gonadotrophin releasing hormone secretory dynamics in the control of the human menstrual cycle. *Human Reproduction*, *8*(suppl 2), 62–65. https://doi.org/10.1093/humrep/8.suppl_2.62

Fillon, A., Sautenet, B., Barbet, C., Moret, L., Thillard, E. M., Jonville-Béra, A. P., & Halimi, J. M. (2022). De novo and relapsing necrotizing vasculitis after COVID-19 vaccination. *Clinical Kidney Journal*, *15*(3), 560–563. https://doi.org/10.1093/ckj/sfab285

Filosto, M., Cotti Piccinelli, S., Gazzina, S., Foresti, C., Frigeni, B., Servalli, M. C., Sessa, M., Cosentino, G., Marchioni, E., Ravaglia, S., Briani, C., Castellani, F., Zara, G., Bianchi, F., Del Carro, U., Fazio, R., Filippi, M., Magni, E., Natalini, G., … Uncini, A. (2021). Guillain-Barré syndrome and COVID-19: an observational multicentre study from two Italian hotspot regions. *Journal of Neurology, Neurosurgery & Psychiatry*, *92*(7), 751–756. https://doi.org/10.1136/jnnp-2020-324837

Finn, R. M., Ellard, K., Eirín-López, J. M., & Ausió, J. (2012). Vertebrate nucleoplasmin and NASP: egg histone storage proteins with multiple chaperone activities. *The FASEB Journal*, *26*(12), 4788–4804. https://doi.org/10.1096/fj.12-216663

Finsterer, J. (2021a). SARS-CoV-2 vaccinations are unsafe for those experiencing post-vaccination Guillain-Barre syndrome. *Annals of Medicine & Surgery*, *68*. https://doi.org/10.1016/j.amsu.2021.102584

Finsterer, J. (2021b). SARS-CoV-2 vaccinations may not only be complicated by GBS but also by distal small fibre neuropathy. *Journal of Neuroimmunology*, *360*, 577703. https://doi.org/10.1016/j.jneuroim.2021.577703

Finsterer, J. (2022). Neuromyelitis optica complicating COVID vaccinations. *Multiple Sclerosis and Related Disorders*, *62*, 103809. https://doi.org/10.1016/j.msard.2022.103809

Finsterer, J. (2023). Neurological Adverse Reactions to SARS-CoV-2 Vaccines. *Clinical Psychopharmacology and Neuroscience*, *21*(2), 222–239. https://doi.org/10.9758/cpn.2023.21.2.222

Finsterer, J., & Scorza, F. A. (2022). A retrospective analysis of clinically confirmed long post-COVID vaccination syndrome. *Journal of Clinical Translational Research, 8*(6), 506–508.

Finsterer, J., Scorza, F. A., & Scorza, C. A. (2021). Post SARS-CoV-2 vaccination Guillain-Barre syndrome in 19 patients. *Clinics, 76*, e3286. https://doi.org/10.6061/clinics/2021/e3286

Fiorillo, G., Pancetti, S., Cortese, A., Toso, F., Manara, S., Costanzo, A., & Borroni, R. G. (2022). Leukocytoclastic vasculitis (cutaneous small-vessel vasculitis) after COVID-19 vaccination. *Journal of Autoimmunity, 127*, 102783. https://doi.org/10.1016/j.jaut.2021.102783

Firak, T. A., & Subramanian, K. N. (1986). Minimal Transcriptional Enhancer of Simian Virus 40 is a 74-Base-Pair Sequence That Has Interacting Domains. *Molecular and Cellular Biology, 6*(11), 3667–3676. https://doi.org/10.1128/mcb.6.11.3667-3676.1986

Flajnik, M. F. (2014). Re-evaluation of the Immunological Big Bang. *Current Biology, 24*(21), R1060–R1065. https://doi.org/10.1016/j.cub.2014.09.070

Flanagan, K. L., Best, E., Crawford, N. W., Giles, M., Koirala, A., Macartney, K., Russell, F., Teh, B. W., & Wen, S. C. (2020). Progress and Pitfalls in the Quest for Effective SARS-CoV-2 (COVID-19) Vaccines. *Frontiers in Immunology, 11*. https://doi.org/10.3389/fimmu.2020.579250

Flannery, P., Yang, I., Keyvani, M., & Sakoulas, G. (2021). Acute Psychosis Due to Anti-N-Methyl D-Aspartate Receptor Encephalitis Following COVID-19 Vaccination: A Case Report. *Frontiers in Neurology, 12*. https://doi.org/10.3389/fneur.2021.764197

Flores-Terry, M. Á., García-Arpa, M., Santiago-Sánchez Mateo, J. L., & Romero Aguilera, G. (2022). Lesiones faciales de vitíligo tras la administración de la vacuna frente a SARS-CoV-2. *Actas Dermo-Sifiliográficas, 113*(7), 721. https://doi.org/10.1016/j.ad.2022.01.030

Folds, A. J., Ullrich, M.-B., Htoo, S., & Chukus, A. (2022). Sporadic Creutzfeldt-Jakob Disease After Receiving the Second Dose of Pfizer-BioNTechCOVID-19 Vaccine. *Internal Medicine., 420*. https://scholarlycommons.hcahealthcare.com/internal-medicine/420

Formeister, E. J., Chien, W., Agrawal, Y., Carey, J. P., Stewart, C. M., & Sun, D. Q. (2021). Preliminary Analysis of Association Between COVID-19 Vaccination and Sudden Hearing Loss Using US Centers for Disease Control and Prevention Vaccine Adverse Events Reporting System Data. *JAMA Otolaryngology–Head & Neck Surgery, 147*(7), 674. https://doi.org/10.1001/jamaoto.2021.0869

Forrester, J. V, Xu, H., Lambe, T., & Cornall, R. (2008). Immune privilege or privileged immunity? *Mucosal Immunology, 1*(5), 372–381. https://doi.org/10.1038/mi.2008.27

Foster, C., & Al-Zubeidi, H. (2018). Menstrual Irregularities. *Pediatric Annals, 47*(1). https://doi.org/10.3928/19382359-20171219-01

Fragiel, M., Miró, Ò., Llorens, P., Jiménez, S., Piñera, P., Burillo, G., Martín, A., Martín-Sánchez, F. J., García-Lamberechts, E. J., Jacob, J., Alquézar-Arbé, A., Juárez, R., Jiménez, B., Del Rio, R., Mateo Roca, M., García, A. H., López Laguna, N., Lopez Diez, M. P., Pedraza García, J., … González del Castillo, J. (2021). Incidence, clinical, risk factors and outcomes of Guillain-Barré in Covid-19. *Annals of Neurology, 89*(3), 598–603. https://doi.org/10.1002/ana.25987

Fragkos, M., Breuleux, M., Clément, N., & Beard, P. (2008). Recombinant adeno-associated viral vectors are deficient in provoking a DNA damage response. *Journal of Virology*, *82*(15), 7379–7387. https://doi.org/10.1128/JVI.00358-08.

Fraiman, J., Erviti, J., Jones, M., Greenland, S., Whelan, P., Kaplan, R. M., & Doshi, P. (2022). Serious adverse events of special interest following mRNA COVID-19 vaccination in randomized trials in adults. *Vaccine*, *40*(40), 5798–5805. https://doi.org/10.1016/j.vaccine.2022.08.036

Frangogiannis, N. G. (2015). Pathophysiology of Myocardial Infarction. *Comprehensive Physiology*, *5*(4), 1841–1875. https://doi.org/10.1002/cphy.c150006

Freeman, M. L., Sheridan, B. S., Bonneau, R. H., & Hendricks, R. L. (2007). Psychological Stress Compromises CD8+ T Cell Control of Latent Herpes Simplex Virus Type 1 Infections. *The Journal of Immunology*, *179*(1), 322–328. https://doi.org/10.4049/jimmunol.179.1.322

Freire de Castro, R., Crema, D., Neiva, F. C., Pinto, R. A. S. R., & Suzuki, F. A. (2022). Prevalence of herpes zoster virus reactivation in patients diagnosed with Bell's palsy. *The Journal of Laryngology & Otology*, *136*(10), 975–978. https://doi.org/10.1017/S0022215121004631

Fu, Y., Xu, H., & Liu, S. (2022). COVID-19 and neurodegenerative diseases. *European Review for Medical and Pharmacological Sciences*, *26*(12), 4535–4544.

Fuchs, J. C., & Tucker, A. S. (2015). *Development and Integration of the Ear* (pp. 213–232). https://doi.org/10.1016/bs.ctdb.2015.07.007

Fujikawa, P., Shah, F. A., Braford, M., Patel, K., & Madey, J. (2021). Neuromyelitis Optica in a Healthy Female After Severe Acute Respiratory Syndrome Coronavirus 2 mRNA-1273 Vaccine. *Cureus*. https://doi.org/10.7759/cureus.17961

Fukushima, T., Tomita, M., Ikeda, S., & Hattori, N. (2022). A case of sensory ataxic Guillain–Barré syndrome with immunoglobulin G anti-GM1 antibodies following the first dose of mRNA COVID-19 vaccine BNT162b2 (Pfizer). *QJM: An International Journal of Medicine*, *115*(1), 25–27. https://doi.org/10.1093/qjmed/hcab296

Fukutomi, Y. (2019). Occupational food allergy. *Current Opinion in Allergy & Clinical Immunology*, *19*(3), 243–248. https://doi.org/10.1097/ACI.0000000000000530

Funabiki, M., Kato, H., Miyachi, Y., Toki, H., Motegi, H., Inoue, M., Minowa, O., Yoshida, A., Deguchi, K., Sato, H., Ito, S., Shiroishi, T., Takeyasu, K., Noda, T., & Fujita, T. (2014). Autoimmune Disorders Associated with Gain of Function of the Intracellular Sensor MDA5. *Immunity*, *40*(2), 199–212. https://doi.org/10.1016/j.immuni.2013.12.014

Fung, M., Thornton, A., Mybeck, K., Wu, J. H.-H., Hornbuckle, K., & Muniz, E. (2001). Evaluation of the Characteristics of Safety Withdrawal of Prescription Drugs from Worldwide Pharmaceutical Markets-1960 to 1999. *Drug Information Journal*, *35*(1), 293–317. https://doi.org/10.1177/009286150103500134

Gale, S. A., Acar, D., & Daffner, K. R. (2018). Dementia. *The American Journal of Medicine*, *131*(10), 1161–1169. https://doi.org/10.1016/j.amjmed.2018.01.022

Gallimore, A., Glithero, A., Godkin, A., Tissot, A. C., Plückthun, A., Elliott, T., Hengartner, H., & Zinkernagel, R. (1998). Induction and Exhaustion of Lymphocytic Choriomeningitis Virus–specific Cytotoxic T Lymphocytes

Visualized Using Soluble Tetrameric Major Histocompatibility Complex Class I–Peptide Complexes. *The Journal of Experimental Medicine*, *187*(9), 1383–1393. https://doi.org/10.1084/jem.187.9.1383

Gallot, D., Seifer, I., Lemery, D., & Bignon, Y. J. (2002). Systemic Diffusion Including Germ Cells after Plasmidic in utero Gene Transfer in the Rat. *Fetal Diagnosis and Therapy*, *17*(3), 157–162. https://doi.org/10.1159/000048030

Gambichler, T., Boms, S., Hessam, S., Tischoff, I., Tannapfel, A., Lüttringhaus, T., Beckman, J., & Stranzenbach, R. (2021). Primary cutaneous anaplastic large-cell lymphoma with marked spontaneous regression of organ manifestation after SARS-CoV-2 vaccination. *British Journal of Dermatology*, *185*(6), 1259–1262. https://doi.org/10.1111/bjd.20630

Gambichler, T., Boms, S., Susok, L., Dickel, H., Finis, C., Abu Rached, N., Barras, M., Stücker, M., & Kasakovski, D. (2022). Cutaneous findings following COVID-19 vaccination: review of world literature and own experience. *Journal of the European Academy of Dermatology and Venereology*, *36*(2), 172–180. https://doi.org/10.1111/jdv.17744

Gamonal, S. B. L., Gamonal, A. C. C., Marques, N. C. V., & Adário, C. L. (2022). Lichen planus and vitiligo occurring after ChAdOx1 nCoV -19 vaccination against SARS-CoV-2. *Dermatologic Therapy*, *35*(5). https://doi.org/10.1111/dth.15422

Gamonal, S. B. L., Marques, N. C. V., Pereira, H. M. B., & Gamonal, A. C. C. (2023). Drug reaction with eosinophilia and systemic symptoms syndrome (DRESS) associated with pancreatitis and hepatitis following Pfizer BioNTech mRNA COVID-19 vaccination. *Journal of the European Academy of Dermatology and Venereology*, *37*(3). https://doi.org/10.1111/jdv.18777

Gang, J., Wang, H., Xue, X., & Zhang, S. (2022). Microbiota and COVID-19: Long-term and complex influencing factors. *Frontiers in Microbiology*, *13*. https://doi.org/10.3389/fmicb.2022.963488

Ganz, P., Heidecker, B., Hveem, K., Jonasson, C., Kato, S., Segal, M. R., Sterling, D. G., & Williams, S. A. (2016). Development and Validation of a Protein-Based Risk Score for Cardiovascular Outcomes Among Patients With Stable Coronary Heart Disease. *JAMA*, *315*(23), 2532. https://doi.org/10.1001/jama.2016.5951

Gao, X., Kouklis, P., Xu, N., Minshall, R. D., Sandoval, R., Vogel, S. M., & Malik, A. B. (2000). Reversibility of increased microvessel permeability in response to VE-cadherin disassembly. *American Journal of Physiology-Lung Cellular and Molecular Physiology*, *279*(6), L1218–L1225. https://doi.org/10.1152/ajplung.2000.279.6.L1218

Gao, X., Zhang, S., Gou, J., Wen, Y., Fan, L., Zhou, J., Zhou, G., Xu, G., & Zhang, Z. (2022). Spike-mediated ACE2 down-regulation was involved in the pathogenesis of SARS-CoV-2 infection. *Journal of Infection*, *85*(4), 418–427. https://doi.org/10.1016/j.jinf.2022.06.030

Garay, R. P., El-Gewely, R., Armstrong, J. K., Garratty, G., & Richette, P. (2012). Antibodies against polyethylene glycol in healthy subjects and in patients treated with PEG-conjugated agents. *Expert Opinion on Drug Delivery*, *9*(11), 1319–1323. https://doi.org/10.1517/17425247.2012.720969

Garg, N., & Smith, T. W. (2015). An update on immunopathogenesis, diagnosis, and treatment of multiple sclerosis. *Brain and Behavior*, *5*(9). https://doi.org/10.1002/brb3.362

Garg, R. K., & Paliwal, V. K. (2022). Spectrum of neurological complications following COVID-19 vaccination. *Neurological Sciences*, *43*(1), 3–40. https://doi.org/10.1007/s10072-021-05662-9

Garg, R., Paliwal, V., Malhotra, H., Singh, B., Rizvi, I., & Kumar, N. (2023). Spectrum of Serious Neurological and Psychiatric Adverse Events in Indian COVID-19 Vaccine Recipients: A Systematic Review of Case Reports and Case Series. *Neurology India*, *71*(2), 209. https://doi.org/10.4103/0028-3886.375420

Garner, S. E., Fidan, D., Frankish, R. R., & Maxwell, L. (2005). Rofecoxib for osteoarthritis. *Cochrane Database of Systematic Reviews*, *2010*(1). https://doi.org/10.1002/14651858.CD005115

Garrido, I., Lopes, S., Simões, M. S., Liberal, R., Lopes, J., Carneiro, F., & Macedo, G. (2021). Autoimmune hepatitis after COVID-19 vaccine – more than a coincidence. *Journal of Autoimmunity*, *125*, 102741. https://doi.org/10.1016/j.jaut.2021.102741

Gartlan, C., Tipton, T., Salguero, F. J., Sattentau, Q., Gorringe, A., & Carroll, M. W. (2022). Vaccine-Associated Enhanced Disease and Pathogenic Human Coronaviruses. *Frontiers in Immunology*, *13*. https://doi.org/10.3389/fimmu.2022.882972

Garwood, J., Heck, N., Reichardt, F., & Faissner, A. (2003). Phosphacan Short Isoform, a Novel Non-proteoglycan Variant of Phosphacan/Receptor Protein Tyrosine Phosphatase-β, Interacts with Neuronal Receptors and Promotes Neurite Outgrowth. *Journal of Biological Chemistry*, *278*(26), 24164–24173. https://doi.org/10.1074/jbc.M211721200

Gasior, S. L., Wakeman, T. P., Xu, B., & Deininger, P. L. (2006). The Human LINE-1 Retrotransposon Creates DNA Double-strand Breaks. *Journal of Molecular Biology*, *357*(5), 1383–1393. https://doi.org/10.1016/j.jmb.2006.01.089

Gat, I., Kedem, A., Dviri, M., Umanski, A., Levi, M., Hourvitz, A., & Baum, M. (2022). Covid-19 vaccination BNT162b2 temporarily impairs semen concentration and total motile count among semen donors. *Andrology*, *10*(6), 1016–1022. https://doi.org/10.1111/andr.13209

Gázquez-Gutiérrez, A., Witteveldt, J., Heras, S. R., & Macias, S. (2021). Sensing of transposable elements by the antiviral innate immune system. *RNA*, *27*(7), 735–752. https://doi.org/10.1261/rna.078721.121

Gedik, B., Bozdogan, Y. C., Yavuz, S., Durmaz, D., & Erol, M. K. (2022). The assesment of retina and optic disc vascular structures in people who received CoronaVac vaccine. *Photodiagnosis and Photodynamic Therapy*, *38*, 102742. https://doi.org/10.1016/j.pdpdt.2022.102742

Gedik, B., Erol, M. K., Suren, E., Yavuz, S., Kucuk, M. F., Bozdogan, Y. C., Ekinci, R., & Akidan, M. (2023). Evaluation of retinal and optic disc vascular structures in individuals before and after Pfizer-BioNTech vaccination. *Microvascular Research*, *147*, 104500. https://doi.org/10.1016/j.mvr.2023.104500

Gee, J., Marquez, P., Su, J., Calvert, G. M., Liu, R., Myers, T., Nair, N., Martin, S., Clark, T., Markowitz, L., Lindsey, N., Zhang, B., Licata, C., Jazwa, A., Sotir, M., & Shimabukuro, T. (2021). First Month of COVID-19 Vaccine Safety Monitoring - United States, December 14, 2020-January 13, 2021. *MMWR Morbidity and Mortality Weekly Report, 70*(8), 283–288. https://doi.org/10.15585/mmwr.mm7008e3.

George, E., Richie, M. B., & Glastonbury, C. M. (2020). Facial Nerve Palsy: Clinical Practice and Cognitive Errors. *The American Journal of Medicine*, *133*(9), 1039–1044. https://doi.org/10.1016/j.amjmed.2020.04.023

Gerhard, A., Raeder, V., Pernice, H. F., Boesl, F., Schroeder, M., Richter, J., Endres, M., Prüß, H., Hahn, K., Audebert, H. J., & Franke, C. (2023). Neurological symptoms after COVID-19 vaccination: a report on the clinical presentation of the first 50 patients. *Journal of Neurology*, *270*(10), 4673–4677. https://doi.org/10.1007/s00415-023-11895-9

Geuking, M. B., Weber, J., Dewannieux, M., Gorelik, E., Heidmann, T., Hengartner, H., Zinkernagel, R. M., & Hangartner, L. (2009). Recombination of Retrotransposon and Exogenous RNA Virus Results in Nonretroviral cDNA Integration. *Science*, *323*(5912), 393–396. https://doi.org/10.1126/science.1167375

Ghaderi, S., Mohammadi, S., Heidari, M., Sharif Jalali, S. S., & Mohammadi, M. (2023). Post-COVID-19 Vaccination CNS Magnetic Resonance Imaging Findings: A Systematic Review. *Canadian Journal of Infectious Diseases and Medical Microbiology*, 1–22. https://doi.org/10.1155/2023/1570830

Gianicolo, E. A. L., Eichler, M., Muensterer, O., Strauch, K., & Blettner, M. (2020). Methods for Evaluating Causality in Observational Studies. *Deutsches Ärzteblatt International*. https://doi.org/10.3238/arztebl.2020.0101

Gibson, E., Li, H., Fruh, V., Gabra, M., Asokan, G., Jukic, A., Baird, D., Curry, C., Fischer-Colbrie, T., Onnela, J., Williams, M., Hauser, R., Coull, B., & Mahalingaiah, S. (2022). Covid-19 vaccination and menstrual cycle length in the Apple Women's Health Study. *NPJ Digital Medicine*. https://doi.org/10.1101/2022.07.07.22277371

Gilbert, S. C. (2002). Bell's palsy and herpesviruses. *Herpes : The Journal of the IHMF*, *9*(3), 70–73.

Gill, J. R., Tashjian, R., & Duncanson, E. (2022). Autopsy Histopathologic Cardiac Findings in 2 Adolescents Following the Second COVID-19 Vaccine Dose. *Archives of Pathology & Laboratory Medicine*, *146*(8), 925–929. https://doi.org/10.5858/arpa.2021-0435-SA

Glenting, J., & Wessels, S. (2005). Ensuring safety of DNA vaccines. *Microbial Cell Factories*, *4*(1), 26. https://doi.org/10.1186/1475-2859-4-26

Goh CY, C., Teng Keat, C., Su Kien, C., & Ai Sim, G. (2022). A probable case of vaccine-induced immune thrombotic thrombocytopenia secondary to Pfizer Comirnaty COVID-19 vaccine. *Journal of the Royal College of Physicians of Edinburgh*, *52*(2), 113–116. https://doi.org/10.1177/14782715221103660

Goldman, S., Bron, D., Tousseyn, T., Vierasu, I., Dewispelaere, L., Heimann, P., Cogan, E., & Goldman, M. (2021). Rapid Progression of Angioimmunoblastic T Cell Lymphoma Following BNT162b2 mRNA Vaccine Booster Shot: A Case Report. *Frontiers in Medicine*, *8*. https://doi.org/10.3389/fmed.2021.798095

Goldsmith, D. R., Rapaport, M. H., & Miller, B. J. (2016). A meta-analysis of blood cytokine network alterations in psychiatric patients: comparisons between schizophrenia, bipolar disorder and depression. *Molecular Psychiatry*, *21*(12), 1696–1709. https://doi.org/10.1038/mp.2016.3

Gonen, M. S., De Bellis, A., Durcan, E., Bellastella, G., Cirillo, P., Scappaticcio, L., Longo, M., Bircan, B. E., Sahin, S., Sulu, C., Ozkaya, H. M., Konukoglu, D., Kartufan, F. F., & Kelestimur, F. (2022). Assessment of Neuroendocrine Changes and Hypothalamo-Pituitary Autoimmunity in Patients with COVID-19. *Hormone and Metabolic Research*, *54*(03), 153–161. https://doi.org/10.1055/a-1764-1260

Gonzalez, D. C., Nassau, D. E., Khodamoradi, K., Ibrahim, E., Blachman-Braun, R., Ory, J., & Ramasamy, R. (2021). Sperm Parameters Before and After COVID-19 mRNA Vaccination. *JAMA*, *326*(3), 273. https://doi.org/10.1001/jama.2021.9976

Gopallawa, I., & Uhal, B. D. (2014). Molecular and cellular mechanisms of the inhibitory effects of ACE-2/ANG1-7/Mas axis on lung injury. *Current Topics in Pharmacology*, *18*(1), 71–80.

Gordon, J. A. (2010). Testing the glutamate hypothesis of schizophrenia. *Nature Neuroscience*, *13*(1), 2–4. https://doi.org/10.1038/nn0110-2

Gorman, C., Lane, D., & Rigby, P. (1984). High efficiency gene transfer into mammalian cells. *Philosophical Transactions of the Royal Society of London. B, Biological Sciences*, *307*(1132), 343–346. https://doi.org/10.1098/rstb.1984.0137

Goswami, T. K., Singh, M., Dhawan, M., Mitra, S., Emran, T. Bin, Rabaan, A. A., Mutair, A. Al, Alawi, Z. Al, Alhumaid, S., & Dhama, K. (2022). Regulatory T cells (Tregs) and their therapeutic potential against autoimmune disorders – Advances and challenges. *Human Vaccines & Immunotherapeutics*, *18*(1). https://doi.org/10.1080/21645515.2022.2035117

Graham, F. L., Smiley, J., Russell, W. C., & Nairn, R. (1977). Characteristics of a human cell line transformed by DNA from human adenovirus type 5. *Journal of General Virology, 36*(1), 59–74. https://doi.org/10.1099/0022-1317-36-1-59.

Grandi, N., & Tramontano, E. (2018). HERV Envelope Proteins: Physiological Role and Pathogenic Potential in Cancer and Autoimmunity. *Frontiers in Microbiology*, *9*. https://doi.org/10.3389/fmicb.2018.00462

Gray, G., Buchbinder, S., & Duerr, A. (2010). Overview of STEP and Phambili trial results: two phase IIb test-of-concept studies investigating the efficacy of MRK adenovirus type 5 gag/pol/nef subtype B HIV vaccine. *Current Opinion in HIV and AIDS*, *5*(5), 357–361. https://doi.org/10.1097/COH.0b013e32833d2d2b

Gray, G. E., Allen, M., Moodie, Z., Churchyard, G., Bekker, L.-G., Nchabeleng, M., Mlisana, K., Metch, B., de Bruyn, G., Latka, M. H., Roux, S., Mathebula, M., Naicker, N., Ducar, C., Carter, D. K., Puren, A., Eaton, N., McElrath, M. J., Robertson, M., … Kublin, J. G. (2011). Safety and efficacy of the HVTN 503/Phambili Study of a clade-B-based HIV-1 vaccine in South Africa: a double-blind, randomised, placebo-controlled test-of-concept phase 2b study. *The Lancet Infectious Diseases*, *11*(7), 507–515. https://doi.org/10.1016/S1473-3099(11)70098-6

Green, M. D., & Al-Humadi, N. H. (2017). Preclinical Toxicology of Vaccines. *In*: A Comprehensive Guide to Toxicology in Nonclinical Drug Development (Second Edition). https://www.sciencedirect.com/book/9780128036204/a-comprehensive-guide-to-toxicology-in-nonclinical-drug-development.

Greenhawt, M., Abrams, E. M., Shaker, M., Chu, D. K., Khan, D., Akin, C., Alqurashi, W., Arkwright, P., Baldwin, J. L., Ben-Shoshan, M., Bernstein, J., Bingemann, T., Blumchen, K., Byrne, A., Bognanni, A., Campbell, D., Campbell, R., Chagla, Z., Chan, E. S., … Golden, D. B. K. (2021). The Risk of Allergic Reaction to SARS-CoV-2 Vaccines and Recommended Evaluation and Management: A Systematic Review, Meta-Analysis, GRADE Assessment, and International Consensus Approach. *The Journal of Allergy and Clinical*

Immunology: In Practice, *9*(10), 3546–3567. https://doi.org/10.1016/j.jaip.2021.06.006
Greinacher, A., Selleng, K., Palankar, R., Wesche, J., Handtke, S., Wolff, M., Aurich, K., Lalk, M., Methling, K., Völker, U., Hentschker, C., Michalik, S., Steil, L., Reder, A., Schönborn, L., Beer, M., Franzke, K., Büttner, A., Fehse, B., … Renné, T. (2021). Insights in ChAdOx1 nCoV-19 vaccine-induced immune thrombotic thrombocytopenia. *Blood*, *138*(22), 2256–2268. https://doi.org/10.1182/blood.2021013231
Greinacher, A., Selleng, K., & Warkentin, T. E. (2017). Autoimmune heparin-induced thrombocytopenia. *Journal of Thrombosis and Haemostasis*, *15*(11), 2099–2114. https://doi.org/10.1111/jth.13813
Greulich, S., Seitz, A., Müller, K. A. L., Grün, S., Ong, P., Ebadi, N., Kreisselmeier, K. P., Seizer, P., Bekeredjian, R., Zwadlo, C., Gräni, C., Klingel, K., Gawaz, M., Sechtem, U., & Mahrholdt, H. (2020). Predictors of Mortality in Patients With Biopsy-Proven Viral Myocarditis: 10-Year Outcome Data. *Journal of the American Heart Association*, *9*(16). https://doi.org/10.1161/JAHA.119.015351
Griffin, J. P. (2004). Venetian treacle and the foundation of medicines regulation. *British Journal of Clinical Pharmacology*, *58*(3), 317–325. https://doi.org/10.1111/j.1365-2125.2004.02147.x
Grifoni, A., Sidney, J., Vita, R., Peters, B., Crotty, S., Weiskopf, D., & Sette, A. (2021). SARS-CoV-2 human T cell epitopes: Adaptive immune response against COVID-19. *Cell Host & Microbe*, *29*(7), 1076–1092. https://doi.org/10.1016/j.chom.2021.05.010
Griscelli, F., Opolon, P., Saulnier, P., Mami-Chouaib, F., Gautier, E., Echchakir, H., Angevin, E., Le Chevalier, T., Bataille, V., Squiban, P., Tursz, T., & Escudier, B. (2003). Recombinant adenovirus shedding after intratumoral gene transfer in lung cancer patients. *Gene Therapy*, *10*(5), 386–395. https://doi.org/10.1038/sj.gt.3301928.
Grover, S., Rani, S., Kohat, K., Kathiravan, S., Patel, G., Sahoo, S., Mehra, A., Singh, S., & Bhadada, S. (2022). First episode psychosis following receipt of first dose of COVID-19 vaccine: A case report. *Schizophrenia Research*, *241*, 70–71. https://doi.org/10.1016/j.schres.2022.01.025
Guardiola, J., Lammert, C., Teal, E., & Chalasani, N. (2022). Unexplained liver test elevations after SARS-CoV-2 vaccination. *Journal of Hepatology*, *77*(1), 251–253. https://doi.org/10.1016/j.jhep.2022.02.014
Guetzkow, J. A. (2022). Effect of mRNA Vaccine Manufacturing Processes on Efficacy and Safety Still an Open Question. Rapid response to: Covid-19: Researchers face wait for patient level data from Pfizer and Moderna vaccine trials. *BMJ*, o1731. https://doi.org/10.1136/bmj.o1731
Guina, J., Barlow, S., & Gutierrez, D. (2022). Bipolar I Disorder Exacerbation Following COVID-19 Vaccination. *Innovations in Clinical Neuroscience*, *19*(7–9), 9–11.
Gunawan, P. Y., Tiffani, P., & Lalisang, L. (2022). Guillain-Barre Syndrome Following SARS-CoV-2 Vaccination: A Case Report. *Clinical Psychopharmacology and Neuroscience*, *20*(4), 777–780. https://doi.org/10.9758/cpn.2022.20.4.777

Gundry, S. R. (2021). Abstract 10712: Observational Findings of PULS Cardiac Test Findings for Inflammatory Markers in Patients Receiving mRNA Vaccines. *Circulation*, *144*(Suppl_1). https://doi.org/10.1161/circ.144.suppl_1.10712
Guo, L., Wu, C., Zhou, H., Wu, C., Paranhos-Baccalà, G., Vernet, G., Jin, Q., Wang, J., & Hung, T. (2013). Identification of a Nonstructural DNA-Binding Protein (DBP) as an Antigen with Diagnostic Potential for Human Adenovirus. *PLoS ONE*, *8*(3), e56708. https://doi.org/10.1371/journal.pone.0056708
Habot-Wilner, Z., Neri, P., Okada, A. A., Agrawal, R., Xin Le, N., Cohen, S., Fischer, N., Kilmartin, F., Coman, A., & Kilmartin, D. (2023). COVID Vaccine-Associated Uveitis. *Ocular Immunology and Inflammation*, *31*(6), 1198–1205. https://doi.org/10.1080/09273948.2023.2200858
Hafner, A. M., Corthésy, B., & Merkle, H. P. (2013). Particulate formulations for the delivery of poly(I:C) as vaccine adjuvant. *Advanced Drug Delivery Reviews*, *65*(10), 1386–1399. https://doi.org/10.1016/j.addr.2013.05.013
Hakroush, S., & Tampe, B. (2021). Case Report: ANCA-Associated Vasculitis Presenting With Rhabdomyolysis and Pauci-Immune Crescentic Glomerulonephritis After Pfizer-BioNTech COVID-19 mRNA Vaccination. *Frontiers in Immunology*, *12*. https://doi.org/10.3389/fimmu.2021.762006
Hall, W. (2023). Austin Bradford Hill's 'Environment and disease: Association or causation.' *Addiction*. https://doi.org/10.1111/add.16329
Halma, M. T. J., Rose, J., & Lawrie, T. (2023a). The Novelty of mRNA Viral Vaccines and Potential Harms: A Scoping Review. *Multidisciplinary Scientific Journal*, *6*(2), 220–235. https://doi.org/10.3390/j6020017.
Halma, M. T. J., Plothe, C., Marik, P., & Lawrie, T. A. (2023b). Strategies for the Management of Spike Protein-Related Pathology. *Microorganisms*, *11*(5), 1308. https://doi.org/10.3390/microorganisms11051308.
Halstead, S. B. (2016). Licensed Dengue Vaccine: Public Health Conundrum and Scientific Challenge. *The American Journal of Tropical Medicine and Hygiene*, *95*(4), 741–745. https://doi.org/10.4269/ajtmh.16-0222
Halstead, S. B., & Katzelnick, L. (2020). COVID-19 Vaccines: Should We Fear ADE? *The Journal of Infectious Diseases*, *222*(12), 1946–1950. https://doi.org/10.1093/infdis/jiaa518
Hampel, H., Hardy, J., Blennow, K., Chen, C., Perry, G., Kim, S. H., Villemagne, V. L., Aisen, P., Vendruscolo, M., Iwatsubo, T., Masters, C. L., Cho, M., Lannfelt, L., Cummings, J. L., & Vergallo, A. (2021). The Amyloid-β Pathway in Alzheimer's Disease. *Molecular Psychiatry*, *26*(10), 5481–5503. https://doi.org/10.1038/s41380-021-01249-0
Hampton, L. M., Aggarwal, R., Evans, S. J. W., & Law, B. (2021). General determination of causation between Covid-19 vaccines and possible adverse events. *Vaccine*, *39*(10), 1478–1480. https://doi.org/10.1016/j.vaccine.2021.01.057
Hanna, N., De Mejia, C. M., Heffes-Doon, A., Lin, X., Botros, B., Gurzenda, E., Clauss-Pascarelli, C., & Nayak, A. (2023). Biodistribution of mRNA COVID-19 vaccines in human breast milk. *EBioMedicine*, *96*, 104800. https://doi.org/10.1016/j.ebiom.2023.104800
Hanna, N., Heffes-Doon, A., Lin, X., Manzano De Mejia, C., Botros, B., Gurzenda, E., & Nayak, A. (2022). Detection of Messenger RNA COVID-19 Vaccines in Human Breast Milk. *JAMA Pediatrics*, *176*(12), 1268. https://doi.org/10.1001/jamapediatrics.2022.3581

Harper, A., Vijayakumar, V., Ouwehand, A. C., ter Haar, J., Obis, D., Espadaler, J., Binda, S., Desiraju, S., & Day, R. (2021). Viral Infections, the Microbiome, and Probiotics. *Frontiers in Cellular and Infection Microbiology, 10*. https://doi.org/10.3389/fcimb.2020.596166

Hartwig, G. W. (1981). Smallpox in the Sudan. *The International Journal of African Historical Studies*, *14*(1), 5–33.

Harvey Sky, N., Jackson, J., Chege, G., Gaymer, J., Kimiti, D., Mutisya, S., Nakito, S., & Shultz, S. (2022). Female reproductive skew exacerbates the extinction risk from poaching in the eastern black rhino. *Proceedings of the Royal Society B: Biological Sciences*, *289*(1972). https://doi.org/10.1098/rspb.2022.0075

Hashimoto, M., Kamphorst, A., Im, S., Kissick, H., Pillai, R., Ramalingam, S., Araki, K., & Ahmed, R. (2018). CD8 T Cell Exhaustion in Chronic Infection and Cancer: Opportunities for Interventions. *Annual Review of Medicine*, *69*, 301–318. https://doi.org/https://doi.org/10.1146/annurev-med-012017-043208

Hashimura, Y., Nozu, K., Kanegane, H., Miyawaki, T., Hayakawa, A., Yoshikawa, N., Nakanishi, K., Takemoto, M., Iijima, K., & Matsuo, M. (2009). Minimal change nephrotic syndrome associated with immune dysregulation, polyendocrinopathy, enteropathy, X-linked syndrome. *Pediatric Nephrology*, *24*(6), 1181–1186. https://doi.org/10.1007/s00467-009-1119-8

Hasnie, A. A., Hasnie, U. A., Patel, N., Aziz, M. U., Xie, M., Lloyd, S. G., & Prabhu, S. D. (2021). Perimyocarditis following first dose of the mRNA-1273 SARS-CoV-2 (Moderna) vaccine in a healthy young male: a case report. *BMC Cardiovascular Disorders*, *21*(1), 375. https://doi.org/10.1186/s12872-021-02183-3

Hatziantoniou, S., Maltezou, H. C., Tsakris, A., Poland, G. A., & Anastassopoulou, C. (2021). Anaphylactic reactions to mRNA COVID-19 vaccines: A call for further study. *Vaccine*, *39*(19), 2605–2607. https://doi.org/10.1016/j.vaccine.2021.03.073

Havenga, M. J., Lemckert, A. A., Ophorst, O. J., van Meijer, M., Germeraad, W. T., Grimbergen, J., van Den Doel, M. A., Vogels, R., van Deutekom, J., Janson, A. A., de Bruijn, J. D., Uytdehaag, F., Quax, P. H., Logtenberg, T., Mehtali, M., & Bout, A. (2002). Exploiting the natural diversity in adenovirus tropism for therapy and prevention of disease. *Journal of Virology*, *76*(9), 4612–4620. https://doi.org/10.1128/jvi.76.9.4612-4620.2002.

Hazan, S., Dave, S., Barrows, B., & Borody, T. J. (2022a). S227 Messenger RNA SARS-CoV-2 Vaccines Affect the Gut Microbiome. *American Journal of Gastroenterology*, *117*(10S), e162–e162. https://doi.org/10.14309/01.ajg.0000857548.07509.09

Hazan, S., Dave, S., Barrows, B., & Borody, T. J. (2022b). S2099 Persistent Damage to the Gut Microbiome Following Messenger RNA SARS-CoV-2 Vaccine. *American Journal of Gastroenterology*, *117*(10S), e1429–e1430. https://doi.org/10.14309/01.ajg.0000865036.78992.16

Hazan, S., Stollman, N., Bozkurt, H. S., Dave, S., Papoutsis, A. J., Daniels, J., Barrows, B. D., Quigley, E. M., & Borody, T. J. (2022). Lost microbes of COVID-19: Bifidobacterium , Faecalibacterium depletion and decreased microbiome diversity associated with SARS-CoV-2 infection severity. *BMJ Open Gastroenterology*, *9*(1), e000871. https://doi.org/10.1136/bmjgast-2022-000871

Hébert, M., Bouhout, S., Vadboncoeur, J., & Aubin, M.-J. (2022). Recurrent and De Novo Toxoplasmosis Retinochoroiditis following Coronavirus Disease 2019

Infection or Vaccination. *Vaccines*, *10*(10), 1692. https://doi.org/10.3390/vaccines10101692
Heinz, F. X., & Stiasny, K. (2021). Distinguishing features of current COVID-19 vaccines: knowns and unknowns of antigen presentation and modes of action. *Npj Vaccines*, *6*(1), 104. https://doi.org/10.1038/s41541-021-00369-6
Helmink, B. A., Khan, M. A. W., Hermann, A., Gopalakrishnan, V., & Wargo, J. A. (2019). The microbiome, cancer, and cancer therapy. *Nature Medicine*, *25*(3), 377–388. https://doi.org/10.1038/s41591-019-0377-7
Henning, A. N., Roychoudhuri, R., & Restifo, N. P. (2018). Epigenetic control of CD8+ T cell differentiation. *Nature Reviews Immunology*, *18*(5), 340–356. https://doi.org/10.1038/nri.2017.146
Herkert, D., Meljen, V., Muasher, L., Price, T. M., Kuller, J. A., & Dotters-Katz, S. (2022). Human Chorionic Gonadotropin—A Review of the Literature. *Obstetrical & Gynecological Survey*, *77*(9), 539–546. https://doi.org/10.1097/OGX.0000000000001053
Herraiz-Adillo, Á., Martínez-Vizcaíno, V., & Pozuelo-Carrascosa, D. P. (2022). Aspiration before intramuscular vaccines injection, should the debate continue? *Enfermería Clínica (English Edition)*, *32*(1), 65–66. https://doi.org/10.1016/j.enfcle.2021.10.002
Hertel, M., Heiland, M., Nahles, S., von Laffert, M., Mura, C., Bourne, P. E., Preissner, R., & Preissner, S. (2022). Real-world evidence from over one million <scp>COVID</scp> -19 vaccinations is consistent with reactivation of the varicella-zoster virus. *Journal of the European Academy of Dermatology and Venereology*, *36*(8), 1342–1348. https://doi.org/10.1111/jdv.18184
Herzum, A., Micalizzi, C., Molle, M. F., & Parodi, A. (2022). New-onset vitiligo following COVID-19 disease. *Skin Health and Disease*, *2*(1). https://doi.org/10.1002/ski2.86
Hey, S. P., London, A. J., Weijer, C., Rid, A., & Miller, F. (2017). Is the concept of clinical equipoise still relevant to research? *BMJ*, j5787. https://doi.org/10.1136/bmj.j5787
Hill, A. B. (1965). The Environment and Disease: Association or Causation? *Proceedings of the Royal Society of Medicine*, *58*(5), 295–300. https://doi.org/10.1177/003591576505800503
Hill, A. B. (2015). The environment and disease: association or causation? *Journal of the Royal Society of Medicine*, *108*(1), 32–37. https://doi.org/10.1177/0141076814562718
Hilts, A., Schreiber, A., & Singh, A. (2022). A Clinical Case of COVID-19 Vaccine-Associated Guillain-Barré Syndrome. *American Journal of Case Reports*, *23*. https://doi.org/10.12659/AJCR.936896
Höfler, M. (2005). The Bradford Hill considerations on causality: a counterfactual perspective. *Emerging Themes in Epidemiology*, *2*(1), 11. https://doi.org/10.1186/1742-7622-2-11
Højsgaard Chow, H., Schreiber, K., Magyari, M., Ammitzbøll, C., Börnsen, L., Romme Christensen, J., Ratzer, R., Soelberg Sørensen, P., & Sellebjerg, F. (2018). Progressive multiple sclerosis, cognitive function, and quality of life. *Brain and Behavior*, *8*(2). https://doi.org/10.1002/brb3.875

Holzworth, A., Couchot, P., Cruz-Knight, W., & Brucculeri, M. (2021). Minimal change disease following the Moderna mRNA-1273 SARS-CoV-2 vaccine. *Kidney International*, *100*(2), 463–464. https://doi.org/10.1016/j.kint.2021.05.007

Hong, L., Wang, Z., Wei, X., Shi, J., & Li, C. (2020). Antibodies against polyethylene glycol in human blood: A literature review. *Journal of Pharmacological and Toxicological Methods*, *102*, 106678. https://doi.org/10.1016/j.vascn.2020.106678

Hou, R., Wu, J., He, D., Yan, Y., & Li, L. (2019). Anti-N-methyl-d-aspartate receptor encephalitis associated with reactivated Epstein–Barr virus infection in pediatric patients. *Medicine*, *98*(20), e15726. https://doi.org/10.1097/MD.0000000000015726

Hromić-Jahjefendić, A., Barh, D., Uversky, V., Aljabali, A. A., Tambuwala, M. M., Alzahrani, K. J., Alzahrani, F. M., Alshammeri, S., & Lundstrom, K. (2023). Can COVID-19 Vaccines Induce Premature Non-Communicable Diseases: Where Are We Heading to? *Vaccines*, *11*(2), 208. https://doi.org/10.3390/vaccines11020208

Hsiao, Y. Y., Liu, L. J., Lin, Y. L. (2023). A case with prolonged headache after COVID-19 vaccination and later developed Bell's palsy. *Acta Neurologica Taiwan, 32*(2), 65–68. *http://www.ant-tnsjournal.com/index_infoN.asp?nn=731*

Hsieh, Y. C., Wu, F. T., Hsiung, C. A., Wu, H. S., Chang, K. Y., & Huang, Y. C. (2014). Comparison of virus shedding after lived attenuated and pentavalent reassortant rotavirus vaccine. *Vaccine*, *32*(10), 1199–1204. https://doi.org/10.1016/j.vaccine.2013.08.041.

Hsiung, S., & Egawa, T. (2023). Population dynamics and gene regulation of T cells in response to chronic antigen stimulation. *International Immunology*, *35*(2), 67–77. https://doi.org/10.1093/intimm/dxac050

Hsu, J. T.-A., Tien, C.-F., Yu, G.-Y., Shen, S., Lee, Y.-H., Hsu, P.-C., Wang, Y., Chao, P.-K., Tsay, H.-J., & Shie, F.-S. (2021). The Effects of Aβ1-42 Binding to the SARS-CoV-2 Spike Protein S1 Subunit and Angiotensin-Converting Enzyme 2. *International Journal of Molecular Sciences*, *22*(15), 8226. https://doi.org/10.3390/ijms22158226

Hu, B., Guo, H., Zhou, P., & Shi, Z.-L. (2021). Characteristics of SARS-CoV-2 and COVID-19. *Nature Reviews Microbiology*, *19*(3), 141–154. https://doi.org/10.1038/s41579-020-00459-7

Huang, F., & MacPherson, G. (2004). Dendritic cells and oral transmission of prion diseases. *Advanced Drug Delivery Reviews*, *56*(6), 901–913. https://doi.org/10.1016/j.addr.2003.09.006

Huang, W., Percie du Sert, N., Vollert, J., & Rice, A. S. C. (2020). General Principles of Preclinical Study Design. *Handbook of Experimental Pharmacology 257,* 55–69. https://doi.org/10.1007/164_2019_277.

Huang, Y., Yang, C., Xu, X., Xu, W., & Liu, S. (2020). Structural and functional properties of SARS-CoV-2 spike protein: potential antivirus drug development for COVID-19. *Acta Pharmacologica Sinica*, *41*(9), 1141–1149. https://doi.org/10.1038/s41401-020-0485-4

Huda, S., Whittam, D., Bhojak, M., Chamberlain, J., Noonan, C., Jacob, A., & Kneen, R. (2019). Neuromyelitis optica spectrum disorders. *Clinical Medicine*, *19*(2), 169–176. https://doi.org/10.7861/clinmedicine.19-2-169

Hudson, B., Mantooth, R., & DeLaney, M. (2021). Myocarditis and pericarditis after vaccination for COVID-19. *Journal of the American College of Emergency Physicians Open*, *2*(4). https://doi.org/10.1002/emp2.12498

Hussain, A., Nduka, C., Moth, P., & Malhotra, R. (2017). Bell's facial nerve palsy in pregnancy: a clinical review. *Journal of Obstetrics and Gynaecology*, *37*(4), 409–415. https://doi.org/10.1080/01443615.2016.1256973

Hwang, B. W., & Bong, J. Bin. (2022). Two possible etiologies of Guillain-Barré syndrome: mRNA-1273 (Moderna) vaccination and scrub typhus: A case report. *Medicine*, *101*(48), e32140. https://doi.org/10.1097/MD.0000000000032140

Iba, T., Levy, J. H., & Warkentin, T. E. (2022). Recognizing Vaccine-Induced Immune Thrombotic Thrombocytopenia. *Critical Care Medicine*, *50*(1), e80–e86. https://doi.org/10.1097/CCM.0000000000005211

Idrees, D., & Kumar, V. (2021). SARS-CoV-2 spike protein interactions with amyloidogenic proteins: Potential clues to neurodegeneration. *Biochemical and Biophysical Research Communications*, *554*, 94–98. https://doi.org/10.1016/j.bbrc.2021.03.100

Ikechi, D., Hashimoto, H., Nakano, H., & Nakamura, K. (2022). A Case of Suspected COVID-19 Vaccine-related Thrombophlebitis. *Internal Medicine*, *61*(10), 8767–21. https://doi.org/10.2169/internalmedicine.8767-21

Ikeda, H., & Togashi, Y. (2022). Aging, cancer, and antitumor immunity. *International Journal of Clinical Oncology*, *27*(2), 316–322. https://doi.org/10.1007/s10147-021-01913-z

Ikewaki, N., Kurosawa, G., Levy, G. A., Preethy, S., & Abraham, S. J. K. (2023). Antibody dependent disease enhancement (ADE) after COVID-19 vaccination and beta glucans as a safer strategy in management. *Vaccine*, *41*(15), 2427–2429. https://doi.org/10.1016/j.vaccine.2023.03.005

Illingworth, J., Butler, N. S., Roetynck, S., Mwacharo, J., Pierce, S. K., Bejon, P., Crompton, P. D., Marsh, K., & Ndungu, F. M. (2013). Chronic exposure to Plasmodium falciparum is associated with phenotypic evidence of B and T cell exhaustion exhaustion. *The Journal of Immunology*, *190*(3), 1038–1047. https://doi.org/10.4049/jimmunol.1202438

Ilyas, U., Umar, Z., Bhangal, R., Shah, D., & Fayman, B. (2022). Guillain-Barré Syndrome: A Sequela of the Original COVID-19 Infection or Vaccination. *Cureus*. https://doi.org/10.7759/cureus.28044

Imai, Y., Kuba, K., & Penninger, J. M. (2007). Angiotensin-converting enzyme 2 in acute respiratory distress syndrome. *Cellular and Molecular Life Sciences*, *64*(15), 2006–2012. https://doi.org/10.1007/s00018-007-6228-6

Imbalzano, G., Ledda, C., Artusi, C. A., Romagnolo, A., Montanaro, E., Rizzone, M. G., Lopiano, L., & Zibetti, M. (2022). SARS-CoV-2 vaccination, Parkinson's disease, and other movement disorders: case series and short literature review. *Neurological Sciences*, *43*(9), 5165–5168. https://doi.org/10.1007/s10072-022-06182-w

Introna, A., Caputo, F., Santoro, C., Guerra, T., Ucci, M., Mezzapesa, D. M., & Trojano, M. (2021). Guillain-Barré syndrome after AstraZeneca COVID-19-vaccination: A causal or casual association? *Clinical Neurology and Neurosurgery*, *208*, 106887. https://doi.org/10.1016/j.clineuro.2021.106887

Ioannidis, J. P. A. (2021). Infection fatality rate of COVID-19 inferred from seroprevalence data. *Bulletin of the World Health Organization*, *99*(1), 19-33F. https://doi.org/10.2471/BLT.20.265892

Irrgang, P., Gerling, J., Kocher, K., Lapuente, D., Steininger, P., Habenicht, K., Wytopil, M., Beileke, S., Schäfer, S., Zhong, J., Ssebyatika, G., Krey, T., Falcone,

V., Schülein, C., Peter, A. S., Nganou-Makamdop, K., Hengel, H., Held, J., Bogdan, C., … Tenbusch, M. (2023). Class switch toward noninflammatory, spike-specific IgG4 antibodies after repeated SARS-CoV-2 mRNA vaccination. *Science Immunology*, *8*(79). https://doi.org/10.1126/sciimmunol.ade2798

Isaak, A., Feisst, A., & Luetkens, J. A. (2021). Myocarditis Following COVID-19 Vaccination. *Radiology*, *301*(1), E378–E379. https://doi.org/10.1148/radiol.2021211766

Ismail, I. I., & Salama, S. (2022). A systematic review of cases of CNS demyelination following COVID-19 vaccination. *Journal of Neuroimmunology*, *362*, 577765. https://doi.org/10.1016/j.jneuroim.2021.577765

Issakov, G., Tzur, Y., Friedman, T., & Tzur, T. (2023). Abnormal Uterine Bleeding Among COVID-19 Vaccinated and Recovered Women: a National Survey. *Reproductive Sciences*, *30*(2), 713–721. https://doi.org/10.1007/s43032-022-01062-2

Jackson, D., Pitcher, M., Hudson, C., Andrews, N., Southern, J., Ellis, J., Höschler, K., Pebody, R., Turner, P. J., Miller, E., & Zambon, M. (2020). Viral Shedding in Recipients of Live Attenuated Influenza Vaccine in the 2016-2017 and 2017-2018 Influenza Seasons in the United Kingdom. *Clinical Infectious Disease*, *70*(12), 2505–2513. https://doi.org/10.1093/cid/ciz719.

Jain, E., Pandav, K., Regmi, P., Michel, G., & Altshuler, I. (2021). Facial Diplegia: A Rare, Atypical Variant of Guillain-Barré Syndrome and Ad26.COV2.S Vaccine. *Cureus*. https://doi.org/10.7759/cureus.16612

Jain, S. S., Steele, J. M., Fonseca, B., Huang, S., Shah, S., Maskatia, S. A., Buddhe, S., Misra, N., Ramachandran, P., Gaur, L., Eshtehardi, P., Anwar, S., Kaushik, N., Han, F., Chaudhuri, N. R., & Grosse-Wortmann, L. (2021). COVID Vaccination-Associated Myocarditis in Adolescents. *Pediatrics*, e2021053427. https://doi.org/10.1542/peds.2021-053427.

James, J., Jose, J., Gafoor, V. A., Smita, B., & Balaram, N. (2021). Guillain-Barré syndrome following ChAdOx1 nCoV-19 COVID-19 vaccination: A case series. *Neurology and Clinical Neuroscience*, *9*(5), 402–405. https://doi.org/10.1111/ncn3.12537

James, M. B., & Giorgio, T. D. (2000). Nuclear-Associated Plasmid, but Not Cell-Associated Plasmid, Is Correlated with Transgene Expression in Cultured Mammalian Cells. *Molecular Therapy*, *1*(4), 339–346. https://doi.org/10.1006/mthe.2000.0054

Jarius, S., & Wildemann, B. (2013). Aquaporin-4 Antibodies (NMO- IgG) as a Serological Marker of Neuromyelitis Optica: A Critical Review of the Literature. *Brain Pathology*, *23*(6), 661–683. https://doi.org/10.1111/bpa.12084

Jasti, A. K., Selmi, C., Sarmiento-Monroy, J. C., Vega, D. A., Anaya, J.-M., & Gershwin, M. E. (2016). Guillain-Barré syndrome: causes, immunopathogenic mechanisms and treatment. *Expert Review of Clinical Immunology*, *12*(11), 1175–1189. https://doi.org/10.1080/1744666X.2016.1193006

Jeet Kaur, R., Dutta, S., Charan, J., Bhardwaj, P., Tandon, A., Yadav, D., Islam, S., & Haque, M. (2021). Cardiovascular Adverse Events Reported from COVID-19 Vaccines: A Study Based on WHO Database. International Journal of Genetic Medicine, 14, 3909–3927. https://doi.org/10.2147/IJGM.S324349.

Jefferis, J., Kassianos, A. J., Grivei, A., Doucet, B., Healy, H., Francis, L., Mon, S. Y., & John, G. T. (2022). SARS-CoV-2 vaccination–associated collapsing glomerulopathy in a kidney transplant recipient. *Kidney International*, *101*(3), 635–636. https://doi.org/10.1016/j.kint.2021.12.018

Jevtović-Todorović, V., Todorovć, S. M., Mennerick, S., Powell, S., Dikranian, K., Benshoff, N., Zorumski, C. F., & Olney, J. W. (1998). Nitrous oxide (laughing gas) is an NMDA antagonist, neuroprotectant and neurotoxin. *Nature Medicine*, *4*(4), 460–463. https://doi.org/10.1038/nm0498-460

Jewett, B. E., & Thapa, B. (2023). *Physiology, NMDA Receptor.*

Jeyanathan, M., Vaseghi-Shanjani, M., Afkhami, S., Grondin, J. A., Kang, A., D'Agostino, M. R., Yao, Y., Jain, S., Zganiacz, A., Kroezen, Z., Shanmuganathan, M., Singh, R., Dvorkin-Gheva, A., Britz-McKibbin, P., Khan, W. I., & Xing, Z. (2022). Parenteral BCG vaccine induces lung-resident memory macrophages and trained immunity via the gut–lung axis. *Nature Immunology*, *23*(12), 1687–1702. https://doi.org/10.1038/s41590-022-01354-4

Jing, Y., Run-Qian, L., Hao-Ran, W., Hao-Ran, C., Ya-Bin, L., Yang, G., & Fei, C. (2020). Potential influence of COVID-19/ACE2 on the female reproductive system. *Molecular Human Reproduction*, *26*(6), 367–373. https://doi.org/10.1093/molehr/gaaa030

John, T. J., & Dharmapalan, D. (2022). Lessons from Vaccine-Related Poliovirus in Israel, UK and USA. *Vaccines* (Basel), *10*(11), 1969. https://doi.org/10.3390/vaccines10111969.

Johnson, P. L. F., Kochin, B. F., McAfee, M. S., Stromnes, I. M., Regoes, R. R., Ahmed, R., Blattman, J. N., & Antia, R. (2011). Vaccination Alters the Balance between Protective Immunity, Exhaustion, Escape, and Death in Chronic Infections. *Journal of Virology*, *85*(11), 5565–5570. https://doi.org/10.1128/JVI.00166-11

Johnston, M. S., Galan, A., Watsky, K. L., & Little, A. J. (2021). Delayed Localized Hypersensitivity Reactions to the Moderna COVID-19 Vaccine. *JAMA Dermatology*, *157*(6), 716. https://doi.org/10.1001/jamadermatol.2021.1214

Jones, K. T., Zhen, J., & Reith, M. E. A. (2012). Importance of cholesterol in dopamine transporter function. *Journal of Neurochemistry*, *123*(5), 700–715. https://doi.org/10.1111/jnc.12007

Joo, C. W., Kim, Y.-K., & Park, S. P. (2022). Vogt-Koyanagi-Harada Disease following mRNA-1273 (Moderna) COVID-19 Vaccination. *Ocular Immunology and Inflammation*, *30*(5), 1250–1254. https://doi.org/10.1080/09273948.2022.2053547

Kadar, N., Romero, R., & Papp, Z. (2018). Ignaz Semmelweis: the "Savior of Mothers." *American Journal of Obstetrics and Gynecology*, *219*(6), 519–522. https://doi.org/10.1016/j.ajog.2018.10.036

Kakoulidis, P., Vlachos, I. S., Thanos, D., Blatch, G. L., Emiris, I. Z., & Anastasiadou, E. (2023). Identifying and profiling structural similarities between Spike of SARS-CoV-2 and other viral or host proteins with Machaon. *Communications Biology*, *6*(1), 752. https://doi.org/10.1038/s42003-023-05076-7

Kalra, R. K., Jayadeep, S., & Ball, A. L. (2022). Acute Pancreatitis in an Adolescent Following COVID Vaccination. *Clinical Pediatrics*, *61*(3), 236–240. https://doi.org/10.1177/00099228211067678

Kaltschmidt, B., & Kaltschmidt, C. (2009). NF-kB in the Nervous System. *Cold Spring Harbor Perspectives in Biology*, *1*(3), a001271–a001271. https://doi.org/10.1101/cshperspect.a001271

Kaminetsky, J., & Rudikoff, D. (2021). New-onset vitiligo following mRNA-1273 (Moderna) COVID-19 vaccination. *Clinical Case Reports*, *9*(9). https://doi.org/10.1002/ccr3.4865

Kamogashira, T., Funayama, H., Asakura, S., & Ishimoto, S. (2022). Vestibular Neuritis Following COVID-19 Vaccination: A Retrospective Study. *Cureus*. https://doi.org/10.7759/cureus.24277

Kanabar, G., & Wilkinson, P. (2021). Guillain-Barré syndrome presenting with facial diplegia following COVID-19 vaccination in two patients. *BMJ Case Reports*, *14*(10), e244527. https://doi.org/10.1136/bcr-2021-244527

Kandel, E. R., Dudai, Y., & Mayford, M. R. (2014). The Molecular and Systems Biology of Memory. *Cell*, *157*(1), 163–186. https://doi.org/10.1016/j.cell.2014.03.001

Kanduc, D. (2023). SARS-CoV-2: The Self-Nonself Issue and Diagnostic Tests. *Journal of Laboratory Physicians*, *15*(01), 056–061. https://doi.org/10.1055/s-0042-1750078

Kanduc, D., & Shoenfeld, Y. (2020). Molecular mimicry between SARS-CoV-2 spike glycoprotein and mammalian proteomes: implications for the vaccine. *Immunologic Research*, *68*(5), 310–313. https://doi.org/10.1007/s12026-020-09152-6

Kang, J. (2022). Unusual arm vein thrombosis after the Moderna (mRNA-1273) COVID-19 vaccination—a case report. *Annals of Palliative Medicine*, *11*(11), 3567–3570. https://doi.org/10.21037/apm-22-343

Kang, M., Chippa, V., & An, J. (2022). Viral Myocarditis. In: StatPearls [Internet]. Treasure Island (FL): StatPearls Publishing; 2023. https://www.ncbi.nlm.nih.gov/books/NBK459259/

Kang, R., & Tang, D. (2012). PKR-Dependent Inflammatory Signals. *Science Signaling*, *5*(247). https://doi.org/10.1126/scisignal.2003511

Kannemeier, C., Shibamiya, A., Nakazawa, F., Trusheim, H., Ruppert, C., Markart, P., Song, Y., Tzima, E., Kennerknecht, E., Niepmann, M., von Bruehl, M.-L., Sedding, D., Massberg, S., Günther, A., Engelmann, B., & Preissner, K. T. (2007). Extracellular RNA constitutes a natural procoagulant cofactor in blood coagulation. *Proceedings of the National Academy of Sciences*, *104*(15), 6388–6393. https://doi.org/10.1073/pnas.0608647104

Kantar, A., Seminara, M., Odoni, M., & Dalla Verde, I. (2021). Acute Mild Pancreatitis Following COVID-19 mRNA Vaccine in an Adolescent. *Children*, *9*(1), 29. https://doi.org/10.3390/children9010029

Kaprara, A., & Huhtaniemi, I. T. (2018). The hypothalamus-pituitary-gonad axis: Tales of mice and men. *Metabolism*, *86*, 3–17. https://doi.org/10.1016/j.metabol.2017.11.018

Karabudak, S., Kurtoğlu, A., Uslu, F., & Gürsoy, A. (2023). A Case Report of Creutzfeldt-Jakob Disease after mRNA COVID-19 Vaccine. *Annals of Clinical Case Reports*, *8*(2408).

Karagöz, I. K., Munk, M. R., Kaya, M., Rückert, R., Yıldırım, M., & Karabaş, L. (2021). Using bioinformatic protein sequence similarity to investigate if SARS CoV-2 infection could cause an ocular autoimmune inflammatory reactions? *Experimental Eye Research*, *203*, 108433. https://doi.org/10.1016/j.exer.2020.108433

Karavani, G., Chill, H. H., Meirman, C., Gutman-Ido, E., Herzberg, S., Tzipora, T., Imbar, T., & Ben-Meir, A. (2022). Sperm quality is not affected by the BNT162b2 mRNA SARS-CoV-2 vaccine: results of a 6–14 months follow-up. *Journal of Assisted Reproduction and Genetics*, *39*(10), 2249–2254. https://doi.org/10.1007/s10815-022-02621-x

Karch, C. P., & Burkhard, P. (2016). Vaccine technologies: From whole organisms to rationally designed protein assemblies. *Biochemical Pharmacology*, *120*, 1–14. https://doi.org/10.1016/j.bcp.2016.05.001

Karikó, K., Muramatsu, H., Ludwig, J., & Weissman, D. (2011). Generating the optimal mRNA for therapy: HPLC purification eliminates immune activation and improves translation of nucleoside-modified, protein-encoding mRNA. *Nucleic Acids Research*, *39*(21), e142–e142. https://doi.org/10.1093/nar/gkr695

Karikó, K., Muramatsu, H., Welsh, F. A., Ludwig, J., Kato, H., Akira, S., & Weissman, D. (2008). Incorporation of Pseudouridine Into mRNA Yields Superior Nonimmunogenic Vector With Increased Translational Capacity and Biological Stability. *Molecular Therapy*, *16*(11), 1833–1840. https://doi.org/10.1038/mt.2008.200

Karthik, K., Senthilkumar, T. M. A., Udhayavel, S., & Raj, G. D. (2020). Role of antibody-dependent enhancement (ADE) in the virulence of SARS-CoV-2 and its mitigation strategies for the development of vaccines and immunotherapies to counter COVID-19. *Human Vaccines & Immunotherapeutics*, *16*(12), 3055–3060. https://doi.org/10.1080/21645515.2020.1796425

Kasahara, M., & Sutoh, Y. (2014). *Two Forms of Adaptive Immunity in Vertebrates* (pp. 59–90). https://doi.org/10.1016/B978-0-12-800267-4.00002-X

Kassab, M., Almomani, B., Nuseir, K., & Alhouary, A. (2020). Efficacy of Sucrose in Reducing Pain during Immunization among 10- to 18-Month-Old Infants and Young Children: A Randomized Controlled Trial. *Journal of Pediatric Nursing*, *50*, e55–e61. https://doi.org/10.1016/j.pedn.2019.11.010

Kaufmann, K. B., Büning, H., Galy, A., Schambach, A., & Grez, M. (2013). Gene therapy on the move. *EMBO Molecular Medicine*, *5*(11), 1642–1661. https://doi.org/10.1002/emmm.201202287

Kawai, T., & Akira, S. (2008). Toll-like Receptor and RIG-1-like Receptor Signaling. *Annals of the New York Academy of Sciences*, *1143*(1), 1–20. https://doi.org/10.1196/annals.1443.020

Kawali, A., Srinivasan, S., Mishra, S. B., Mahendradas, P., & Shetty, B. (2023). Epidemic retinitis during the COVID-19 pandemic. *Indian Journal of Ophthalmology*, *71*(7), 2779–2783. https://doi.org/10.4103/IJO.IJO_3349_22

Kawano, H., Hamaguchi, E., Kawahito, S., Tsutsumi, Y. M., Tanaka, K., Kitahata, H., & Oshita, S. (2011). Anaesthesia for a patient with paraneoplastic limbic encephalitis with ovarian teratoma: relationship to anti-N-methyl-d-aspartate receptor antibodies. *Anaesthesia*, *66*(6), 515–518. https://doi.org/10.1111/j.1365-2044.2011.06707.x

Kayser, M. S., & Dalmau, J. (2016). Anti-NMDA receptor encephalitis, autoimmunity, and psychosis. *Schizophrenia Research*, *176*(1), 36–40. https://doi.org/10.1016/j.schres.2014.10.007

Keddie, S., Pakpoor, J., Mousele, C., Pipis, M., Machado, P. M., Foster, M., Record, C. J., Keh, R. Y. S., Fehmi, J., Paterson, R. W., Bharambe, V., Clayton, L. M., Allen, C., Price, O., Wall, J., Kiss-Csenki, A., Rathnasabapathi, D. P., Geraldes,

R., Yermakova, T., … Lunn, M. P. (2021). Epidemiological and cohort study finds no association between COVID-19 and Guillain-Barré syndrome. *Brain*, *144*(2), 682–693. https://doi.org/10.1093/brain/awaa433

Keithley, E. M. (2022). Inner ear immunity. *Hearing Research*, *419*, 108518. https://doi.org/10.1016/j.heares.2022.108518

Kempf, W., Kettelhack, N., Kind, F., Courvoisier, S., Galambos, J., & Pfaltz, K. (2021). 'COVID arm' – histological features of a delayed-type hypersensitivity reaction to Moderna mRNA-1273 SARS-CoV2 vaccine. *Journal of the European Academy of Dermatology and Venereology*, *35*(11). https://doi.org/10.1111/jdv.17506

Kerbl, R. (2021). Myokarditis nach COVID-19-mRNA-Impfung. *Monatsschrift Kinderheilkunde*, *169*(10), 893–894. https://doi.org/10.1007/s00112-021-01283-w

Kerneis, M., Bihan, K., & Salem, J.-E. (2021). COVID-19 vaccines and myocarditis. *Archives of Cardiovascular Diseases*, *114*(6–7), 515–517. https://doi.org/10.1016/j.acvd.2021.06.001

Kervella, D., Jacquemont, L., Chapelet-Debout, A., Deltombe, C., & Ville, S. (2021). Minimal change disease relapse following SARS-CoV-2 mRNA vaccine. *Kidney International*, *100*(2), 457–458. https://doi.org/10.1016/j.kint.2021.04.033

Khan, E., Shrestha, A. K., Colantonio, M. A., Liberio, R. N., & Sriwastava, S. (2022). Acute transverse myelitis following SARS-CoV-2 vaccination: a case report and review of literature. *Journal of Neurology*, *269*(3), 1121–1132. https://doi.org/10.1007/s00415-021-10785-2

Khan, S., Shafiei, M. S., Longoria, C., Schoggins, J. W., Savani, R. C., & Zaki, H. (2021). SARS-CoV-2 spike protein induces inflammation via TLR2-dependent activation of the NF-κB pathway. *ELife*, *10*. https://doi.org/10.7554/eLife.68563

Khandelwal, S., Ravi, J., Rauova, L., Johnson, A., Lee, G. M., Gilner, J. B., Gunti, S., Notkins, A. L., Kuchibhatla, M., Frank, M., Poncz, M., Cines, D. B., & Arepally, G. M. (2018). Polyreactive IgM initiates complement activation by PF4/heparin complexes through the classical pathway. *Blood*, *132*(23), 2431–2440. https://doi.org/10.1182/blood-2018-03-834598

Khanmohammadi, S., Malekpour, M., Jabbari, P., & Rezaei, N. (2021). Genetic basis of Guillain-Barre syndrome. *Journal of Neuroimmunology*, *358*, 577651. https://doi.org/10.1016/j.jneuroim.2021.577651

Khanna, U., Oprea, Y., Mir, A., & Halverstam, C. (2022). New diagnosis of systemic lupus erythematosus after COVID-19 vaccination: A case report and review of literature. *JAAD Case Reports*, *30*, 30–34. https://doi.org/10.1016/j.jdcr.2022.09.026

Khavinson, V., Terekhov, A., Kormilets, D., & Maryanovich, A. (2021). Homology between SARS CoV-2 and human proteins. *Scientific Reports*, *11*(1), 17199. https://doi.org/10.1038/s41598-021-96233-7

Khayat-Khoei, M., Bhattacharyya, S., Katz, J., Harrison, D., Tauhid, S., Bruso, P., Houtchens, M. K., Edwards, K. R., & Bakshi, R. (2022). COVID-19 mRNA vaccination leading to CNS inflammation: a case series. *Journal of Neurology*, *269*(3), 1093–1106. https://doi.org/10.1007/s00415-021-10780-7

Kho, M. M. L., Reinders, M. E. J., Baan, C. C., van Baarle, D., Bemelman, F. J., Diavatopoulos, D. A., Gansevoort, R. T., van der Klis, F. R. M., Koopmans, M. P. G., Messchendorp, A. L., van der Molen, R. G., Remmerswaal, E. B. M., Rots, N., Vart, P., de Vries, R. D., Hilbrands, L. B., Sanders, J.-S. F., Abrahams, A. C.,

Hemmelder, M. H., … Malahé, S. R. K. (2021). The RECOVAC IR study: the immune response and safety of the mRNA-1273 COVID-19 vaccine in patients with chronic kidney disease, on dialysis or living with a kidney transplant. *Nephrology Dialysis Transplantation*, *36*(9), 1761–1764. https://doi.org/10.1093/ndt/gfab186

Khogali, F., & Abdelrahman, R. (2021). Unusual Presentation of Acute Perimyocarditis Following SARS-COV-2 mRNA-1237 Moderna Vaccination. *Cureus*. https://doi.org/10.7759/cureus.16590

Kiecolt-Glaser, J. K., & Glaser, R. (2002). Depression and immune function. *Journal of Psychosomatic Research*, *53*(4), 873–876. https://doi.org/10.1016/S0022-3999(02)00309-4

Kikuchi, K., Shibahara, H., Hirano, Y., Kohno, T., Hirashima, C., Suzuki, T., Takamizawa, S., & Suzuki, M. (2003). Antinuclear Antibody Reduces the Pregnancy Rate in the First IVF-ET Treatment Cycle but Not the Cumulative Pregnancy Rate without Specific Medication. *American Journal of Reproductive Immunology*, *50*(4), 363–367. https://doi.org/10.1034/j.1600-0897.2003.00088.x

Kim, E., & Reig, B. (2022). Breast Inflammatory Change Is Transient Following COVID-19 Vaccination. *Radiology*, *304*(3), 533–533. https://doi.org/10.1148/radiol.220321

Kim, H. W., Canchola, J. G., Brandt, C. D., Pyles, G., Chanock, R. M., Jensen, K., & Parrott, R. H. (1969). Respiratory syncytial virus disease in infants despite prior administration of antigenic inactivated vaccine. *American Journal of Epidemiology*, *89*(4), 422–434. https://doi.org/10.1093/oxfordjournals.aje.a120955

Kim, H. W., Jenista, E. R., Wendell, D. C., Azevedo, C. F., Campbell, M. J., Darty, S. N., Parker, M. A., & Kim, R. J. (2021). Patients With Acute Myocarditis Following mRNA COVID-19 Vaccination. *JAMA Cardiology*, *6*(10), 1196. https://doi.org/10.1001/jamacardio.2021.2828

Kim, I.-C., Kim, H., Lee, H. J., Kim, J. Y., & Kim, J.-Y. (2021). Cardiac Imaging of Acute Myocarditis Following COVID-19 mRNA Vaccination. *Journal of Korean Medical Science*, *36*(32). https://doi.org/10.3346/jkms.2021.36.e229

Kim, J. H., Chae, H. B., Woo, S., Song, M. S., Kim, H.-J., & Woo, C. G. (2023). Clinicopathological Characteristics of Autoimmune-Like Hepatitis Induced by COVID-19 mRNA Vaccine (Pfizer-BioNTech, BNT162b2): A Case Report and Literature Review. *International Journal of Surgical Pathology*, *31*(6), 1156–1162. https://doi.org/10.1177/10668969231177877

Kim, J. W., Kim, Y. G., Park, Y. C., Choi, S., Lee, S., Min, H. J., & Kim, M. J. (2022). Guillain-Barre Syndrome After Two COVID-19 Vaccinations: Two Case Reports With Follow-up Electrodiagnostic Study. *Journal of Korean Medical Science*, *37*(7). https://doi.org/10.3346/jkms.2022.37.e58

Kim, N., Kim, J.-H., & Park, J.-S. (2022). Guillain–Barré syndrome associated with BNT162b2 COVID vaccination: a first case report from South Korea. *Neurological Sciences*, *43*(3), 1491–1493. https://doi.org/10.1007/s10072-021-05849-0

King, W. W., Petersen, M. R., Matar, R. M., Budweg, J. B., Cuervo Pardo, L., & Petersen, J. W. (2021). Myocarditis following mRNA vaccination against SARS-CoV-2, a case series. *American Heart Journal Plus: Cardiology Research and Practice*, *8*, 100042. https://doi.org/10.1016/j.ahjo.2021.100042

Kircheis, R., & Planz, O. (2022). Could a Lower Toll-like Receptor (TLR) and NF-κB Activation Due to a Changed Charge Distribution in the Spike Protein Be the Reason for the Lower Pathogenicity of Omicron? *International Journal of Molecular Sciences*, *23*(11), 5966. https://doi.org/10.3390/ijms23115966

Kis, Z., Kontoravdi, C., Shattock, R., & Shah, N. (2020). Resources, Production Scales and Time Required for Producing RNA Vaccines for the Global Pandemic Demand. *Vaccines*, *9*(1), 3. https://doi.org/10.3390/vaccines9010003

Kitikoon, P., Knetter, S. M., Mogler, M. A., Morgan, C. L., Hoehn, A., Puttamreddy, S., Strait, E. L., & Segers, R. P. A. M. (2023). Quadrivalent neuraminidase RNA particle vaccine protects pigs against homologous and heterologous strains of swine influenza virus infection. *Vaccine*, *41*(47), 6941–6951. https://doi.org/10.1016/j.vaccine.2023.10.005

Kizawa, M., & Iwasaki, Y. (2022). Amyloid β-related angiitis of the central nervous system occurring after COVID-19 vaccination: A case report. *World Journal of Clinical Cases*, *10*(34), 12617–12622. https://doi.org/10.12998/wjcc.v10.i34.12617

Klinman, D. M., Klaschik, S., Tross, D., Shirota, H., & Steinhagen, F. (2010). FDA guidance on prophylactic DNA vaccines: Analysis and recommendations. *Vaccine*, *28*(16), 2801–2805. https://doi.org/10.1016/j.vaccine.2009.11.025

Kobayashi, H., Fukuda, S., Matsukawa, R., Asakura, Y., Kanno, Y., Hatta, T., Saito, Y., Shimizu, Y., Kawarasaki, S., Kihara, M., Kinoshita, N., Umeda, H., Noda, T., Imamura, T., Nishioka, Y., Yamaguchi, T., Hayashi, S., & Iguchi, T. (2023). Risks of Myocarditis and Pericarditis Following Vaccination with SARS-CoV-2 mRNA Vaccines in Japan: An Analysis of Spontaneous Reports of Suspected Adverse Events. *Therapeutic Innovation & Regulatory Science*, *57*(2), 329–342. https://doi.org/10.1007/s43441-022-00466-1

Koç Yıldırım, S. (2022). A new-onset vitiligo following the inactivated COVID-19 vaccine. *Journal of Cosmetic Dermatology*, *21*(2), 429–430. https://doi.org/10.1111/jocd.14677

Kohli, U., Desai, L., Chowdhury, D., Harahsheh, A. S., Yonts, A. B., Ansong, A., Sabati, A., Nguyen, H. H., Hussain, T., Khan, D., Parra, D. A., Su, J. A., Patel, J. K., Ronai, C., Bohun, M., Freij, B. J., O'Connor, M. J., Rosanno, J. W., Gupta, A., … Ang, J. Y. (2022). mRNA Coronavirus Disease 2019 Vaccine-Associated Myopericarditis in Adolescents: A Survey Study. *The Journal of Pediatrics*, *243*, 208-213.e3. https://doi.org/10.1016/j.jpeds.2021.12.025

Kohlrausch, F. B., Berteli, T. S., Wang, F., Navarro, P. A., & Keefe, D. L. (2022). Control of LINE-1 Expression Maintains Genome Integrity in Germline and Early Embryo Development. *Reproductive Sciences*, *29*(2), 328–340. https://doi.org/10.1007/s43032-021-00461-1

Komaba, H., Wada, T., & Fukagawa, M. (2021). Relapse of Minimal Change Disease Following the Pfizer-BioNTech COVID-19 Vaccine. *American Journal of Kidney Diseases*, *78*(3), 469–470. https://doi.org/10.1053/j.ajkd.2021.05.006

Kovesdi, I., & Hedley, S. J. (2010). Adenoviral Producer Cells. *Viruses*, *2*(8), 1681–1703. https://doi.org/10.3390/v2081681

Kovesdy, C. P. (2022). Epidemiology of chronic kidney disease: an update 2022. *Kidney International Supplements*, *12*(1), 7–11. https://doi.org/10.1016/j.kisu.2021.11.003

Kowalski, P. S., Rudra, A., Miao, L., & Anderson, D. G. (2019). Delivering the Messenger: Advances in Technologies for Therapeutic mRNA Delivery. *Molecular Therapy*, *27*(4), 710–728. https://doi.org/10.1016/j.ymthe.2019.02.012

Kozma, G. T., Shimizu, T., Ishida, T., & Szebeni, J. (2020). Anti-PEG antibodies: Properties, formation, testing and role in adverse immune reactions to PEGylated nano-biopharmaceuticals. *Advanced Drug Delivery Reviews*, *154–155*, 163–175. https://doi.org/10.1016/j.addr.2020.07.024

Krauson, A. J., Casimero, F. V. C., Siddiquee, Z., & Stone, J. R. (2023). Duration of SARS-CoV-2 mRNA vaccine persistence and factors associated with cardiac involvement in recently vaccinated patients. *Npj Vaccines*, *8*(1), 141. https://doi.org/10.1038/s41541-023-00742-7

Kripalani, Y., Lakkappan, V., Parulekar, L., Shaikh, A., Singh, R., & Vyas, P. (2021). A Rare Case of Guillain-Barré Syndrome following COVID-19 Vaccination. *European Journal of Case Reports in Internal Medicine*. https://doi.org/10.12890/2021_002797

Kronzer, V. L., Bridges, S. L. Jr, & Davis, J. M. 3rd. (2020). Why women have more autoimmune diseases than men: An evolutionary perspective. *Evolutionary Applications, 14*(3), 629–633. https://doi.org/10.1111/eva.1316

Krug, A., Stevenson, J., & Høeg, T. B. (2022). BNT162b2 Vaccine-Associated Myo/Pericarditis in Adolescents: A Stratified Risk-Benefit Analysis. *European Journal of Clinical Investigation*, *52*(5). https://doi.org/10.1111/eci.13759

Krumholz, H. M., Wi, Y., Sawano, M., Shah, R., Zhou, T., Arun, A. S., Kholsa, P., Kaleen, S., Vashist, A., Bhattacharjee, B., Ding., Q., Lu, Y., Caraballo, C., Warner, F., Huang., C., Herrin, J., Putrino, D., Hertz, D., Dressen, B., & Iwasaki, A. (2023). Post-vaccination syndrome: A descriptive analysis of reported symptoms and patient experiences after Covid-19 immunization. *MedRxiv : The Preprint Server for Health Sciences*. https://doi.org/10.1101/2023.11.09.23298266

Krutzke, L., Rösler, R., Allmendinger, E., Engler, T., Wiese, S., & Kochanek, S. (2022). Process- and product-related impurities in the ChAdOx1 nCov-19 vaccine. *ELife*, *11*. https://doi.org/10.7554/eLife.78513

Kuhn, C. C., Basnet, N., Bodakuntla, S., Alvarez-Brecht, P., Nichols, S., Martinez-Sanchez, A., Agostini, L., Soh, Y.-M., Takagi, J., Biertümpfel, C., & Mizuno, N. (2023). Direct Cryo-ET observation of platelet deformation induced by SARS-CoV-2 spike protein. *Nature Communications*, *14*(1), 620. https://doi.org/10.1038/s41467-023-36279-5

Kulanayake, S., & Tikoo, S. (2021). Adenovirus Core Proteins: Structure and Function. *Viruses*, *13*(3), 388. https://doi.org/10.3390/v13030388

Kulhankova, K., George, C. L. S., Kline, J. N., Snyder, J. M., Darling, M., Field, E. H., & Thorne, P. S. (2009). Early-life co-administration of cockroach allergen and endotoxin augments pulmonary and systemic responses. *Clinical & Experimental Allergy*, *39*(7), 1069–1079. https://doi.org/10.1111/j.1365-2222.2009.03254.x

Kunal, S., Ray, I., & Ish, P. (2021). Global implication of booster doses of COVID-19 vaccine. *Le Infezioni in Medicina*, *29*(4), 643–647. https://doi.org/10.53854/liim-2904-20

Kundi, M. (2007). Causality and the interpretation of epidemiologic evidence. *Ciência & Saúde Coletiva*, *12*(2), 419–428. https://doi.org/10.1590/S1413-81232007000200018

Kurachi, M. (2019). CD8+ T cell exhaustion. *Seminars in Immunopathology*, *41*(3), 327–337. https://doi.org/10.1007/s00281-019-00744-5

Kurth, R. (1995). Risk Potential of the Chromosomal Insertion of Foreign DNA. *Annals of the New York Academy of Sciences*, *772*(1), 140–151. https://doi.org/10.1111/j.1749-6632.1995.tb44739.x

Kuwabara, S. (2004). Guillain-Barr?? Syndrome. *Drugs*, *64*(6), 597–610. https://doi.org/10.2165/00003495-200464060-00003

Kyriakopoulos, A. M., Nigh, G., McCullough, P. A., Olivier, M. D., & Seneff, S. (2023). *Bell's palsy or an aggressive infiltrating basaloid carcinoma post-mRNA vaccination for covid-19? A case report and review of the literature. 22*, 992–1011.

Kyriakopoulos, A. M., Nigh, G., McCullough, P. A., Seneff, S. (2022). Mitogen Activated Protein Kinase (MAPK) Activation, p53, and Autophagy Inhibition Characterize the Severe Acute Respiratory Syndrome Coronavirus 2 (SARS-CoV-2) Spike Protein Induced Neurotoxicity. *Cureus, 14*(12), e32361. https://doi.org/10.7759/cureus.32361.

Laganà, A. S., Veronesi, G., Ghezzi, F., Ferrario, M. M., Cromi, A., Bizzarri, M., Garzon, S., & Cosentino, M. (2022). Evaluation of menstrual irregularities after COVID-19 vaccination: Results of the MECOVAC survey. *Open Medicine*, *17*(1), 475–484. https://doi.org/10.1515/med-2022-0452

Lai, C. M., Lai, Y. K., & Rakoczy, P. E. (2002). Adenovirus and adeno-associated virus vectors. *DNA Cellular Biology*, *21*(12), 895–913. https://doi.org/10.1089/104454902762053855.

Lai, M., Huijbers, M. G., Lancaster, E., Graus, F., Bataller, L., Balice-Gordon, R., Cowell, J. K., & Dalmau, J. (2010). Investigation of LGI1 as the antigen in limbic encephalitis previously attributed to potassium channels: a case series. *The Lancet Neurology*, *9*(8), 776–785. https://doi.org/10.1016/S1474-4422(10)70137-X

Laisuan, W. (2021). COVID-19 Vaccine Anaphylaxis: Current Evidence and Future Approaches. *Frontiers in Allergy*, *2*. https://doi.org/10.3389/falgy.2021.801322

Lally, C., Jones, C., Farwell, W., Reyna, S. P., Cook, S. F., & Flanders, W. D. (2017). Indirect estimation of the prevalence of spinal muscular atrophy Type I, II, and III in the United States. *Orphanet Journal of Rare Diseases, 12*(1), 175. https://doi.org/10.1186/s13023-017-0724-z.

Laman, J. D., Huizinga, R., Boons, G.-J., & Jacobs, B. C. (2022). Guillain-Barré syndrome: expanding the concept of molecular mimicry. *Trends in Immunology*, *43*(4), 296–308. https://doi.org/10.1016/j.it.2022.02.003

Lambert, P.-H., Ambrosino, D. M., Andersen, S. R., Baric, R. S., Black, S. B., Chen, R. T., Dekker, C. L., Didierlaurent, A. M., Graham, B. S., Martin, S. D., Molrine, D. C., Perlman, S., Picard-Fraser, P. A., Pollard, A. J., Qin, C., Subbarao, K., & Cramer, J. P. (2020). Consensus summary report for CEPI/BC March 12–13, 2020 meeting: Assessment of risk of disease enhancement with COVID-19 vaccines. *Vaccine*, *38*(31), 4783–4791. https://doi.org/10.1016/j.vaccine.2020.05.064

Langer, B., Renner, M., Scherer, J., Schüle, S., & Cichutek, K. (2013). *Safety Assessment of Biolistic DNA Vaccination* (pp. 371–388). https://doi.org/10.1007/978-1-62703-110-3_27

Lanman, T. A., Wu, C., Cheung, H., Goyal, N., & Greene, M. (2022). Guillain-Barré Syndrome with Rapid Onset and Autonomic Dysfunction Following First Dose of

Pfizer-BioNTech COVID-19 Vaccine: A Case Report. *The Neurohospitalist*, *12*(2), 388–390. https://doi.org/10.1177/19418744211065242
Lapébie, F.-X., Kennel, C., Magy, L., Projetti, F., Honnorat, J., Pichon, N., Vignon, P., & François, B. (2014). Potential side effect of propofol and sevoflurane for anesthesia of anti-NMDA-R encephalitis. *BMC Anesthesiology*, *14*(1), 5. https://doi.org/10.1186/1471-2253-14-5
Larsen, S., Hansen, J., Hansen, E., Clausen, P., & Nielsen, G. (2007). Airway inflammation and adjuvant effect after repeated airborne exposures to di-(2-ethylhexyl)phthalate and ovalbumin in BALB/c mice. *Toxicology*, *235*(1–2), 119–129. https://doi.org/10.1016/j.tox.2007.03.010
Larson, K. F., Ammirati, E., Adler, E. D., Cooper, L. T., Hong, K. N., Saponara, G., Couri, D., Cereda, A., Procopio, A., Cavalotti, C., Oliva, F., Sanna, T., Ciconte, V. A., Onyango, G., Holmes, D. R., & Borgeson, D. D. (2021). Myocarditis After BNT162b2 and mRNA-1273 Vaccination. *Circulation*, *144*(6), 506–508. https://doi.org/10.1161/CIRCULATIONAHA.121.055913
Larson, V., Seidenberg, R., Caplan, A., Brinster, N. K., Meehan, S. A., & Kim, R. H. (2022). Clinical and histopathological spectrum of delayed adverse cutaneous reactions following COVID-19 vaccination. *Journal of Cutaneous Pathology*, *49*(1), 34–41. https://doi.org/10.1111/cup.14104
Laudicella, R., Burger, I. A., Panasiti, F., Longo, C., Scalisi, S., Minutoli, F., Baldari, S., Grimaldi, L. M. E., & Alongi, P. (2021). Subcutaneous Uptake on [18F]Florbetaben PET/CT: a Case Report of Possible Amyloid-Beta Immune-Reactivity After COVID-19 Vaccination. *SN Comprehensive Clinical Medicine*, *3*(12), 2626–2628. https://doi.org/10.1007/s42399-021-01058-0
Lázaro Hernández, C., Llauradó Gayete, A., Sánchez-Tejerina San José, D., Cabirta, A., Carpio, C., Sotoca, J., Salvadó Figueras, M., Raguer Sanz, N., Restrepo, J., & Juntas Morales, R. (2022). Síndrome de Guillain-Barré y trombocitopenia tras la vacunación contra el SARS-CoV-2 con Moderna. Descripción de un caso. *Revista de Neurología*, *75*(08), 247. https://doi.org/10.33588/rn.7508.2022138
Lazzerini, P. E., Laghi-Pasini, F., Boutjdir, M., & Capecchi, P. L. (2019). Cardioimmunology of arrhythmias: the role of autoimmune and inflammatory cardiac channelopathies. *Nature Reviews Immunology*, *19*(1), 63–64. https://doi.org/10.1038/s41577-018-0098-z
Le, T., Sun, C., Chang, J., Zhang, G., & Yin, X. (2022). mRNA Vaccine Development for Emerging Animal and Zoonotic Diseases. *Viruses*, *14*(2), 401. https://doi.org/10.3390/v14020401.
Lebedev, L., Sapojnikov, M., Wechsler, A., Varadi-Levi, R., Zamir, D., Tobar, A., Levin-Iaina, N., Fytlovich, S., & Yagil, Y. (2021). Minimal Change Disease Following the Pfizer-BioNTech COVID-19 Vaccine. *American Journal of Kidney Diseases*, *78*(1), 142–145. https://doi.org/10.1053/j.ajkd.2021.03.010
Leccese, D., Cornacchini, S., Nacmias, B., Sorbi, S., & Bessi, V. (2023). Creutzfeldt-Jakob Disease in a Patient with Previous COVID-19 Infection: "The Virus Caused the Derangement in My Brain." *Journal of Alzheimer's Disease Reports*, *7*(1), 129–134. https://doi.org/10.3233/ADR-220095
Leclerc, S., Royal, V., Lamarche, C., & Laurin, L.-P. (2021). Minimal Change Disease With Severe Acute Kidney Injury Following the Oxford-AstraZeneca COVID-19 Vaccine: A Case Report. *American Journal of Kidney Diseases*, *78*(4), 607–610. https://doi.org/10.1053/j.ajkd.2021.06.008

Ledford, H. (2021). COVID vaccines and blood clots: five key questions. *Nature*, *592*(7855), 495–496. https://doi.org/10.1038/d41586-021-00998-w

Ledgerwood, J. E., Costner, P., Desai, N., Holman, L., Enama, M. E., Yamshchikov, G., Mulangu, S., Hu, Z., Andrews, C. A., Sheets, R. A., Koup, R. A., Roederer, M., Bailer, R., Mascola, J. R., Pau, M. G., Sullivan, N. J., Goudsmit, J., Nabel, G. J., & Graham, B. S. (2010). A replication defective recombinant Ad5 vaccine expressing Ebola virus GP is safe and immunogenic in healthy adults. *Vaccine*, *29*(2), 304–313. https://doi.org/10.1016/j.vaccine.2010.10.037

Lednicky, J. A., & Butel, J. S. (2001). Simian virus 40 regulatory region structural diversity and the association of viral archetypal regulatory regions with human brain tumors. *Seminars in Cancer Biology*, *11*(1), 39–47. https://doi.org/10.1006/scbi.2000.0345

Ledwith, B. J., Manam, S., Troilo, P. J., Barnum, A. B., Pauley, C. J., Griffiths II, T. G., Harper, L. B., Beare, C. M., Bagdon, W. J., & Nichols, W. W. (2000). Plasmid DNA Vaccines: Investigation of Integration into Host Cellular DNA following Intramuscular Injection in Mice. *Intervirology*, *43*(4–6), 258–272. https://doi.org/10.1159/000053993

Lee, G. M., & Arepally, G. M. (2013). Heparin-induced thrombocytopenia. *Hematology*, *2013*(1), 668–674. https://doi.org/10.1182/asheducation-2013.1.668

Lee, H. Y., & Lien, W.-C. (2023). Effects of COVID-19 vaccine type on Guillain-Barré syndrome: Two cases and a literature review. *Human Vaccines & Immunotherapeutics*, *19*(1). https://doi.org/10.1080/21645515.2023.2171231

Lee, K. M. N., Junkins, E. J., Luo, C., Fatima, U. A., Cox, M. L., & Clancy, K. B. H. (2022). Investigating trends in those who experience menstrual bleeding changes after SARS-CoV-2 vaccination. *Science Advances*, *8*(28). https://doi.org/10.1126/sciadv.abm7201

Lee, M. H., Perl, D. P., Nair, G., Li, W., Maric, D., Murray, H., Dodd, S. J., Koretsky, A. P., Watts, J. A., Cheung, V., Masliah, E., Horkayne-Szakaly, I., Jones, R., Stram, M. N., Moncur, J., Hefti, M., Folkerth, R. D., & Nath, A. (2021). Microvascular Injury in the Brains of Patients with COVID. New England Journal of Medicine, 384(5), 481–483. https://doi.org/10.1056/NEJMc2033369

Lee, W. S., Wheatley, A. K., Kent, S. J., & DeKosky, B. J. (2020). Antibody-dependent enhancement and SARS-CoV-2 vaccines and therapies. *Nature Microbiology*, *5*(10), 1185–1191. https://doi.org/10.1038/s41564-020-00789-5

Lee, Y. F., Chen, S. J., Chung, Y. M., Liu, J. H., & Wong, W. W. (2000). Diffuse toxoplasmic retinochoroiditis as the initial manifestation of acquired immunodeficiency syndrome. *Journal of the Formosan Medical Association = Taiwan Yi Zhi*, *99*(3), 219–223.

Lehnhardt, E. (1984). [Clinical aspects of labyrinthine hearing loss]. *Archives of Oto-Rhino-Laryngology. Supplement = Archiv Fur Ohren-, Nasen- Und Kehlkopfheilkunde. Supplement*, *1*, 58–218.

Lei, Y., Zhang, J., Schiavon, C. R., He, M., Chen, L., Shen, H., Zhang, Y., Yin, Q., Cho, Y., Andrade, L., Shadel, G. S., Hepokoski, M., Lei, T., Wang, H., Zhang, J., Yuan, J. X.-J., Malhotra, A., Manor, U., Wang, S., … Shyy, J. Y.-J. (2021). SARS-CoV-2 Spike Protein Impairs Endothelial Function via Downregulation of ACE 2. *Circulation Research*, *128*(9), 1323–1326. https://doi.org/10.1161/CIRCRESAHA.121.318902

Leitão, M. J., Baldeiras, I., Almeida, M. R., Ribeiro, M. H., Santos, A. C., Ribeiro, M., Tomás, J., Rocha, S., Santana, I., & Oliveira, C. R. (2016). Sporadic Creutzfeldt–Jakob disease diagnostic accuracy is improved by a new CSF ELISA 14-3-3γ assay. *Neuroscience*, *322*, 398–407. https://doi.org/10.1016/j.neuroscience.2016.02.057

Lemus, H. N., Warrington, A. E., & Rodriguez, M. (2018). Multiple Sclerosis. *Neurologic Clinics*, *36*(1), 1–11. https://doi.org/10.1016/j.ncl.2017.08.002

Leong, S., Teh, B. M., & Kim, A. H. (2023). Characterization of otologic symptoms appearing after COVID-19 vaccination. *American Journal of Otolaryngology*, *44*(2), 103725. https://doi.org/10.1016/j.amjoto.2022.103725

Lesch, H. P., Heikkilä, K. M., Lipponen, E. M., Valonen, P., Müller, A., Räsänen, E., Tuunanen, T., Hassinen, M. M., Parker, N., Karhinen, M., Shaw, R., & Ylä-Herttuala, S. (2015). Process Development of Adenoviral Vector Production in Fixed Bed Bioreactor: From Bench to Commercial Scale. *Human Gene Therapy*, *26*(8), 560–571. https://doi.org/10.1089/hum.2015.081

Lessans, N., Rottenstreich, A., Stern, S., Gilan, A., Saar, T. D., Porat, S., & Dior, U. P. (2023). The effect of BNT162b2 SARS-CoV-2 mRNA vaccine on menstrual cycle symptoms in healthy women. *International Journal of Gynecology & Obstetrics*, *160*(1), 313–318. https://doi.org/10.1002/ijgo.14356

Levi, M., & Sivapalaratnam, S. (2018). Disseminated intravascular coagulation: an update on pathogenesis and diagnosis. *Expert Review of Hematology*, *11*(8), 663–672. https://doi.org/10.1080/17474086.2018.1500173

Levine, H., Jørgensen, N., Martino-Andrade, A., Mendiola, J., Weksler-Derri, D., Mindlis, I., Pinotti, R., & Swan, S. H. (2017). Temporal trends in sperm count: a systematic review and meta-regression analysis. *Human Reproduction Update*, *23*(6), 646–659. https://doi.org/10.1093/humupd/dmx022

Li, C., Jiang, M., Pan, C., Li, J., & Xu, L. (2021). The global, regional, and national burden of acute pancreatitis in 204 countries and territories, 1990–2019. *BMC Gastroenterology*, *21*(1), 332. https://doi.org/10.1186/s12876-021-01906-2

Li, H., Dai, B., Fan, J., Chen, C., Nie, X., Yin, Z., Zhao, Y., Zhang, X., & Wang, D. W. (2019). The Different Roles of miRNA-92a-2-5p and let-7b-5p in Mitochondrial Translation in db/db Mice. *Molecular Therapy - Nucleic Acids*, *17*, 424–435. https://doi.org/10.1016/j.omtn.2019.06.013

Li, J.-X., Wang, Y.-H., Bair, H., Hsu, S.-B., Chen, C., Wei, J. C.-C., & Lin, C.-J. (2023). Risk assessment of retinal vascular occlusion after COVID-19 vaccination. *Npj Vaccines*, *8*(1), 64. https://doi.org/10.1038/s41541-023-00661-7

Li, S., Ho, M., Mak, A., Lai, F., Brelen, M., Chong, K., & Young, A. (2023). Intraocular inflammation following COVID-19 vaccination: the clinical presentations. *International Ophthalmology*, *43*(8), 2971–2981. https://doi.org/10.1007/s10792-023-02684-4

Li, X., & Chen, W. (2019). Mechanisms of failure of chimeric antigen receptor T-cell therapy. *Current Opinion in Hematology*, *26*(6), 427–433. https://doi.org/10.1097/MOH.0000000000000548

Li, X., Yuan, J., Liu, L., & Hu, W. (2019). Antibody-LGI 1 autoimmune encephalitis manifesting as rapidly progressive dementia and hyponatremia: a case report and literature review. *BMC Neurology*, *19*(1), 19. https://doi.org/10.1186/s12883-019-1251-4

Li, Z., Hu, F., Li, Q., Wang, S., Chen, C., Zhang, Y., Mao, Y., Shi, X., Zhou, H., Cao, X., & Peng, X. (2022). Ocular Adverse Events after Inactivated COVID-19 Vaccination. *Vaccines*, *10*(6), 918. https://doi.org/10.3390/vaccines10060918

Liang, H., Cao, Y., Zhong, W., Ma, Z., Liu, J., & Chen, H. (2022). Miller-Fisher syndrome and Guillain–Barre syndrome overlap syndrome following inactivated COVID-19 vaccine: Case report and scope review. *Human Vaccines & Immunotherapeutics*, *18*(6). https://doi.org/10.1080/21645515.2022.2125753

Lichtenstein, D. L., & Wold, W. S. (2004). Experimental infections of humans with wild-type adenoviruses and with replication-competent adenovirus vectors: replication, safety, and transmission. *Cancer Gene Therapy, 11*(12), 819–829. https://doi.org/10.1038/sj.cgt.7700765.

Lien, Y.-L., Wei, C.-Y., & Liang, J.-S. (2023). Acute psychosis induced by mRNA-based COVID-19 vaccine in adolescents: A pediatric case report. *Pediatrics & Neonatology*, *64*(3), 364–365. https://doi.org/10.1016/j.pedneo.2022.10.007

Lim, J.-H., Han, M.-H., Kim, Y.-J., Kim, M.-S., Jung, H.-Y., Choi, J.-Y., Cho, J.-H., Kim, C.-D., Kim, Y.-L., & Park, S.-H. (2021). New-onset Nephrotic Syndrome after Janssen COVID-19 Vaccination: a Case Report and Literature Review. *Journal of Korean Medical Science*, *36*(30). https://doi.org/10.3346/jkms.2021.36.e218

Lin, C.-Y., & Chien, H.-J. (2023). Acute exacerbation of ocular graft-versus-host disease and anterior uveitis after COVID-19 vaccination. *BMC Ophthalmology*, *23*(1), 360. https://doi.org/10.1186/s12886-023-03103-z

Lin, D., & Selleck, A. M. (2023). Tinnitus cases after COVID-19 vaccine administration, one institution's observations. *American Journal of Otolaryngology*, *44*(4), 103863. https://doi.org/10.1016/j.amjoto.2023.103863

Lindgren, A. L., Austin, A. H., & Welsh, K. M. (2021). COVID Arm: Delayed Hypersensitivity Reactions to SARS-CoV-2 Vaccines Misdiagnosed as Cellulitis. *Journal of Primary Care & Community Health*, *12*, 215013272110244. https://doi.org/10.1177/21501327211024431

Ling, L., Bagshaw, S. M., & Villeneuve, P.-M. (2021). Guillain–Barré syndrome after SARS-CoV-2 vaccination in a patient with previous vaccine-associated Guillain–Barré syndrome. *Canadian Medical Association Journal*, *193*(46), E1766–E1769. https://doi.org/10.1503/cmaj.210947

Ling, V. W. T., Fan, B. E., Lau, S. L., Lee, X. H., Tan, C. W., & Lee, S. Y. (2022). Severe Thrombocytopenia, Thrombosis and Anti-PF4 Antibody after Pfizer-BioNTech COVID-19 mRNA Vaccine Booster—Is It Vaccine-Induced Immune Thrombotic Thrombocytopenia? *Vaccines*, *10*(12), 2023. https://doi.org/10.3390/vaccines10122023

Little, D. T., Šeman, E. I., & Walsh, A. L. (2021). COVID-19 Vaccination: Guidance for Ethical, Informed Consent in a National Context. *Issues in Law & Medicine*, *36*(2), 127–162.

Litviňuková, M., Talavera-López, C., Maatz, H., Reichart, D., Worth, C. L., Lindberg, E. L., Kanda, M., Polanski, K., Heinig, M., Lee, M., Nadelmann, E. R., Roberts, K., Tuck, L., Fasouli, E. S., DeLaughter, D. M., McDonough, B., Wakimoto, H., Gorham, J. M., Samari, S., … Teichmann, S. A. (2020). Cells of the adult human heart. *Nature*, *588*(7838), 466–472. https://doi.org/10.1038/s41586-020-2797-4

Liu, C., Martins, A. J., Lau, W. W., Rachmaninoff, N., Chen, J., Imberti, L., Mostaghimi, D., Fink, D. L., Burbelo, P. D., Dobbs, K., Delmonte, O. M., Bansal,

N., Failla, L., Sottini, A., Quiros-Roldan, E., Han, K. L., Sellers, B. A., Cheung. T.-W., … Tsang, J. S. (2021). Time-resolved systems immunology reveals a late juncture linked to fatal COVID. *Cell, 184*,1836–1857.e22.

Liu, J., Zhou, F., Guan, Y., Meng, F., Zhao, Z., Su, Q., Bao, W., Wang, X., Zhao, J., Huo, Z., Zhang, L., Zhou, S., Chen, Y., & Wang, X. (2022). The Biogenesis of miRNAs and Their Role in the Development of Amyotrophic Lateral Sclerosis. *Cells*, *11*(3), 572. https://doi.org/10.3390/cells11030572

Liu, K., & Tirado, C. A. (2019). MECOM: A Very Interesting Gene Involved also in Lymphoid Malignancies. *Journal of the Association of Genetic Technologists*, *45*(3), 109–114.

Liu, R., Du, S., Zhao, L., Jain, S., Sahay, K., Rizvanov, A., Lezhnyova, V., Khaibullin, T., Martynova, E., Khaiboullina, S., & Baranwal, M. (2022). Autoreactive lymphocytes in multiple sclerosis: Pathogenesis and treatment target. *Frontiers in Immunology*, *13*. https://doi.org/10.3389/fimmu.2022.996469

Liu, S., Hossinger, A., Heumüller, S.-E., Hornberger, A., Buravlova, O., Konstantoulea, K., Müller, S. A., Paulsen, L., Rousseau, F., Schymkowitz, J., Lichtenthaler, S. F., Neumann, M., Denner, P., & Vorberg, I. M. (2021). Highly efficient intercellular spreading of protein misfolding mediated by viral ligand-receptor interactions. *Nature Communications*, *12*(1), 5739. https://doi.org/10.1038/s41467-021-25855-2

Liu, Y., Soh, W. T., Kishikawa, J., Hirose, M., Nakayama, E. E., Li, S., Sasai, M., Suzuki, T., Tada, A., Arakawa, A., Matsuoka, S., Akamatsu, K., Matsuda, M., Ono, C., Torii, S., Kishida, K., Jin, H., Nakai, W., Arase, N., … Arase, H. (2021). An infectivity-enhancing site on the SARS-CoV-2 spike protein targeted by antibodies. *Cell*, *184*(13), 3452-3466.e18. https://doi.org/10.1016/j.cell.2021.05.032

Lockett, L. J., & Both, G. W. (2002). Complementation of a defective human adenovirus by an otherwise incompatible ovine adenovirus recombinant carrying a functional E1A gene. *Virology*, *294*(2), 333–341. https://doi.org/10.1006/viro.2001.1327. PMID: 12009875.

Logunov, D. Y., Dolzhikova, I. V, Shcheblyakov, D. V, Tukhvatulin, A. I., Zubkova, O. V, Dzharullaeva, A. S., Kovyrshina, A. V, Lubenets, N. L., Grousova, D. M., Erokhova, A. S., Botikov, A. G., Izhaeva, F. M., Popova, O., Ozharovskaya, T. A., Esmagambetov, I. B., Favorskaya, I. A., Zrelkin, D. I., Voronina, D. V, Shcherbinin, D. N., … Gintsburg, A. L. (2021). Safety and efficacy of an rAd26 and rAd5 vector-based heterologous prime-boost COVID-19 vaccine: an interim analysis of a randomised controlled phase 3 trial in Russia. *The Lancet*, *397*(10275), 671–681. https://doi.org/10.1016/S0140-6736(21)00234-8

Loli-Ausejo, D., Gómez-Armayones, S., Sáez-Peñataro, J., González-Matamala, M., Mascaró, B., Muñoz-Cano, R., & Bartra, J. (2023). COVID-19 Vaccine Tolerability in a Patient With a Delayed Allergic Reaction to Polyethylene Glycol: A Case Report. *Journal of Investigational Allergy and Clinical Immunology*, *33*(3), 232–233. https://doi.org/10.18176/jiaci.0843

López Riquelme, I., Fernández Ballesteros, M. D., Serrano Ordoñez, A., & Godoy Díaz, D. J. (2022). COVID and autoimmune phenomena: Vitiligo after Astrazeneca vaccine. *Dermatologic Therapy*, *35*(7). https://doi.org/10.1111/dth.15502

Lorentzen, C. L., Haanen, J. B., Met, Ö., & Svane, I. M. (2022). Clinical advances and ongoing trials on mRNA vaccines for cancer treatment. *Lancet Oncology, 23*(10), e450–e458. https://doi.org/10.1016/S1470-2045(22)00372-2

Lu, J.-C., Huang, Y.-F., & Lu, N.-Q. (2008). Antisperm immunity and infertility. *Expert Review of Clinical Immunology*, *4*(1), 113–126. https://doi.org/10.1586/1744666X.4.1.113

Lu, S., Xie, X., Zhao, L., Wang, B., Zhu, J., Yang, T., Yang, G., Ji, M., Lv, C., Xue, J., Dai, E., Fu, X., Liu, D., Zhang, L., Hou, S., Yu, X., Wang, Y., Gao, H., Shi, X., … Liu, R. (2021). The immunodominant and neutralization linear epitopes for SARS-CoV-2. *Cell Reports*, *34*(4), 108666. https://doi.org/10.1016/j.celrep.2020.108666

Lucas, R. M., & McMichael, A. J. (2005). Association or causation: evaluating links between "environment and disease". *Bulletin of the World Health Organization*, *83*(10), 792–795.

Lucchese, G., & Flöel, A. (2020). SARS-CoV-2 and Guillain-Barré syndrome: molecular mimicry with human heat shock proteins as potential pathogenic mechanism. *Cell Stress and Chaperones*, *25*(5), 731–735. https://doi.org/10.1007/s12192-020-01145-6

Luciano, P. Q., Binatti, R., Sodré, A. R., Zajac, S. R., Marson, F. A. L., & Ortega, M. M. (2022). Vaccine-induced immune thrombotic thrombocytopenia after ChAdOx1 nCoV-19 vaccine in an older patient: Minireview and a case report. *Journal of Infection and Public Health*, *15*(6), 638–642. https://doi.org/10.1016/j.jiph.2022.04.008

Luisetto, M., Tarro, G., Almukthar, N., Ahmadabadi, N. B., Sahu, R., Khan, A. F., Rasool, M. G., Cabianca, L., Fiazza, C., Prince, G. G., & Latyshew, O. Y. (2023). Bio-Pharmaceutical Manufacturing Large Scale Production Process: The Graphene Derivates Role and mRNA Vaccine. *Journal of Current Chemical and Pharmaceutical Sciences*, *13*(1). https://doi.org/10.37532/2277-2871.23.13.002

Luk, A., Clarke, B., Dahdah, N., Ducharme, A., Krahn, A., McCrindle, B., Mizzi, T., Naus, M., Udell, J. A., Virani, S., Zieroth, S., & McDonald, M. (2021). Myocarditis and Pericarditis After COVID-19 mRNA Vaccination: Practical Considerations for Care Providers. *Canadian Journal of Cardiology*, *37*(10), 1629–1634. https://doi.org/10.1016/j.cjca.2021.08.001

Lukashev, A. N., & Zamyatnin, A. A. (2016). Viral vectors for gene therapy: Current state and clinical perspectives. *Biochemistry (Moscow)*, *81*(7), 700–708. https://doi.org/10.1134/S0006297916070063

Lurie, N., Saville, M., Hatchett, R., & Halton, J. (2020). Developing Covid-19 Vaccines at Pandemic Speed. *New England Journal of Medicine*, *382*(21), 1969–1973. https://doi.org/10.1056/NEJMp2005630

Lyon, A. R., Rees, P. S., Prasad, S., Poole-Wilson, P. A., & Harding, S. E. (2008). Stress (Takotsubo) cardiomyopathy—a novel pathophysiological hypothesis to explain catecholamine-induced acute myocardial stunning. *Nature Clinical Practice Cardiovascular Medicine*, *5*(1), 22–29. https://doi.org/10.1038/ncpcardio1066

M M Al-Mehaisen, L., A Mahfouz, I., Khamaiseh, K., N AL-Beitawe, S., & Al-Kuran, O. A. H. (2022). Short Term Effect of Corona Virus Diseases Vaccine on the Menstrual Cycles. *International Journal of Women's Health, Volume 14*, 1385–1394. https://doi.org/10.2147/IJWH.S376950

Ma, J., Han, W., & Jiang, L. (2020). Japanese encephalitis-induced anti-N-methyl-d-aspartate receptor encephalitis: A hospital-based prospective study. *Brain and Development*, *42*(2), 179–184. https://doi.org/10.1016/j.braindev.2019.09.003

Ma, K. C., Shirk, P., Lambrou, A. S., Hassell, N., Zheng, X., Payne, A. B., Ali, A. R., Batra, D., Caravas, J., Chau, R., Cook, P. W., Howard, D., Kovacs, N. A., Lacek, K. A., Lee, J. S., MacCannell, D. R., Malapati, L., Mathew, S., Mittal, N., … Paden, C. R. (2023). Genomic Surveillance for SARS-CoV-2 Variants: Circulation of Omicron Lineages — United States, January 2022–May 2023. *MMWR. Morbidity and Mortality Weekly Report*, *72*(24), 651–656. https://doi.org/10.15585/mmwr.mm7224a2

Maas, R. J., Gianotten, S., & van der Meijden, W. A. G. (2021). An Additional Case of Minimal Change Disease Following the Pfizer-BioNTech COVID-19 Vaccine. *American Journal of Kidney Diseases*, *78*(2), 312. https://doi.org/10.1053/j.ajkd.2021.05.003

Macca, L., Peterle, L., Ceccarelli, M., Ingrasciotta, Y., Nunnari, G., & Guarneri, C. (2022). Vitiligo-like Lesions and COVID-19: Case Report and Review of Vaccination- and Infection-Associated Vitiligo. *Vaccines*, *10*(10), 1647. https://doi.org/10.3390/vaccines10101647

Macchietto, M. G., Langlois, R. A., & Shen, S. S. (2020). Virus-induced transposable element expression up-regulation in human and mouse host cells. *Life Science Alliance*, *3*(2), e201900536. https://doi.org/10.26508/lsa.201900536

Madike, R., & Lee, A. (2023). A case of acute transverse myelitis following the AstraZeneca COVID-19 vaccine. *Global Journal of Medical and Clinical Case Reports*, *10*(1), 011–012. https://doi.org/10.17352/2455-5282.000169

Magen, E., & Landman, S. (2023). New Onset of Vitiligo and Atopic Dermatitis–Like Eczematous Dermatitis After Pfizer BioNTech's BNT162b2 Vaccination. *Dermatitis®*, *34*(4), 339–340. https://doi.org/10.1097/DER.0000000000000877

Magen, E., Mukherjee, S., Bhattacharya, M., Detroja, R., Merzon, E., Blum, I., Livoff, A., Shlapobersky, M., Baum, G., Talisman, R., Cherniavsky, E., Dori, A., & Frenkel-Morgenstern, M. (2022). Clinical and Molecular Characterization of a Rare Case of BNT162b2 mRNA COVID-19 Vaccine-Associated Myositis. *Vaccines*, *10*(7), 1135. https://doi.org/10.3390/vaccines10071135

Maggioni, A. Pietro, & Andreotti, F. (2021). Efficacy of COVID-19 Vaccines Against Active Comparators or Inert Placebos. *JAMA Internal Medicine*, *181*(9), 1257. https://doi.org/10.1001/jamainternmed.2021.2124

Magnaterra, E., Magliulo, M., Mariotti, E. B., Ruffo Di Calabria, V., Quintarelli, L., Corrà, A., Aimo, C., Verdelli, A., & Caproni, M. (2023). Subacute cutaneous lupus erythematosus induced by Pfizer COVID-19 vaccine. *Italian Journal of Dermatology and Venereology*, *158*(3). https://doi.org/10.23736/S2784-8671.23.07373-5

Mahajan, A., Nayak, M., Gaikwad, S., Sharma, K., Padma Srivastava, Mv., Anand, P., Oinam, R., & Mishra, B. (2023). Post-Vaccination/Post-COVID Immune-Mediated Demyelination of the Brain and Spinal Cord: A Novel Neuroimaging Finding. *Neurology India*, *71*(1), 86. https://doi.org/10.4103/0028-3886.370449

Mahendradas, P., Mishra, S. B., Mangla, R., Sanjay, S., Kawali, A., Shetty, R., & Dharmanand, B. (2022). Reactivation of juvenile idiopathic arthritis associated uveitis with posterior segment manifestations following anti-SARS-CoV-2 vaccination. *Journal of Ophthalmic Inflammation and Infection*, *12*(1), 15. https://doi.org/10.1186/s12348-022-00294-2

Mahendradas, P., Parmar, Y., Mishra, S. B., Patil, A., Kawali, A., Sanjay, S., & Shetty, B. (2023). Pole-to-pole involvement of varicella zoster virus reactivation following COVID-19 vaccination. *Indian Journal of Ophthalmology*, *71*(5), 2001–2007. https://doi.org/10.4103/IJO.IJO_2942_22

Makrides, S. C. (2003). *Vectors for gene expression in mammalian cells* (pp. 9–26). https://doi.org/10.1016/S0167-7306(03)38002-0

Malamud, E., Otallah, S. I., Caress, J. B., & Lapid, D. J. (2022). Guillain-Barré Syndrome After COVID-19 Vaccination in an Adolescent. *Pediatric Neurology*, *126*, 9–10. https://doi.org/10.1016/j.pediatrneurol.2021.10.003

Mallapaty, S., & Ledford, H. (2020). COVID-vaccine results are on the way — and scientists' concerns are growing. *Nature*, *586*(7827), 16–17. https://doi.org/10.1038/d41586-020-02706-6

Mancha, D., Antunes, J., Soares de Almeida, L., Borges-da-Costa, J., & Filipe, P. (2023). Localized Vitiligo and Post-Inflammatory Hypopigmentation at the Injection Site of a COVID-19 mRNA Vaccine. *Dermatology Practical & Conceptual*, e2023023. https://doi.org/10.5826/dpc.1301a23

Mancianti, N., Guarnieri, A., Tripodi, S., Salvo, D. P., & Garosi, G. (2021). Minimal change disease following vaccination for SARS-CoV-2. *Journal of Nephrology*, *34*(4), 1039–1040. https://doi.org/10.1007/s40620-021-01091-1

Mansour, J., Short, R. G., Bhalla, S., Woodard, P. K., Verma, A., Robinson, X., & Raptis, D. A. (2021). Acute myocarditis after a second dose of the mRNA COVID-19 vaccine: a report of two cases. *Clinical Imaging*, *78*, 247–249. https://doi.org/10.1016/j.clinimag.2021.06.019

Maoz-Segal, R., Shavit, R., Kidon, M. I., Offengenden, I., Machnes-Maayan, D., Lifshitz-Tunitsky, Y., Niznik, S., & Agmon-Levin, N. (2022). Late Hypersensitivity Reactions to the BNT162b2 SARS-CoV-2 Vaccine Are Linked to Delayed Skin Sensitization and Prior Exposure to Hyaluronic Acid. *Life*, *12*(12), 2021. https://doi.org/10.3390/life12122021

Maramattom, B. V., Krishnan, P., Paul, R., Padmanabhan, S., Cherukudal Vishnu Nampoothiri, S., Syed, A. A., & Mangat, H. S. (2021). Guillain-Barré Syndrome following ChAdOx1-S/nCoV-19 Vaccine. *Annals of Neurology*, *90*(2), 312–314. https://doi.org/10.1002/ana.26143

Marasca, F., Sinha, S., Vadalà, R., Polimeni, B., Ranzani, V., Paraboschi, E. M., Burattin, F. V., Ghilotti, M., Crosti, M., Negri, M. L., Campagnoli, S., Notarbartolo, S., Sartore-Bianchi, A., Siena, S., Prati, D., Montini, G., Viale, G., Torre, O., Harari, S., … Bodega, B. (2022). LINE1 are spliced in non-canonical transcript variants to regulate T cell quiescence and exhaustion. *Nature Genetics*, *54*(2), 180–193. https://doi.org/10.1038/s41588-021-00989-7

Marietta, M., Coluccio, V., & Luppi, M. (2022). Potential mechanisms of vaccine-induced thrombosis. *European Journal of Internal Medicine*, *105*, 1–7. https://doi.org/10.1016/j.ejim.2022.08.002

Marino Gammazza, A., Légaré, S., Lo Bosco, G., Fucarino, A., Angileri, F., Conway de Macario, E., Macario, A. J., & Cappello, F. (2020). Human molecular chaperones share with SARS-CoV-2 antigenic epitopes potentially capable of eliciting autoimmunity against endothelial cells: possible role of molecular

mimicry in COVID-19. *Cell Stress and Chaperones*, *25*(5), 737–741. https://doi.org/10.1007/s12192-020-01148-3
Marshall, M., Ferguson, I. D., Lewis, P., Jaggi, P., Gagliardo, C., Collins, J. S., Shaughnessy, R., Caron, R., Fuss, C., Corbin, K. J. E., Emuren, L., Faherty, E., Hall, E. K., Di Pentima, C., Oster, M. E., Paintsil, E., Siddiqui, S., Timchak, D. M., & Guzman-Cottrill, J. A. (2021). Symptomatic Acute Myocarditis in 7 Adolescents After Pfizer-BioNTech COVID-19 Vaccination. *Pediatrics*, *148*(3). https://doi.org/10.1542/peds.2021-052478
Martignoni, M., Groothuis, G. M. M., & de Kanter, R. (2006). Species differences between mouse, rat, dog, monkey and human CYP-mediated drug metabolism, inhibition and induction. *Expert Opinion on Drug Metabolism & Toxicology*, *2*(6), 875–894. https://doi.org/10.1517/17425255.2.6.875
Martinez, C. V., Old, M. O., Kwock, D. K., Khan, S. S., Garcia, J. J., Chan, C. S., Webster, R., Falkovitz-Halpern, M. S., & Maldonado, Y. A. (2004). Shedding of sabin poliovirus Type 3 containing the nucleotide 472 uracil-to-cytosine point mutation after administration of oral poliovirus vaccine. *Journal of Infectious Diseases*, *190*(2), 409–416. https://doi.org/10.1086/421703.
Martínez-Cué, C., & Rueda, N. (2020). Cellular Senescence in Neurodegenerative Diseases. *Frontiers in Cellular Neuroscience*, *14*. https://doi.org/10.3389/fncel.2020.00016
Martínez-Zamora, M. Á., Feixas, G., Gracia, M., Rius, M., Quintas, L., de Guirior, C., & Carmona, F. (2023). Evaluation of menstrual symptoms after Coronavirus disease 2019 vaccination in women with endometriosis. *Women's Health*, *19*, 174550572311767. https://doi.org/10.1177/17455057231176751
Maruggi, G., Mallett, C. P., Westerbeck, J. W., Chen, T., Lofano, G., Friedrich, K., Qu, L., Sun, J. T., McAuliffe, J., Kanitkar, A., Arrildt, K. T., Wang, K.-F., McBee, I., McCoy, D., Terry, R., Rowles, A., Abrahim, M. A., Ringenberg, M. A., Gains, M. J., … Yu, D. (2022). A self-amplifying mRNA SARS-CoV-2 vaccine candidate induces safe and robust protective immunity in preclinical models. *Molecular Therapy*, *30*(5), 1897–1912. https://doi.org/10.1016/j.ymthe.2022.01.001
Massari, M., Spila Alegiani, S., Morciano, C., Spuri, M., Marchione, P., Felicetti, P., Belleudi, V., Poggi, F. R., Lazzeretti, M., Ercolanoni, M., Clagnan, E., Bovo, E., Trifirò, G., Moretti, U., Monaco, G., Leoni, O., Da Cas, R., Petronzelli, F., Tartaglia, L., … Menniti Ippolito, F. (2022). Postmarketing active surveillance of myocarditis and pericarditis following vaccination with COVID-19 mRNA vaccines in persons aged 12 to 39 years in Italy: A multi-database, self-controlled case series study. *PLOS Medicine*, *19*(7), e1004056. https://doi.org/10.1371/journal.pmed.1004056
Mastora, E., Christodoulaki, A., Papageorgiou, K., Zikopolous, A., & Georgiou, I. (2021). Expression of Retroelements in Mammalian Gametes and Embryos. *In Vivo*, *35*(4), 1921–1927. https://doi.org/10.21873/invivo.12458
Masuccio, F. G., Comi, C., & Solaro, C. (2022). Guillain–Barrè syndrome following COVID-19 vaccine mRNA-1273: a case report. *Acta Neurologica Belgica*, *122*(5), 1369–1371. https://doi.org/10.1007/s13760-021-01838-4
Matar, E., Manser, D., Spies, J. M., Worthington, J. M., & Parratt, K. L. (2021). Acute Hemichorea-Hemiballismus Following COVID-19 (AZD1222) Vaccination. *Movement Disorders*, *36*(12), 2714–2715. https://doi.org/10.1002/mds.28796

Matarneh, A. S., Al-battah, A. H., Farooqui, K., Ghamoodi, M., & Alhatou, M. (2021). COVID-19 vaccine causing Guillain-Barre syndrome, a rare potential side effect. *Clinical Case Reports*, *9*(9). https://doi.org/10.1002/ccr3.4756

Mathieu, E., Ritchie, H., Rodés-Guirao, L., Appel, C., Giattino, C., Hasell, J., Macdonald, B., Dattani, S., Beltekian. D., Ortiz-Ospina, E., & Roser, R. (2020). Coronavirus Pandemic (COVID-19). Published online at OurWorldInData.org. Retrieved from: https://ourworldindata.org/coronavirus [Online Resource].

Matsumoto, M., Tsuneyama, K., Morimoto, J., Hosomichi, K., Matsumoto, M., & Nishijima, H. (2020). Tissue-specific autoimmunity controlled by Aire in thymic and peripheral tolerance mechanisms. *International Immunology, 32*(2):117-131. https://doi.org/10.1093/intimm/dxz066.

Mazereel, V., Van Assche, K., Detraux, J., & De Hert, M. (2021). COVID-19 vaccination for people with severe mental illness: why, what, and how? *The Lancet Psychiatry*, *8*(5), 444–450. https://doi.org/10.1016/S2215-0366(20)30564-2

Mazraani, M., & Barbari, A. (2021). Anti-Coronavirus Disease 2019 Vaccines: Need for Informed Consent. *Experimental and Clinical Transplantation, 19*(8), 753–762. https://doi.org/10.6002/ect.2021.0235

Mazzeo, A. T., Noto, A., Asmundo, A., Granata, F., Galletta, K., Mallamace, R., De Gregorio, C., Puliatti, F., Fazio, M. C., Germano', A., Musolino, C., & Ferlazzo, G. (2021). Cerebral venous sinus thrombosis (CVST) associated with SARS-CoV-2 vaccines: clues for an immunopathogenesis common to CVST observed in COVID-19. *Journal of Anesthesia, Analgesia and Critical Care, 1*(1), 15. https://doi.org/10.1186/s44158-021-00020-9

McCabe, B. F. (1979). Autoimmune Sensorineural Hearing Loss. *Annals of Otology, Rhinology & Laryngology*, *88*(5), 585–589. https://doi.org/10.1177/000348947908800501

McCafferty, S., Haque, A. K. M. A., Vandierendonck, A., Weidensee, B., Plovyt, M., Stuchlíková, M., François, N., Valembois, S., Heyndrickx, L., Michiels, J., Ariën, K. K., Vandekerckhove, L., Abdelnabi, R., Foo, C. S., Neyts, J., Sahu, I., & Sanders, N. N. (2022). A dual-antigen self-amplifying RNA SARS-CoV-2 vaccine induces potent humoral and cellular immune responses and protects against SARS-CoV-2 variants through T cell-mediated immunity. *Molecular Therapy*, *30*(9), 2968–2983. https://doi.org/10.1016/j.ymthe.2022.04.014

McCaul, J. A., Cascarini, L., Godden, D., Coombes, D., Brennan, P. A., & Kerawala, C. J. (2014). Evidence based management of Bell's palsy. *British Journal of Oral and Maxillofacial Surgery*, *52*(5), 387–391. https://doi.org/10.1016/j.bjoms.2014.03.001

McCullough, P. A., Wynn, C., & Procter, B. C. (2023). Clinical Rationale for SARS-CoV-2 Base Spike Protein Detoxification in Post COVID-19 and Vaccine Injury Syndromes. *Journal of American Physicians and Surgeons,* 28(3), 90–93. https://doi.org/10.5281/zenodo.8286459.

McKernan, K., Helbert, Y., Kane, L. T., & McLaughlin, S. (2023). Sequencing of bivalent Moderna and Pfizer mRNA vaccines reveals nanogram to microgram quantities of expression vector dsDNA per dose . *Medicinal Genomics*. https://cdn-ceo-ca.s3.amazonaws.com/1i4tp3q-Sequencing%20of%20bivalent_4-11-23.pdf

McKerrow, W., Wang, X., Mendez-Dorantes, C., Mita, P., Cao, S., Grivainis, M., Ding, L., LaCava, J., Burns, K. H., Boeke, J. D., & Fenyö, D. (2022). LINE-1 expression in cancer correlates with p53 mutation, copy number alteration, and S phase checkpoint. *Proceedings of the National Academy of Sciences*, *119*(8). https://doi.org/10.1073/pnas.2115999119

McLane, L. M., Abdel-Hakeem, M. S., & Wherry, E. J. (2019). CD8 T Cell Exhaustion During Chronic Viral Infection and Cancer. *Annual Review of Immunology*, *37*(1), 457–495. https://doi.org/10.1146/annurev-immunol-041015-055318

McLean, K., & Johnson, T. J. (2021). Myopericarditis in a previously healthy adolescent male following COVID-19 vaccination: A case report. *Academic Emergency Medicine*, *28*(8), 918–921. https://doi.org/10.1111/acem.14322

McLendon, K., Goyal, A., & Attia, M. (2023). *Deep Venous Thrombosis Risk Factors*.

McMahon, D. E., Kovarik, C. L., Damsky, W., Rosenbach, M., Lipoff, J. B., Tyagi, A., Chamberlin, G., Fathy, R., Nazarian, R. M., Desai, S. R., Lim, H. W., Thiers, B. H., Hruza, G. J., French, L. E., Blumenthal, K., Fox, L. P., & Freeman, E. E. (2022). Clinical and pathologic correlation of cutaneous COVID-19 vaccine reactions including V-REPP: A registry-based study. *Journal of the American Academy of Dermatology*, *86*(1), 113–121. https://doi.org/10.1016/j.jaad.2021.09.002

McNeil, M. M., Weintraub, E. S., Duffy, J., Sukumaran, L., Jacobsen, S. J., Klein, N. P., Hambidge, S. J., Lee, G. M., Jackson, L. A., Irving, S. A., King, J. P., Kharbanda, E. O., Bednarczyk, R. A., & DeStefano, F. (2016). Risk of anaphylaxis after vaccination in children and adults. *Journal of Allergy and Clinical Immunology*, *137*(3), 868–878. https://doi.org/10.1016/j.jaci.2015.07.048

McSharry, B. P., Burgert, H.-G., Owen, D. P., Stanton, R. J., Prod'homme, V., Sester, M., Koebernick, K., Groh, V., Spies, T., Cox, S., Little, A.-M., Wang, E. C. Y., Tomasec, P., & Wilkinson, G. W. G. (2008). Adenovirus E3/19K Promotes Evasion of NK Cell Recognition by Intracellular Sequestration of the NKG2D Ligands Major Histocompatibility Complex Class I Chain-Related Proteins A and B. *Journal of Virology*, *82*(9), 4585–4594. https://doi.org/10.1128/JVI.02251-07

Mederos, M. A., Reber, H. A., & Girgis, M. D. (2021). Acute Pancreatitis. *JAMA*, *325*(4), 382. https://doi.org/10.1001/jama.2020.20317

Medjitna, T. D. E., Stadler, C., Bruckner, L., Griot, C., & Ottiger, H. P. (2006). DNA vaccines: safety aspect assessment and regulation. *Developments in Biologicals*, *126*, 261–270; discussion 327.

Melenotte, C., Silvin, A., Goubet, A.-G., Lahmar, I., Dubuisson, A., Zumla, A., Raoult, D., Merad, M., Gachot, B., Hénon, C., Solary, E., Fontenay, M., André, F., Maeurer, M., Ippolito, G., Piacentini, M., Wang, F.-S., Ginhoux, F., Marabelle, A., … Zitvogel, L. (2020). Immune responses during COVID-19 infection. *OncoImmunology*, *9*(1). https://doi.org/10.1080/2162402X.2020.1807836

Mema, E., Lane, E. G., Drotman, M. B., Eisen, C. S., Thomas, C., Prince, M. R., & Dodelzon, K. (2023). Axillary Lymphadenopathy After a COVID-19 Vaccine Booster Dose: Time to Resolution on Ultrasound Follow-Up and Associated Factors. *American Journal of Roentgenology*, *221*(2), 175–183. https://doi.org/10.2214/AJR.22.28970

Merad, M., Blish, C. A., Sallusto, F., & Iwasaki, A. (2022). The immunology and immunopathology of COVID-19. *Science*, *375*(6585), 1122–1127. https://doi.org/10.1126/science.abm8108

Merchant, H. (2021). Thrombosis after covid-19 vaccination. *BMJ*. https://doi.org/10.1136/bmj.n958

Merchant, H. (2022). Inadvertent injection of COVID-19 vaccine into deltoid muscle vasculature may result in vaccine distribution to distance tissues and consequent adverse reactions. *Postgraduate Medical Journal*, *98*(1161), e5–e5. https://doi.org/10.1136/postgradmedj-2021-141119

Michels, C., Perrier, D., Kunadhasan, J., Clark, E., Gehrett, J., Gehrett, B., Kwiatek, K., Adams, S., Chandler, R., Stagno, L., Damian, T., Delph, E., & Flowers, C. (2023). Forensic analysis of the 38 subject deaths in the 6-Month Interim Report of the Pfizer/BioNTech BNT162b2 mRNA Vaccine Clinical Trial. *International Journal of Vaccine Theory, Practice, and Research*, *3*(1), 973–1008. https://doi.org/10.56098/ijvtpr.v3i1.85

Miesbach, W., & Makris, M. (2020). COVID-19: Coagulopathy, Risk of Thrombosis, and the Rationale for Anticoagulation. *Clinical and Applied Thrombosis/Hemostasis*, *26*, 107602962093814. https://doi.org/10.1177/1076029620938149

Mikasova, L., De Rossi, P., Bouchet, D., Georges, F., Rogemond, V., Didelot, A., Meissirel, C., Honnorat, J., & Groc, L. (2012). Disrupted surface cross-talk between NMDA and Ephrin-B2 receptors in anti-NMDA encephalitis. *Brain*, *135*(5), 1606–1621. https://doi.org/10.1093/brain/aws092

Militello, M., Ambur, A. B., & Steffes, W. (2022). Vitiligo Possibly Triggered by COVID-19 Vaccination. *Cureus*. https://doi.org/10.7759/cureus.20902

Min, Y. G., Ju, W., Ha, Y.-E., Ban, J.-J., Lee, S. A., Sung, J.-J., & Shin, J.-Y. (2021). Sensory Guillain-Barre syndrome following the ChAdOx1 nCov-19 vaccine: Report of two cases and review of literature. *Journal of Neuroimmunology*, *359*, 577691. https://doi.org/10.1016/j.jneuroim.2021.577691

Minocha, P. K., Better, D., Singh, R. K., & Hoque, T. (2021). Recurrence of Acute Myocarditis Temporally Associated with Receipt of the mRNA Coronavirus Disease 2019 (COVID-19) Vaccine in a Male Adolescent. *The Journal of Pediatrics*, *238*, 321–323. https://doi.org/10.1016/j.jpeds.2021.06.035

Mir, T. H., Zargar, P. A., Sharma, A., Jabeen, B., Sharma, S., Parvaiz, M. O., Bashir, S., & Javeed, R. (2023). Post COVID-19 AA amyloidosis of the kidneys with rapidly progressive renal failure. *Prion*, *17*(1), 111–115. https://doi.org/10.1080/19336896.2023.2201151

Mishra, R., & Banerjea, A. C. (2021). SARS-CoV-2 Spike Targets USP33-IRF9 Axis via Exosomal miR-148a to Activate Human Microglia. *Frontiers in Immunology*, *12*. https://doi.org/10.3389/fimmu.2021.656700

Mishra, S. B., Mahendradas, P., Kawali, A., Sanjay, S., & Shetty, R. (2023). Reactivation of varicella zoster infection presenting as acute retinal necrosis post COVID 19 vaccination in an Asian Indian male. *European Journal of Ophthalmology*, *33*(1), NP32–NP36. https://doi.org/10.1177/11206721211046485

Miyashita, Y., Yoshida, T., Takagi, Y., Tsukamoto, H., Takashima, K., Kouwaki, T., Makino, K., Fukushima, S., Nakamura, K., & Oshiumi, H. (2022). Circulating extracellular vesicle microRNAs associated with adverse reactions, pro-

inflammatory cytokine, and antibody production after COVID-19 vaccination. *Npj Vaccines*, *7*(1), 16. https://doi.org/10.1038/s41541-022-00439-3
Moghimi, S. M. (2021). Allergic Reactions and Anaphylaxis to LNP-Based COVID-19 Vaccines. *Molecular Therapy*, *29*(3), 898–900. https://doi.org/10.1016/j.ymthe.2021.01.030
Moghimi, S. M., Simberg, D., Papini, E., & Farhangrazi, Z. S. (2020). Complement activation by drug carriers and particulate pharmaceuticals: Principles, challenges and opportunities. *Advanced Drug Delivery Reviews*, *157*, 83–95. https://doi.org/10.1016/j.addr.2020.04.012
Mogilyansky, E., & Rigoutsos, I. (2013). The miR-17/92 cluster: a comprehensive update on its genomics, genetics, functions and increasingly important and numerous roles in health and disease. *Cell Death & Differentiation*, *20*(12), 1603–1614. https://doi.org/10.1038/cdd.2013.125
Mohta, A., & Sharma, M. K. (2022). Development of delayed dermal hypersensitivity reaction following the second dose of COVID -19 vaccine – A series of 37 cases. *Journal of the European Academy of Dermatology and Venereology*, *36*(9). https://doi.org/10.1111/jdv.18206
Montes-Grajales, D., & Olivero-Verbel, J. (2021). Bioinformatics Prediction of SARS-CoV-2 Epitopes as Vaccine Candidates for the Colombian Population. *Vaccines*, *9*(7), 797. https://doi.org/10.3390/vaccines9070797
Montgomery, J., Ryan, M., Engler, R., Hoffman, D., McClenathan, B., Collins, L., Loran, D., Hrncir, D., Herring, K., Platzer, M., Adams, N., Sanou, A., & Cooper, L. T. (2021). Myocarditis Following Immunization With mRNA COVID-19 Vaccines in Members of the US Military. *JAMA Cardiology*, *6*(10), 1202. https://doi.org/10.1001/jamacardio.2021.2833
Mopuru, R., & Menon, V. (2023). COVID-19 vaccine-related psychiatric adverse events: Mechanisms and considerations. *Asian Journal of Psychiatry*, *79*, 103329. https://doi.org/10.1016/j.ajp.2022.103329
Morais, P., Adachi, H., & Yu, Y.-T. (2021). The Critical Contribution of Pseudouridine to mRNA COVID-19 Vaccines. *Frontiers in Cell and Developmental Biology*, *9*. https://doi.org/10.3389/fcell.2021.789427
Morehouse, Z. P., Paulus, A., Jasti, S. A., & Bing, X. (2021). A Rare Variant of Guillain-Barre Syndrome Following Ad26.COV2.S Vaccination. *Cureus*. https://doi.org/10.7759/cureus.18153
Morlidge, C., El-Kateb, S., Jeevaratnam, P., & Thompson, B. (2021). Relapse of minimal change disease following the AstraZeneca COVID-19 vaccine. *Kidney International*, *100*(2), 459. https://doi.org/10.1016/j.kint.2021.06.005
Morohoshi, K., Goodwin, A. M., Ohbayashi, M., & Ono, S. J. (2009). Autoimmunity in retinal degeneration: Autoimmune retinopathy and age-related macular degeneration. *Journal of Autoimmunity*, *33*(3–4), 247–254. https://doi.org/10.1016/j.jaut.2009.09.003
Morris, R. S., Morris, A. J., & IL, N. (2021). Exposure of ovaries to COVID-19 vaccination does not impair fertility. *Fertility and Sterility*, *116*(3), e473. https://doi.org/10.1016/j.fertnstert.2021.08.027
Mörz, M. (2022). A Case Report: Multifocal Necrotizing Encephalitis and Myocarditis after BNT162b2 mRNA Vaccination against COVID-19. *Vaccines*, *10*(10), 1651. https://doi.org/10.3390/vaccines10101651

Mosleh, W., Chen, K., Pfau, S. E., & Vashist, A. (2020). Endotheliitis and Endothelial Dysfunction in Patients with COVID-19: Its Role in Thrombosis and Adverse Outcomes. *Journal of Clinical Medicine*, *9*(6), 1862. https://doi.org/10.3390/jcm9061862

Motta-Mena, N. V., & Puts, D. A. (2017). Endocrinology of human female sexuality, mating, and reproductive behavior. *Hormones and Behavior*, *91*, 19–35. https://doi.org/10.1016/j.yhbeh.2016.11.012

Mousa, N., Saleh, A. M., Khalid, A., Alshaya, A. K., & Alanazi, S. M. M. (2022). Systemic lupus erythematosus with acute pancreatitis and vasculitic rash following COVID-19 vaccine: a case report and literature review. *Clinical Rheumatology*, *41*(5), 1577–1582. https://doi.org/10.1007/s10067-022-06097-z

Moutinho, S., & Wadman, M. (2021). Brazil and Russia face off over vaccine contamination charge. *Science*, *372*(6542), 554–554. https://doi.org/10.1126/science.372.6542.554a

Mtimkulu-Eyde, L., Denholm, J., Narain, A., Fatima, R., Sagili, K. D., Perumal, R., & Padayatchi, N. (2022). Mandatory COVID-19 Vaccination: Lessons from Tuberculosis and HIV. *Health and Human Rights, 24*(1), 85–91.

Muchtar, E., Dispenzieri, A., Magen, H., Grogan, M., Mauermann, M., McPhail, E. D., Kurtin, P. J., Leung, N., Buadi, F. K., Dingli, D., Kumar, S. K., & Gertz, M. A. (2021). Systemic amyloidosis from A (AA) to T (ATTR): a review. *Journal of Internal Medicine*, *289*(3), 268–292. https://doi.org/10.1111/joim.13169

Mufti, Z., Dietz, N., Pearson, L., Fortuny, E., Mettille, J., Ding, D., Brown, M., & Mufti, H. (2023). Immune-Mediated Necrotizing Myopathy With Concurrent Statin Use After Routine COVID-19 Inoculation: A Case Report. *Cureus*. https://doi.org/10.7759/cureus.37876

Muhaidat, N., Alshrouf, M. A., Azzam, M. I., Karam, A. M., Al-Nazer, M., & Al-Ani, A. (2022). Menstrual Symptoms After COVID-19 Vaccine: A Cross-Sectional Investigation in the MENA Region. *International Journal of Women's Health*, *14*, 395–404. https://doi.org/10.2147/IJWH.S352167

Müller, F., Gailani, D., & Renné, T. (2011). Factor XI and XII as antithrombotic targets. *Current Opinion in Hematology*, *18*(5), 349–355. https://doi.org/10.1097/MOH.0b013e3283497e61

Müller, M. M., & Griesmacher, A. (2022). Markers of endothelial dysfunction. *Clinical Chemistry Laboratory Medicine*, *38*(2), 77–85. https://doi.org/10.1515/CCLM.2000.013.

Mungmunpuntipantip, R., & Wiwanitkit, V. (2022). Post SARS-CoV-2 Vaccine Chilblains-like Lesions. *The Journal of Rheumatology*, *49*(7), 859–859. https://doi.org/10.3899/jrheum.210996

Murgova, S., & Balchev, G. (2022). Ophthalmic manifestation after SARS-CoV-2 vaccination: a case series. *Journal of Ophthalmic Inflammation and Infection*, *12*(1), 20. https://doi.org/10.1186/s12348-022-00298-y

Murphy, F. A., Poland, C. A., Duffin, R., Al-Jamal, K. T., Ali-Boucetta, H., Nunes, A., Byrne, F., Prina-Mello, A., Volkov, Y., Li, S., Mather, S. J., Bianco, A., Prato, M., MacNee, W., Wallace, W. A., Kostarelos, K., & Donaldson, K. (2011). Length-Dependent Retention of Carbon Nanotubes in the Pleural Space of Mice Initiates Sustained Inflammation and Progressive Fibrosis on the Parietal Pleura. *The American Journal of Pathology*, *178*(6), 2587–2600. https://doi.org/10.1016/j.ajpath.2011.02.040

Murphy, M. P., & LeVine, H. (2010). Alzheimer's Disease and the Amyloid-β Peptide. *Journal of Alzheimer's Disease*, *19*(1), 311–323. https://doi.org/10.3233/JAD-2010-1221

Muthukumar, A., Narasimhan, M., Li, Q.-Z., Mahimainathan, L., Hitto, I., Fuda, F., Batra, K., Jiang, X., Zhu, C., Schoggins, J., Cutrell, J. B., Croft, C. L., Khera, A., Drazner, M. H., Grodin, J. L., Greenberg, B. M., Mammen, P. P. A., Morrison, S. J., & de Lemos, J. A. (2021). In-Depth Evaluation of a Case of Presumed Myocarditis After the Second Dose of COVID-19 mRNA Vaccine. *Circulation*, *144*(6), 487–498. https://doi.org/10.1161/CIRCULATIONAHA.121.056038

N, A. M., Saleh, A. M., Khalid, A., Alshaya, A. K., & Alanazi, S. M. M. (2022). Systemic lupus erythematosus with acute pancreatitis and vasculitic rash following COVID vaccine: a case report and literature review. *Clinical Rheumatology, 41*(5):1577–1582. https://doi.org/10.1007/s10067-022-06097-z.

Nabizadeh, F., Ramezannezhad, E., Kazemzadeh, K., Khalili, E., Ghaffary, E. M., & Mirmosayyeb, O. (2022). Multiple sclerosis relapse after COVID-19 vaccination: A case report-based systematic review. *Journal of Clinical Neuroscience*, *104*, 118–125. https://doi.org/10.1016/j.jocn.2022.08.012

Nagalli, S., & Shankar Kikkeri, N. (2022). Sub-acute Onset of Guillain-Barré Syndrome Post-mRNA-1273 Vaccination: a Case Report. *SN Comprehensive Clinical Medicine*, *4*(1), 41. https://doi.org/10.1007/s42399-022-01124-1

Naharci, M. I., & Tasci, I. (2021). Delirium in a patient with Alzheimer's dementia following COVID-19 vaccination. *Psychogeriatrics*, *21*(5), 846–847. https://doi.org/10.1111/psyg.12747

Nakahara, T., Iwabuchi, Y., Miyazawa, R., Tonda, K., Shiga, T., Strauss, H. W., Antoniades, C., Narula, J., & Jinzaki, M. (2023). Assessment of Myocardial 18F-FDG Uptake at PET/CT in Asymptomatic SARS-CoV-2-vaccinated and Nonvaccinated Patients. . *Radiology*, *308*(3). https://doi.org/10.1148/radiol.230743

Nakano, R., Nakano, A., Yano, H., & Okamoto, R. (2017). Role of AmpR in the High Expression of the Plasmid-Encoded AmpC β-Lactamase CFE-1. *MSphere*, *2*(4). https://doi.org/10.1128/mSphere.00192-17

Nanatsue, K., Takahashi, M., Itaya, S., Abe, K., & Inaba, A. (2022). A case of Miller Fisher syndrome with delayed onset peripheral facial nerve palsy after COVID-19 vaccination: a case report. *BMC Neurology*, *22*(1), 309. https://doi.org/10.1186/s12883-022-02838-4

Nance, K. D., & Meier, J. L. (2021). Modifications in an Emergency: The Role of N1-Methylpseudouridine in COVID-19 Vaccines. *ACS Central Science*, *7*(5), 748–756. https://doi.org/10.1021/acscentsci.1c00197

Nanji, A. A., & Fraunfelder, F. T. (2022). Anterior Uveitis following COVID Vaccination: A Summary of Cases from Global Reporting Systems. *Ocular Immunology and Inflammation*, *30*(5), 1244–1246. https://doi.org/10.1080/09273948.2022.2042316

Nappi, E., Racca, F., Piona, A., Messina, M., Ferri, S., Lamacchia, D., Cataldo, G., Costanzo, G., Del Moro, L., Puggioni, F., Canonica, G., Heffler, E., & Paoletti, G. (2023). Polyethylene Glycol and Polysorbate 80 Skin Tests in the Context of an Allergic Risk Assessment for Hypersensitivity Reactions to Anti-SARS-CoV-2 mRNA Vaccines. *Vaccines*, *11*(5), 915. https://doi.org/10.3390/vaccines11050915

Narayanan, S., de Mores, A. R., Cohen, L., Anwar, M. M., Lazar, F., Hicklen, R., Lopez, G., Yang, P., & Bruera, E. (2023). Medicinal Mushroom Supplements in Cancer: A Systematic Review of Clinical Studies. *Current Oncology Reports*, *25*(6), 569–587. https://doi.org/10.1007/s11912-023-01408-2

Nassar, M., Nso, N., Gonzalez, C., Lakhdar, S., Alshamam, M., Elshafey, M., Abdalazeem, Y., Nyein, A., Punzalan, B., Durrance, R. J., Alfishawy, M., Bakshi, S., & Rizzo, V. (2021). COVID-19 vaccine-induced myocarditis: Case report with literature review. *Diabetes & Metabolic Syndrome: Clinical Research & Reviews*, *15*(5), 102205. https://doi.org/10.1016/j.dsx.2021.102205

Nasuelli, N. A., De Marchi, F., Cecchin, M., De Paoli, I., Onorato, S., Pettinaroli, R., Savoini, G., & Godi, L. (2021). A case of acute demyelinating polyradiculoneuropathy with bilateral facial palsy after ChAdOx1 nCoV-19 vaccine. *Neurological Sciences*, *42*(11), 4747–4749. https://doi.org/10.1007/s10072-021-05467-w

Nau, H. (1986). Species differences in pharmacokinetics and drug teratogenesis. *Environmental Health Perspectives*, *70*, 113–129. https://doi.org/10.1289/ehp.8670113

Navar, A. M., McNally, E., Yancy, C. W., O'Gara, P. T., & Bonow, R. O. (2021). Temporal Associations Between Immunization With the COVID-19 mRNA Vaccines and Myocarditis. *JAMA Cardiology*, *6*(10), 1117. https://doi.org/10.1001/jamacardio.2021.2853

Navarrete, S., Solar, C., Tapia, R., Pereira, J., Fuentes, E., & Palomo, I. (2022). Pathophysiology of deep vein thrombosis. *Clinical and Experimental Medicine*, *23*(3), 645–654. https://doi.org/10.1007/s10238-022-00829-w

Negrea, L., & Rovin, B. H. (2021). Gross hematuria following vaccination for severe acute respiratory syndrome coronavirus 2 in 2 patients with IgA nephropathy. *Kidney International*, *99*(6), 1487. https://doi.org/10.1016/j.kint.2021.03.002

Nevet, A. (2021). Acute myocarditis associated with anti-COVID-19 vaccination. *Clinical and Experimental Vaccine Research*, *10*(2), 196. https://doi.org/10.7774/cevr.2021.10.2.196

Ng, S. C., Peng, Y., Zhang, L., Mok, C. K., Zhao, S., Li, A., Ching, J. Y., Liu, Y., Yan, S., Chan, D. L. S., Zhu, J., Chen, C., Fung, A. C., Wong, K. K., Hui, D. S., Chan, F. K., & Tun, H. M. (2022). Gut microbiota composition is associated with SARS-CoV-2 vaccine immunogenicity and adverse events. *Gut*, *71*(6), 1106–1116. https://doi.org/10.1136/gutjnl-2021-326563

Nishimi, K., Neylan, T. C., Bertenthal, D., Seal, K. H., & O'Donovan, A. (2022). Association of Psychiatric Disorders With Incidence of SARS-CoV-2 Breakthrough Infection Among Vaccinated Adults. *JAMA Network Open*, *5*(4), e227287. https://doi.org/10.1001/jamanetworkopen.2022.7287

Noé, A., Dang, T. D., Axelrad, C., Burrell, E., Germano, S., Elia, S., Burgner, D., Perrett, K. P., Curtis, N., & Messina, N. L. (2023). BNT162b2 COVID-19 vaccination in children alters cytokine responses to heterologous pathogens and Toll-like receptor agonists. *Frontiers in Immunology*, *14*. https://doi.org/10.3389/fimmu.2023.1242380

Nosadini, M., Mohammad, S. S., Corazza, F., Ruga, E. M., Kothur, K., Perilongo, G., Frigo, A. C., Toldo, I., Dale, R. C., & Sartori, S. (2017). Herpes simplex virus-induced anti- N -methyl- d -aspartate receptor encephalitis: a systematic literature review with analysis of 43 cases. *Developmental Medicine & Child Neurology, 59*(8), 796–805. https://doi.org/10.1111/dmcn.13448

Notghi, A. A., Atley, J., & Silva, M. (2021). Lessons of the month 1: Longitudinal extensive transverse myelitis following AstraZeneca COVID-19 vaccination. *Clinical Medicine, 21*(5), e535–e538. https://doi.org/10.7861/clinmed.2021-0470

Nunez-Castilla, J., Stebliankin, V., Baral, P., Balbin, C. A., Sobhan, M., Cickovski, T., Mondal, A. M., Narasimhan, G., Chapagain, P., Mathee, K., & Siltberg-Liberles, J. (2022). Potential Autoimmunity Resulting from Molecular Mimicry between SARS-CoV-2 Spike and Human Proteins. *Viruses, 14*(7), 1415. https://doi.org/10.3390/v14071415

Núñez-Gil, I. J., Molina, M., Bernardo, E., Ibañez, B., Ruiz-Mateos, B., García-Rubira, J. C., Vivas, D., Feltes, G., Luaces, M., Alonso, J., Zamorano, J., Macaya, C., & Fernández-Ortiz, A. (2012). Síndrome de tako-tsubo e insuficiencia cardiaca: seguimiento a largo plazo. *Revista Española de Cardiología, 65*(11), 996–1002. https://doi.org/10.1016/j.recesp.2012.04.016

Nuovo, G. J., Suster, D., Sawant, D., Mishra, A., Michaille, J.-J., & Tili, E. (2022). The amplification of CNS damage in Alzheimer's disease due to SARS-CoV2 infection. *Annals of Diagnostic Pathology, 61*, 152057. https://doi.org/10.1016/j.anndiagpath.2022.152057

Nyström, S., & Hammarström, P. (2022). Amyloidogenesis of SARS-CoV-2 Spike Protein. *Journal of the American Chemical Society, 144*(20), 8945–8950. https://doi.org/10.1021/jacs.2c03925

Obando-Pereda, G. (2021). Can molecular mimicry explain the cytokine storm of SARS-CoV-2?: An in silico approach. *Journal of Medical Virology, 93*(9), 5350–5357. https://doi.org/10.1002/jmv.27040

O'Brien, B. C. V., Weber, L., Hueffer, K., & Weltzin, M. M. (2023). SARS-CoV-2 spike ectodomain targets α7 nicotinic acetylcholine receptors. *Journal of Biological Chemistry, 299*(5), 104707. https://doi.org/10.1016/j.jbc.2023.104707

Odeh-Natour, R., Shapira, M., Estrada, D., Freimann, S., Tal, Y., Atzmon, Y., Bilgory, A., Aslih, N., Abu-Raya, Y. S., & Shalom-Paz, E. (2022). Does mRNA SARS-CoV-2 vaccine in the follicular fluid impact follicle and oocyte performance in IVF treatments? *American Journal of Reproductive Immunology, 87*(5). https://doi.org/10.1111/aji.13530

Oertelt-Prigione, S. (2012). Immunology and the menstrual cycle. *Autoimmunity Reviews, 11*(6–7), A486–A492. https://doi.org/10.1016/j.autrev.2011.11.023

Ogbebor, O., Seth, H., Min, Z., & Bhanot, N. (2021). Guillain-Barré syndrome following the first dose of SARS-CoV-2 vaccine: A temporal occurrence, not a causal association. *IDCases, 24*, e01143. https://doi.org/10.1016/j.idcr.2021.e01143

Ogino, Y., Namba, K., Iwata, D., Suzuki, K., Mizuuchi, K., Hiraoka, M., Kitaichi, N., & Ishida, S. (2023). A case of APMPPE-like panuveitis presenting with extensive outer retinal layer impairment following COVID-19 vaccination. *BMC Ophthalmology, 23*(1), 233. https://doi.org/10.1186/s12886-023-02978-2

Ogunjimi, O. B., Tsalamandris, G., Paladini, A., Varrassi, G., & Zis, P. (2023). Guillain-Barré Syndrome Induced by Vaccination Against COVID-19: A Systematic Review and Meta-Analysis. *Cureus*. https://doi.org/10.7759/cureus.37578

Okan, G., & Vural, P. (2022). Worsening of the vitiligo following the second dose of the BNT162B2 mRNA COVID-19 vaccine. *Dermatologic Therapy*, *35*(3). https://doi.org/10.1111/dth.15280

Okayasu, H., Sutter, R. W., Czerkinsky, C., Ogra, P. L. (2011). Mucosal immunity and poliovirus vaccines: impact on wild poliovirus infection and transmission. *Vaccine*, *29*(46), 8205–8214. https://doi.org/10.1016/j.vaccine.2011.08.059.

Oldenburg, J., Klamroth, R., Langer, F., Albisetti, M., von Auer, C., Ay, C., Korte, W., Scharf, R. E., Pötzsch, B., & Greinacher, A. (2021). Diagnosis and Management of Vaccine-Related Thrombosis following AstraZeneca COVID-19 Vaccination: Guidance Statement from the GTH. *Hämostaseologie*, *41*(03), 184–189. https://doi.org/10.1055/a-1469-7481

Oldfield, P. R., Hibberd, J., & Bridle, B. W. (2021). How Does Severe Acute Respiratory Syndrome-Coronavirus-2 Affect the Brain and Its Implications for the Vaccines Currently in Use. *Vaccines*, *10*(1), 1. https://doi.org/10.3390/vaccines10010001

Omidi, N., Azaran, A., Makvandi, M., Khataminia, G., Ahmadi Angali, K., & Jalilian, S. (2022). Characterization of the conserved regions of E1A protein from human adenovirus for reinforcement of cytotoxic T lymphocytes responses to all genogroups causes ocular manifestation through an in silico approach. *Iran Journal of Microbiology*, *14*(5), 746–758. https://doi.org/10.18502/ijm.v14i5.10971.

Onishi, N., Konishi, Y., Kaneko, T., Maekawa, N., Suenaga, A., Nomura, S., Kobayashi, T., Kyo, S., Okabayashi, M., Higami, H., Oi, M., Higashitani, N., Saijo, S., Nakazeki, F., Oyamada, N., Jinnai, T., Okuno, T., Shirase, T., & Kaitani, K. (2023). Fulminant myocarditis with complete atrioventricular block after mRNA COVID-19 vaccination: A case report. *Journal of Cardiology Cases*, *27*(5), 229–232. https://doi.org/10.1016/j.jccase.2023.01.004

Onoda, K., Sashida, R., Fujiwara, R., Wakamiya, T., Michiwaki, Y., Tanaka, T., Shimoji, K., Suehiro, E., Yamane, F., Kawashima, M., & Matsuno, A. (2022). Trigeminal neuropathy after tozinameran vaccination against COVID-19 in postmicrovascular decompression for trigeminal neuralgia: illustrative case. *Journal of Neurosurgery: Case Lessons*, *3*(16). https://doi.org/10.3171/CASE22101

Oo, W. M., Giri, P., & de Souza, A. (2021). AstraZeneca COVID-19 vaccine and Guillain- Barré Syndrome in Tasmania: A causal link? *Journal of Neuroimmunology*, *360*, 577719. https://doi.org/10.1016/j.jneuroim.2021.577719

Ooi, X. T., Choi, E. C., & Lee, J. S. (2022). Manifestation of a cancer-associated TIF - 1 gamma dermatomyositis after COVID -19 vaccine. *International Journal of Dermatology*, *61*(11), 1425–1426. https://doi.org/10.1111/ijd.16358

Orlikowski, D., Prigent, H., Sharshar, T., Lofaso, F., & Claude Raphael, J. (2004). Respiratory Dysfunction in Guillain-Barré Syndrome. *Neurocritical Care*, *1*(4), 415–422. https://doi.org/10.1385/NCC:1:4:415

Ormundo, L. F., Machado, C. F., Sakamoto, E. D., Simões, V., & Armelin-Correa, L. (2020). LINE-1 specific nuclear organization in mice olfactory sensory neurons. *Molecular and Cellular Neuroscience*, *105*, 103494. https://doi.org/10.1016/j.mcn.2020.103494

Ortiz Balbuena, J., Tutor de Ureta, P., Rivera Ruiz, E., & Mellor Pita, S. (2016). Enfermedad de Vogt-Koyanagi-Harada. *Medicina Clínica*, *146*(2), 93–94. https://doi.org/10.1016/j.medcli.2015.04.005

Ortiz-Egea, J. M., Sánchez, C. G., López-Jiménez, A., & Navarro, O. D. (2022). Herpetic anterior uveitis following Pfizer–BioNTech coronavirus disease 2019 vaccine: two case reports. *Journal of Medical Case Reports*, *16*(1), 127. https://doi.org/10.1186/s13256-022-03350-6

Ortiz-Millán, G. (2021). Placebo-controlled trials of Covid-19 vaccines – Are they still ethical? *Indian Journal of Medical Ethics*, *06*(02), 96–99. https://doi.org/10.20529/IJME.2021.015

Osowicki, J., Morgan, H., Harris, A., Crawford, N. W., Buttery, J. P., & Kiers, L. (2021). Guillain-Barré Syndrome in an Australian State Using Both mRNA and Adenovirus-Vector SARS-CoV-2 Vaccines. *Annals of Neurology*, *90*(5), 856–858. https://doi.org/10.1002/ana.26218

Oster, M. E., Shay, D. K., Su, J. R., Gee, J., Creech, C. B., Broder, K. R., Edwards, K., Soslow, J. H., Dendy, J. M., Schlaudecker, E., Lang, S. M., Barnett, E. D., Ruberg, F. L., Smith, M. J., Campbell, M. J., Lopes, R. D., Sperling, L. S., Baumblatt, J. A., Thompson, D. L., … Shimabukuro, T. T. (2022). Myocarditis Cases Reported After mRNA-Based COVID-19 Vaccination in the US From December 2020 to August 2021. *JAMA*, *327*(4), 331. https://doi.org/10.1001/jama.2021.24110

Ozaka, S., Kodera, T., Ariki, S., Kobayashi, T., & Murakami, K. (2022). Acute pancreatitis soon after COVID-19 vaccination. *Medicine*, *101*(2), e28471. https://doi.org/10.1097/MD.0000000000028471

Özkan, G., Bayrakçı, N., Karabağ, S., Güzel, E., & Ulusoy, S. (2022). Relapse of minimal change disease after inactivated SARS-CoV-2 vaccination: case report. *International Urology and Nephrology*, *54*(4), 971–972. https://doi.org/10.1007/s11255-021-02889-5

Pagenkopf, C., & Südmeyer, M. (2021). A case of longitudinally extensive transverse myelitis following vaccination against Covid-19. *Journal of Neuroimmunology*, *358*, 577606. https://doi.org/10.1016/j.jneuroim.2021.577606

Paladino, L., Vitale, A. M., Caruso Bavisotto, C., Conway de Macario, E., Cappello, F., Macario, A. J. L., & Marino Gammazza, A. (2020). The Role of Molecular Chaperones in Virus Infection and Implications for Understanding and Treating COVID-19. *Journal of Clinical Medicine*, *9*(11), 3518. https://doi.org/10.3390/jcm9113518

Pandey, A., Madan, R., & Singh, S. (2022). Immunology to Immunotherapeutics of SARS-CoV-2: Identification of Immunogenic Epitopes for Vaccine Development. *Current Microbiology*, *79*(10), 306. https://doi.org/10.1007/s00284-022-03003-3

Panou, E., Nikolaou, V., Marinos, L., Kallambou, S., Sidiropoulou, P., Gerochristou, M., & Stratigos, A. (2022). Recurrence of cutaneous T-cell lymphoma post viral vector COVID-19 vaccination. *Journal of the European Academy of Dermatology and Venereology*, *36*(2). https://doi.org/10.1111/jdv.17736

Paoletti, P., Bellone, C., & Zhou, Q. (2013). NMDA receptor subunit diversity: impact on receptor properties, synaptic plasticity and disease. *Nature Reviews Neuroscience*, *14*(6), 383–400. https://doi.org/10.1038/nrn3504

Paolilo, R. B., Deiva, K., Neuteboom, R., Rostásy, K., & Lim, M. (2020). Acute Disseminated Encephalomyelitis: Current Perspectives. *Children*, *7*(11), 210. https://doi.org/10.3390/children7110210

Papadimitriou, I., Bakirtzi, K., Sotiriou, E., Vakirlis, E., Hatzibougias, D., & Ioannides, D. (2022). Delayed localized hypersensitivity reactions to COVID-19 mRNA vaccines: a 6-month retrospective study. *Clinical and Experimental Dermatology*, *47*(1), 157–158. https://doi.org/10.1111/ced.14856

Pappano, A., & Wier, WG. (2019). *Cardiovascular Physiology* (11 th edition). Elsevier Health Sciences.

Pardi, N., Hogan, M. J., Naradikian, M. S., Parkhouse, K., Cain, D. W., Jones, L., Moody, M. A., Verkerke, H. P., Myles, A., Willis, E., LaBranche, C. C., Montefiori, D. C., Lobby, J. L., Saunders, K. O., Liao, H. X., Korber BT, Sutherland LL, Scearce RM, Hraber PT, Tombácz I., … Weissman D. (2018a). Nucleoside-modified mRNA vaccines induce potent T follicular helper and germinal center B cell responses. *Journal of Experimental Medicine, 215*(6), 1571–1588. https://doi.org/10.1084/jem.20171450.

Pardi, N., Hogan, M. J., Porter, F. W., & Weissman, D. (2018b). mRNA vaccines — a new era in vaccinology. *Nature Reviews Drug Discovery*, *17*(4), 261–279. https://doi.org/10.1038/nrd.2017.243

Park, H. J., Montgomery, J. R., & Boggs, N. A. (2022). Anaphylaxis After the Covid-19 Vaccine in a Patient With Cholinergic Urticaria. *Military Medicine*, *187*(Special Issue_13), e1556–e1558. https://doi.org/10.1093/milmed/usab138

Park, H., Yun, K. W., Kim, K.-R., Song, S. H., Ahn, B., Kim, D. R., Kim, G. B., Huh, J., Choi, E. H., & Kim, Y.-J. (2021). Epidemiology and Clinical Features of Myocarditis/Pericarditis before the Introduction of mRNA COVID-19 Vaccine in Korean Children: a Multicenter Study. *Journal of Korean Medical Science*, *36*(32). https://doi.org/10.3346/jkms.2021.36.e232

Park, J., Brekke, D. R., & Bratincsak, A. (2022). Self-limited myocarditis presenting with chest pain and ST segment elevation in adolescents after vaccination with the BNT162b2 mRNA vaccine. *Cardiology in the Young*, *32*(1), 146–149. https://doi.org/10.1017/S1047951121002547

Parkash, O., Sharko, A., Farooqi, A., Ying, G. W., & Sura, P. (2021). Acute Pancreatitis: A Possible Side Effect of COVID-19 Vaccine. *Cureus*. https://doi.org/10.7759/cureus.14741

Parr, C. J. C., Wada, S., Kotake, K., Kameda, S., Matsuura, S., Sakashita, S., Park, S., Sugiyama, H., Kuang, Y., & Saito, H. (2020). N 1-Methylpseudouridine substitution enhances the performance of synthetic mRNA switches in cells. *Nucleic Acids Research*, *48*(6), e35–e35. https://doi.org/10.1093/nar/gkaa070

Parrino, D., Frosolini, A., Gallo, C., De Siati, R. D., Spinato, G., & de Filippis, C. (2022). Tinnitus following COVID-19 vaccination: report of three cases. *International Journal of Audiology*, *61*(6), 526–529. https://doi.org/10.1080/14992027.2021.1931969

Parry, P. I., Lefringhausen, A., Turni, C., Neil, C. J., Cosford, R., Hudson, N. J., & Gillespie, J. (2023). 'Spikeopathy': COVID-19 Spike Protein Is Pathogenic, from Both Virus and Vaccine mRNA. *Biomedicines*, *11*(8), 2287. https://doi.org/10.3390/biomedicines11082287

Pascual-Ramírez, J., Muñoz-Torrero, J. J., Bacci, L., Trujillo, S. G., & García-Serrano, N. (2011). Anesthetic management of ovarian teratoma excision associated with anti-N-methyl-D-aspartate receptor encephalitis. *International Journal of Gynecology & Obstetrics*, *115*(3), 291–292. https://doi.org/10.1016/j.ijgo.2011.07.028

Pastore, A., Martin, S. R., Politou, A., Kondapalli, K. C., Stemmler, T., & Temussi, P. A. (2007). Unbiased Cold Denaturation: Low- and High-Temperature Unfolding of Yeast Frataxin under Physiological Conditions. *Journal of the American Chemical Society*, *129*(17), 5374–5375. https://doi.org/10.1021/ja0714538

Patel, A. H. (2022). Acute Liver Injury and IgG4-related Autoimmune Pancreatitis following mRNA based COVID-19 vaccination. *Hepatology Forum*. https://doi.org/10.14744/hf.2022.2022.0019

Patel, K. G., Hilton, T., Choi, R. Y., & Abbey, A. M. (2022). Uveitis and Posterior Ophthalmic Manifestations Following the SARS-CoV-2 (COVID-19) Vaccine. *Ocular Immunology and Inflammation*, *30*(5), 1142–1148. https://doi.org/10.1080/09273948.2022.2079533

Patel, V. B., Zhong, J.-C., Grant, M. B., & Oudit, G. Y. (2016). Role of the ACE2/Angiotensin 1-7 Axis of the Renin-Angiotensin System in Heart Failure. *Circulation Research*, *118*(8), 1313–1326. https://doi.org/10.1161/CIRCRESAHA.116.307708

Patel, Y. R., Louis, D. W., Atalay, M., Agarwal, S., & Shah, N. R. (2021). Cardiovascular magnetic resonance findings in young adult patients with acute myocarditis following mRNA COVID vaccination: a case series. *Journal of Cardiovascular Magnetic Resonance, 23*(1),101. https://doi.org/10.1186/s12968-021-00795-4.

Patel, Y. R., Shah, N. R., Lombardi, K., Agarwal, S., Salber, G., Patel, R., Poppas, A., & Atalay, M. K. (2022). Follow-Up Cardiovascular Magnetic Resonance Findings in Patients With COVID-19 Vaccination-Associated Acute Myocarditis. *JACC: Cardiovascular Imaging*, *15*(11), 2007–2010. https://doi.org/10.1016/j.jcmg.2022.06.009

Paterni, I., Granchi, C., Katzenellenbogen, J. A., & Minutolo, F. (2014). Estrogen receptors alpha (ERα) and beta (ERβ): Subtype-selective ligands and clinical potential. *Steroids*, *90*, 13–29. https://doi.org/10.1016/j.steroids.2014.06.012

Paterson, R. W., Brown, R. L., Benjamin, L., Nortley, R., Wiethoff, S., Bharucha, T., Jayaseelan, D. L., Kumar, G., Raftopoulos, R. E., Zambreanu, L., Vivekanandam, V., Khoo, A., Geraldes, R., Chinthapalli, K., Boyd, E., Tuzlali, H., Price, G., Christofi, G., Morrow, J., … Zandi, M. S. (2020). The emerging spectrum of COVID-19 neurology: clinical, radiological and laboratory findings. *Brain*, *143*(10), 3104–3120. https://doi.org/10.1093/brain/awaa240

Patrignani, A., Schicchi, N., Calcagnoli, F., Falchetti, E., Ciampani, N., Argalia, G., & Mariani, A. (2021). Acute myocarditis following Comirnaty vaccination in a healthy man with previous SARS-CoV-2 infection. *Radiology Case Reports*, *16*(11), 3321–3325. https://doi.org/10.1016/j.radcr.2021.07.082.

Patrizio, A., Ferrari, S. M., Antonelli, A., & Fallahi, P. (2021). A case of Graves' disease and type 1 diabetes mellitus following SARS-CoV-2 vaccination. *Journal of Autoimmunity*, *125*, 102738. https://doi.org/10.1016/j.jaut.2021.102738

Paz, J., Yao, H., Lim, H. S., Lu, X.-Y., & Zhang, W. (2007). The neuroprotective role of attractin in neurodegeneration. *Neurobiology of Aging*, *28*(9), 1446–1456. https://doi.org/10.1016/j.neurobiolaging.2006.06.014

Pearce, N. (1999). Epidemiology as a population science. *International Journal of Epidemiology*, *28*(5), S1015–S1018. https://doi.org/10.1093/oxfordjournals.ije.a019904
Pegat, A., Vogrig, A., Khouri, C., Masmoudi, K., Vial, T., & Bernard, E. (2022). Adenovirus COVID-19 Vaccines and Guillain-Barré Syndrome with Facial Paralysis. *Annals of Neurology*, *91*(1), 162–163. https://doi.org/10.1002/ana.26258
Pelletier, J., Thomas, G., & Volarević, S. (2018). Ribosome biogenesis in cancer: new players and therapeutic avenues. *Nature Reviews Cancer*, *18*(1), 51–63. https://doi.org/10.1038/nrc.2017.104
Pelliccia, M., Andreozzi, P., Paulose, J., D'Alicarnasso, M., Cagno, V., Donalisio, M., Civra, A., Broeckel, R. M., Haese, N., Jacob Silva, P., Carney, R. P., Marjomäki, V., Streblow, D. N., Lembo, D., Stellacci, F., Vitelli, V., & Krol, S. (2016). Additives for vaccine storage to improve thermal stability of adenoviruses from hours to months. *Nature Communications*, *7*(1), 13520. https://doi.org/10.1038/ncomms13520
Pepe, S., Gregory, A. T., & Denniss, A. R. (2021). Myocarditis, Pericarditis and Cardiomyopathy After COVID-19 Vaccination. *Heart, Lung and Circulation*, *30*(10), 1425–1429. https://doi.org/10.1016/j.hlc.2021.07.011
Percharde, M., Lin, C.-J., Yin, Y., Guan, J., Peixoto, G. A., Bulut-Karslioglu, A., Biechele, S., Huang, B., Shen, X., & Ramalho-Santos, M. (2018). A LINE1-Nucleolin Partnership Regulates Early Development and ESC Identity. *Cell*, *174*(2), 391-405.e19. https://doi.org/10.1016/j.cell.2018.05.043
Pereira, V. M., Reis, F. M., Santos, R. A. S., Cassali, G. D., Santos, S. H. S., Honorato-Sampaio, K., & dos Reis, A. M. (2009). Gonadotropin Stimulation Increases the Expression of Angiotensin-(1–7) and Mas Receptor in the Rat Ovary. *Reproductive Sciences*, *16*(12), 1165–1174. https://doi.org/10.1177/1933719109343309
Perico, L., Morigi, M., Galbusera, M., Pezzotta, A., Gastoldi, S., Imberti, B., Perna, A., Ruggenenti, P., Donadelli, R., Benigni, A., & Remuzzi, G. (2022). SARS-CoV-2 Spike Protein 1 Activates Microvascular Endothelial Cells and Complement System Leading to Platelet Aggregation. *Frontiers in Immunology*, *13*. https://doi.org/10.3389/fimmu.2022.827146
Pfueller, S. L., Logan, D., Tran, T. T., & Bilston, R. A. (1990). Naturally occurring human IgG antibodies to intracellular and cytoskeletal components of human platelets. *Clinical and Experimental Immunology*, *79*(3), 367–373. https://doi.org/10.1111/j.1365-2249.1990.tb08097.x
Phumsatitpong, C., Wagenmaker, E. R., & Moenter, S. M. (2021). Neuroendocrine interactions of the stress and reproductive axes. *Frontiers in Neuroendocrinology*, *63*, 100928. https://doi.org/10.1016/j.yfrne.2021.100928
Piantadosi, S. (1997). *Clinical trials : a methodologic perspective*. Wiley-Interscience.
Piantadosi, , S., Byar, D. P., & Green, S. B. (1988). The ecological fallacy. *American Journal of Epidemiology*, *127*(5), 893–904. https://doi.org/10.1093/oxfordjournals.aje.a114892
Picard, M., Stone, C. A., & Greenhawt, M. (2023). Management of patients with immediate reactions to COVID-19 vaccines. *Journal of Allergy and Clinical Immunology*, *151*(2), 413–415. https://doi.org/10.1016/j.jaci.2022.09.003
Piccolo, V., Mazzatenta, C., Bassi, A., Argenziano, G., Cutrone, M., Grimalt, R., & Russo, T. (2022). COVID vaccine-induced lichen planus on areas previously

affected by vitiligo. *Journal of the European Academy of Dermatology and Venereology*, *36*(1). https://doi.org/10.1111/jdv.17687

Picken, M. M. (2020). The Pathology of Amyloidosis in Classification: A Review. *Acta Haematologica*, *143*(4), 322–334. https://doi.org/10.1159/000506696

Pignatti, P., Ramirez, G. A., Russo, M., Marraccini, P., Nannipieri, S., Asperti, C., Torre, F. Della, Tiri, A., Gatti, B. M., Gurrado, A., Meriggi, A., Benanti, G., Cilona, M. B., Pigatto, P., Burastero, S. E., Dagna, L., & Yacoub, M.-R. (2023). Hypersensitivity reactions to anti-SARS-CoV-2 vaccines: Basophil reactivity to excipients. *Vaccine*, *41*(32), 4693–4699. https://doi.org/10.1016/j.vaccine.2023.06.039

Pino, V., Sanz, A., Valdés, N., Crosby, J., & Mackenna, A. (2020). The effects of aging on semen parameters and sperm DNA fragmentation. *JBRA Assisted Reproduction*. https://doi.org/10.5935/1518-0557.20190058

Pirola, F. J. C., Santos, B. A. M., Sapienza, G. F., Cetrangolo, L. Y., Geranutti, C. H. W. G., & de Aguiar, P. H. P. (2022). Miller–Fisher syndrome after first dose of Oxford/AstraZeneca coronavirus disease 2019 vaccine: a case report. *Journal of Medical Case Reports*, *16*(1), 437. https://doi.org/10.1186/s13256-022-03592-4

Pisetsky, D. S. (2016). Anti-DNA antibodies — quintessential biomarkers of SLE. *Nature Reviews Rheumatology*, *12*(2), 102–110. https://doi.org/10.1038/nrrheum.2015.151

Pisetsky, D. S., Garza Reyna, A., Belina, M. E., & Spencer, D. M. (2022). The Interaction of Anti-DNA Antibodies with DNA: Evidence for Unconventional Binding Mechanisms. *International Journal of Molecular Sciences*, *23*(9), 5227. https://doi.org/10.3390/ijms23095227

Pitlick, M. M., Joshi, A. Y., Gonzalez-Estrada, A., & Chiarella, S. E. (2022). Delayed systemic urticarial reactions following mRNA COVID-19 vaccination. *Allergy and Asthma Proceedings*, *43*(1), 40–43. https://doi.org/10.2500/aap.2022.43.210101

Planty, C., Chevalier, G., Duclos, M., Chalmey, C., Thirion-Delalande, C., Sobry, C., Steff, A., & Destexhe, E. (2020). Nonclinical safety assessment of repeated administration and biodistribution of ChAd3-EBO-Z Ebola candidate vaccine. *Journal of Applied Toxicology*, *40*(6), 748–762. https://doi.org/10.1002/jat.3941

Pniewska, E., & Pawliczak, R. (2013). The involvement of phospholipases A2 in asthma and chronic obstructive pulmonary disease. *Mediators of Inflammation*, 1–12. https://doi.org/10.1155/2013/793505

Polack, F. P., Thomas, S. J., Kitchin, N., Absalon, J., Gurtman, A., Lockhart, S., Perez, J. L., Pérez Marc, G., Moreira, E. D., Zerbini, C., Bailey, R., Swanson, K. A., Roychoudhury, S., Koury, K., Li, P., Kalina, W. V., Cooper, D., Frenck, R. W., Hammitt, L. L., … Gruber, W. C. (2020). Safety and Efficacy of the BNT162b2 mRNA Covid-19 Vaccine. *New England Journal of Medicine*, *383*(27), 2603–2615. https://doi.org/10.1056/NEJMoa2034577

Popa, C. C., Badiu, D. C., Rusu, O. C., Grigorean, V. T., Neagu, S. I., & Strugaru, C. R. (2016). Mortality prognostic factors in acute pancreatitis. *Journal of Medicine and Life*, *9*(4), 413–418.

Pothiawala, S. (2021). Bell's Palsy After Second Dose of Moderna COVID-19 Vaccine: Coincidence or Causation? *Acta Medica Lituanica*, *28*(2), 7. https://doi.org/10.15388/Amed.2021.28.2.7

Poudel, S., Nepali, P., Baniya, S., Shah, S., Bogati, S., Nepal, G., Ojha, R., Edaki, O., Lazovic, G., & Kara, S. (2022). Bell's palsy as a possible complication of mRNA-1273 (Moderna) vaccine against COVID-19. *Annals of Medicine & Surgery*, *78*. https://doi.org/10.1016/j.amsu.2022.103897

Prado, M. B., & Adiao, K. J. B. (2022). Facial Diplegia as the Sole Manifestation of Post-Vaccination Guillain-Barre Syndrome: A Case Report and Literature Review. *The Neurohospitalist*, *12*(3), 508–511. https://doi.org/10.1177/19418744221097350

Prasad, A., Hurlburt, G., Podury, S., Tandon, M., Kingree, S., & Sriwastava, S. (2021). A Novel Case of Bifacial Diplegia Variant of Guillain-Barré Syndrome Following Janssen COVID-19 Vaccination. *Neurology International*, *13*(3), 404–409. https://doi.org/10.3390/neurolint13030040

Prasad, T. K., & Rao, N. M. (2005). The role of plasmid constructs containing the SV40 DNA nuclear-targeting sequence in cationic lipid-mediated DNA delivery. *Cellular & Molecular Biology Letters*, *10*(2), 203–215.

Prinz, A. L. (2020). Chocolate consumption and Noble laureates. *Social Sciences & Humanities Open*, *2*(1), 100082. https://doi.org/10.1016/j.ssaho.2020.100082

Puangpet, P., Lai-Cheong, J., & McFadden, J. P. (2013). Chemical atopy. *Contact Dermatitis*, *68*(4), 208–213. https://doi.org/10.1111/cod.12029

Puranik, A., Lenehan, P. J., Silvert, E., Niesen, M. J. M., Corchado-Garcia, J., O'Horo, J. C., Virk, A., Swift, M. D., Halamka, J., Badley, A. D., Venkatakrishnan, A. J., & Soundararajan, V. (2021). Comparison of two highly-effective mRNA vaccines for COVID-19 during periods of Alpha and Delta variant prevalence. *MedRxiv : The Preprint Server for Health Sciences*. https://doi.org/10.1101/2021.08.06.21261707

Putaala, J., Metso, A. J., Metso, T. M., Konkola, N., Kraemer, Y., Haapaniemi, E., Kaste, M., & Tatlisumak, T. (2009). Analysis of 1008 Consecutive Patients Aged 15 to 49 With First-Ever Ischemic Stroke. *Stroke*, *40*(4), 1195–1203. https://doi.org/10.1161/STROKEAHA.108.529883

Qureshi, Z. P., Seoane-Vazquez, E., Rodriguez-Monguio, R., Stevenson, K. B., & Szeinbach, S. L. (2011). Market withdrawal of new molecular entities approved in the United States from 1980 to 2009. *Pharmacoepidemiology and Drug Safety*, *20*(7), 772–777. https://doi.org/10.1002/pds.2155

Raddi, N., Vigant, F., Wagner-Ballon, O., Giraudier, S., Custers, J., Hemmi, S., & Benihoud, K. (2016). Pseudotyping Serotype 5 Adenovirus with the Fiber from Other Serotypes Uncovers a Key Role of the Fiber Protein in Adenovirus 5-Induced Thrombocytopenia. *Human Gene Therapy*, *27*(2), 193–201. https://doi.org/10.1089/hum.2015.154

Rägo, L., & Santoso, B. (2008). Drug Regulation: History, Present and Future. In C. van Boxtel, B. Santoso, & I. Edwards (Eds.), *Drug Benefits and Risks: International Textbook of Clinical Pharmacology* (2nd edition, pp. 65–77). IOS Press and Uppsala Monitoring Centre.

Rahamimov, N., Baturov, V., Shani, A., Ben Zoor, I., Fischer, D., & Chernihovsky, A. (2021). Inadequate deltoid muscle penetration and concerns of improper COVID mRNA vaccine administration can be avoided by injection technique modification. *Vaccine*, *39*(37), 5326–5330. https://doi.org/10.1016/j.vaccine.2021.06.081

Raj, S., Ogola, G., & Han, J. (2022). COVID-19 Vaccine-Associated Subclinical Axillary Lymphadenopathy on Screening Mammogram. *Academic Radiology, 29*(4), 501–507. https://doi.org/10.1016/j.acra.2021.11.010

Rajpurkar, M., O'Brien, S. H., Haamid, F. W., Cooper, D. L., Gunawardena, S., & Chitlur, M. (2016). Heavy Menstrual Bleeding as a Common Presenting Symptom of Rare Platelet Disorders: Illustrative Case Examples. *Journal of Pediatric and Adolescent Gynecology, 29*(6), 537–541. https://doi.org/10.1016/j.jpag.2016.02.002

Rancourt, D. G., Baudin, M., Hickey, J., & Mercier, J. (2023). *COVID-19 vaccine-associated mortality in the Southern Hemisphere*. https://correlation-canada.org/covid-19-vaccine-associated-mortality-in-the-Southern-Hemisphere/

Ransing, R., Dashi, E., Rehman, S., Chepure, A., Mehta, V., & Kundadak, G. K. (2021). COVID-19 anti-vaccine movement and mental health: Challenges and the way forward. *Asian Journal of Psychiatry, 58*, 102614. https://doi.org/10.1016/j.ajp.2021.102614

Rao, S. J., Khurana, S., Murthy, G., Dawson, E. T., Jazebi, N., & Haas, C. J. (2021). A case of Guillain–Barre syndrome following Pfizer COVID-19 vaccine. *Journal of Community Hospital Internal Medicine Perspectives, 11*(5), 597–600. https://doi.org/10.1080/20009666.2021.1954284

Rastegar, T., Feryduni, L., & Fakhraei, M. (2023). COVID-19 vaccine side effects on menstrual disturbances among Iranian women. *New Microbes and New Infections, 53*,101114. https://doi.org/10.1016/j.nmni.2023.101114.

Ravi, V., Saxena, S., & Panda, P. S. (2022). Basic virology of SARS-CoV 2. *Indian Journal of Medical Microbiology, 40*(2), 182–186. https://doi.org/10.1016/j.ijmmb.2022.02.005

Reddy, Y. M., Murthy, J. M., Osman, S., Jaiswal, S. K., Gattu, A. K., Pidaparthi, L., Boorgu, S. K., Chavan, R., Ramakrishnan, B., & Yeduguri, S. R. (2023). Guillain-Barré syndrome associated with SARS-CoV-2 vaccination: how is it different? a systematic review and individual participant data meta-analysis. *Clinical and Experimental Vaccine Research, 12*(2), 143. https://doi.org/10.7774/cevr.2023.12.2.143

Reed, B. G., & Carr, B. R. (2000). *The Normal Menstrual Cycle and the Control of Ovulation . [Updated 2018 Aug 5]*. Endotext [Internet]. https://www.ncbi.nlm.nih.gov/books/NBK279054/

Reina-Campos, M., Scharping, N. E., & Goldrath, A. W. (2021). CD8+ T cell metabolism in infection and cancer. *Nature Reviews Immunology, 21*(11), 718–738. https://doi.org/10.1038/s41577-021-00537-8

Reinfeld, S., Cáceda, R., Gil, R., Strom, H., & Chacko, M. (2021). Can new onset psychosis occur after mRNA based COVID-19 vaccine administration? A case report. *Psychiatry Research, 304*, 114165. https://doi.org/10.1016/j.psychres.2021.114165

Reis, F. M., Bouissou, D. R., Pereira, V. M., Camargos, A. F., dos Reis, A. M., & Santos, R. A. (2011). Angiotensin-(1-7), its receptor Mas, and the angiotensin-converting enzyme type 2 are expressed in the human ovary. *Fertility and Sterility, 95*(1), 176–181. https://doi.org/10.1016/j.fertnstert.2010.06.060

Renemane, L., Vrublevska, J., & Cera, I. (2022). First Episode Psychosis Following COVID-19 Vaccination: a Case Report. *Psychiatria Danubina, 34*(Suppl 8), 56–59.

Rha, M.-S., & Shin, E.-C. (2021). Activation or exhaustion of CD8+ T cells in patients with COVID-19. *Cellular & Molecular Immunology*, *18*(10), 2325–2333. https://doi.org/10.1038/s41423-021-00750-4

Rhazouani, A., Gamrani, H., El Achaby, M., Aziz, K., Gebrati, L., Uddin, M. S., & AZIZ, F. (2021). Synthesis and Toxicity of Graphene Oxide Nanoparticles: A Literature Review of In Vitro and In Vivo Studies. *BioMed Research International*, 1–19. https://doi.org/10.1155/2021/5518999

Rhea, E. M., Logsdon, A. F., Hansen, K. M., Williams, L. M., Reed, M. J., Baumann, K. K., Holden, S. J., Raber, J., Banks, W. A., & Erickson, M. A. (2021). The S1 protein of SARS-CoV-2 crosses the blood–brain barrier in mice. *Nature Neuroscience*, *24*(3), 368–378. https://doi.org/10.1038/s41593-020-00771-8

Richardson, R. T., Alekseev, O. M., Grossman, G., Widgren, E. E., Thresher, R., Wagner, E. J., Sullivan, K. D., Marzluff, W. F., & O'Rand, M. G. (2006). Nuclear Autoantigenic Sperm Protein (NASP), a Linker Histone Chaperone That Is Required for Cell Proliferation. *Journal of Biological Chemistry*, *281*(30), 21526–21534. https://doi.org/10.1074/jbc.M603816200

Richardson, R. T., Batova, I. N., Widgren, E. E., Zheng, L.-X., Whitfield, M., Marzluff, W. F., & O'Rand, M. G. (2000). Characterization of the Histone H1-binding Protein, NASP, as a Cell Cycle-regulated Somatic Protein. *Journal of Biological Chemistry*, *275*(39), 30378–30386. https://doi.org/10.1074/jbc.M003781200

Richardson-May, J., Purcaru, E., Campbell, C., Hillier, C., & Parkin, B. (2022). Guillain-Barré Syndrome and Unilateral Optic Neuritis Following Vaccination for COVID-19: A Case Report and Literature Review. *Neuro-Ophthalmology*, *46*(6), 413–419. https://doi.org/10.1080/01658107.2022.2048861

Richie, T. L., & Villasante, E. F. (2013). Use of Adenovirus Serotype 5 Vaccine Vectors in Seropositive, Uncircumcised Men: Safety Lessons from the Step Trial. *Journal of Infectious Diseases*, *207*(4), 689–690. https://doi.org/10.1093/infdis/jis737

Robb, M., & Robb, L. (2021). Delayed-type hypersensitivity skin reaction to Covid-19 vaccine. *Journal of Family Medicine and Primary Care*, *10*(10), 3908. https://doi.org/10.4103/jfmpc.jfmpc_361_21

Roberge, G., Côté, B., Calabrino, A., Gilbert, N., & Gagnon, N. (2022). Acute lower limb ischemia caused by vaccine-induced immune thrombotic thrombocytopenia: focus on perioperative considerations for 2 cases. *Thrombosis Journal*, *20*(1), 38. https://doi.org/10.1186/s12959-022-00398-8

Roberts, K., Sidhu, N., Russel, M., & Abbas, M. (2021). Psychiatric pathology potentially induced by COVID-19 vaccine. . *Progress in Neurology and Psychiatry*, *25*(4), 8–10. https://doi.org/https://doi.org/10.1002/pnp.723

Robles, J. P., Zamora, M., Adan-Castro, E., Siqueiros-Marquez, L., Martinez de la Escalera, G., & Clapp, C. (2022). The spike protein of SARS-CoV-2 induces endothelial inflammation through integrin α5β1 and NF-κB signaling. *Journal of Biological Chemistry*, *298*(3), 101695. https://doi.org/10.1016/j.jbc.2022.101695

Rocha Cabrero, F., & Morrison, E. H. (2023). *Miller Fisher Syndrome*. StatPearls Publishing. https://www.ncbi.nlm.nih.gov/books/NBK507717/

Rocha, S. (2013). Targeted Drug Delivery Across the Blood Brain Barrier in Alzheimer's Disease. *Current Pharmaceutical Design*, *19*(37), 6635–6646. https://doi.org/10.2174/1381612811319990613

Rodrigues Silva, N. (2010). Chocolate Consumption and Effects on Serotonin Synthesis. *Archives of Internal Medicine*, *170*(17), 1604. https://doi.org/10.1001/archinternmed.2010.331
Rodríguez Quejada, L., Toro Wills, M. F., Martínez-Ávila, M. C., & Patiño-Aldana, A. F. (2022). Menstrual cycle disturbances after COVID-19 vaccination. *Women's Health*, *18*, 174550572211093. https://doi.org/10.1177/17455057221109375
Roesler, E., Weiss, R., Weinberger, E. E., Fruehwirth, A., Stoecklinger, A., Mostböck, S., Ferreira, F., Thalhamer, J., & Scheiblhofer, S. (2009). Immunize and disappear—Safety-optimized mRNA vaccination with a panel of 29 allergens. *Journal of Allergy and Clinical Immunology*, *124*(5), 1070-1077.e11. https://doi.org/10.1016/j.jaci.2009.06.036
Röltgen, K., Nielsen, S. C. A., Silva, O., Younes, S. F., Zaslavsky, M., Costales, C., Yang, F., Wirz, O. F., Solis, D., Hoh, R. A., Wang, A., Arunachalam, P. S., Colburg, D., Zhao, S., Haraguchi, E., Lee, A. S., Shah, M. M., Manohar, M., Chang, I., … Boyd, S. D. (2022). Immune imprinting, breadth of variant recognition, and germinal center response in human SARS-CoV-2 infection and vaccination. *Cell*, *185*(6), 1025-1040.e14. https://doi.org/10.1016/j.cell.2022.01.018
Román, G. C., Gracia, F., Torres, A., Palacios, A., Gracia, K., & Harris, D. (2021). Acute Transverse Myelitis (ATM):Clinical Review of 43 Patients With COVID-19-Associated ATM and 3 Post-Vaccination ATM Serious Adverse Events With the ChAdOx1 nCoV-19 Vaccine (AZD1222). *Frontiers in Immunology*, *12*. https://doi.org/10.3389/fimmu.2021.653786
Rona, R. J., Keil, T., Summers, C., Gislason, D., Zuidmeer, L., Sodergren, E., Sigurdardottir, S. T., Lindner, T., Goldhahn, K., Dahlstrom, J., McBride, D., & Madsen, C. (2007). The prevalence of food allergy: A meta-analysis. *Journal of Allergy and Clinical Immunology*, *120*(3), 638–646. https://doi.org/10.1016/j.jaci.2007.05.026
Roncati, L., Manenti, A., & Corsi, L. (2022). A Three-Case Series of Thrombotic Deaths in Patients over 50 with Comorbidities Temporally after modRNA COVID-19 Vaccination. *Pathogens*, *11*(4), 435. https://doi.org/10.3390/pathogens11040435
Rosa Silva, J. P., Santiago Júnior, J. B., dos Santos, E. L., de Carvalho, F. O., de França Costa, I. M. P., & Mendonça, D. M. F. de. (2020). Quality of life and functional independence in amyotrophic lateral sclerosis: A systematic review. *Neuroscience & Biobehavioral Reviews*, *111*, 1–11. https://doi.org/10.1016/j.neubiorev.2019.12.032
Rose, J. (2021). Critical Appraisal of VAERS Pharmacovigilance: Is the U.S. Vaccine Adverse Events Reporting System (VAERS) a Functioning Pharmacovigilance System? *Science, Public Health Policy and the Law*, *3*, 100–129.
Rose, J., Hulscher, N., & McCullough, P. (2023). Determinants of COVID-19 vaccine induced myocarditis. *Zenodo*. https://doi.org/10.5281/zenodo.8356800
Rosner, C. M., Genovese, L., Tehrani, B. N., Atkins, M., Bakhshi, H., Chaudhri, S., Damluji, A. A., de Lemos, J. A., Desai, S. S., Emaminia, A., Flanagan, M. C., Khera, A., Maghsoudi, A., Mekonnen, G., Muthukumar, A., Saeed, I. M., Sherwood, M. W., Sinha, S. S., O'Connor, C. M., & deFilippi, C. R. (2021). Myocarditis Temporally Associated With COVID-19 Vaccination. *Circulation*, *144*(6), 502–505. https://doi.org/10.1161/CIRCULATIONAHA.121.055891

Rossetti, A., Gheihman, G., O'Hare, M., & Kosowsky, J. M. (2021). Guillain-Barré Syndrome Presenting as Facial Diplegia after COVID-19 Vaccination: A Case Report. *The Journal of Emergency Medicine*, *61*(6), e141–e145. https://doi.org/10.1016/j.jemermed.2021.07.062

Rothman, K. J., & Greenland, S. (2005). Causation and Causal Inference in Epidemiology. *American Journal of Public Health*, *95*(S1), S144–S150. https://doi.org/10.2105/AJPH.2004.059204

Ruiz Rodríguez, A., lavijo Grimaldi, D., Mejía, O., Ruiz, M., García Cardona, A., García, G., & Casadiego, C. (2006). Bases biológicas y patobiológicas humanas de la esclerosis lateral amiotrófica. *Universitas Médica*, *47*(1).

Russell, R., & Quinn, B. (2022). Acute Worsening of Atypical Parkinson's Syndrome After Receiving Second Dose of Moderna COVID-19 Vaccine. *WMJ : Official Publication of the State Medical Society of Wisconsin*, *121*(3), E46–E49.

Russell, W. C., Graham, F. L., Smiley, J., & Nairn, R. (1977). Characteristics of a Human Cell Line Transformed by DNA from Human Adenovirus Type 5. *Journal of General Virology*, *36*(1), 59–72. https://doi.org/10.1099/0022-1317-36-1-59

Ryterska, K., Kordek, A., & Załęska, P. (2021). Has Menstruation Disappeared? Functional Hypothalamic Amenorrhea—What Is This Story about? *Nutrients*, *13*(8), 2827. https://doi.org/10.3390/nu13082827

Ryu, D.-W., Lim, E.-Y., & Cho, A.-H. (2022). A case of hemichorea following administration of the Pfizer-BioNTech COVID-19 vaccine. *Neurological Sciences*, *43*(2), 771–773. https://doi.org/10.1007/s10072-021-05763-5

Rzymski, P. (2023). Guillain-Barré syndrome and COVID-19 vaccines: focus on adenoviral vectors. *Frontiers in Immunology*, *14*. https://doi.org/10.3389/fimmu.2023.1183258

Saadi, F., Pal, D., & Sarma, J. D. (2021). Spike Glycoprotein Is Central to Coronavirus Pathogenesis-Parallel Between m-CoV and SARS-CoV-2. *Annals of Neuroscience, 28*(3-4), 201–218. https://doi.org/10.1177/09727531211023755.

Sabat, R., Dayton, O. L., Agarwal, A., & Vedam-Mai, V. (2023). Analyzing the effect of the COVID-19 vaccine on Parkinson's disease symptoms. *Frontiers in Immunology*, *14*. https://doi.org/10.3389/fimmu.2023.1158364

Sadeghi, E., Mahmoudzadeh, R., Garg, S. J., & Nowroozzadeh, M. H. (2023). Ocular posterior segment complications following COVID-19 vaccination. *International Ophthalmology*, *43*(11), 4343–4357. https://doi.org/10.1007/s10792-023-02795-y

Sadelain, M. (2004). Insertional oncogenesis in gene therapy: how much of a risk? *Gene Therapy*, *11*(7), 569–573. https://doi.org/10.1038/sj.gt.3302243

Sadoff, J., Gray, G., Vandebosch, A., Cárdenas, V., Shukarev, G., Grinsztejn, B., Goepfert, P. A., Truyers, C., Fennema, H., Spiessens, B., Offergeld, K., Scheper, G., Taylor, K. L., Robb, M. L., Treanor, J., Barouch, D. H., Stoddard, J., Ryser, M. F., Marovich, M. A., … Douoguih, M. (2021). Safety and Efficacy of Single-Dose Ad26.COV2.S Vaccine against Covid-19. *New England Journal of Medicine*, *384*(23), 2187–2201. https://doi.org/10.1056/NEJMoa2101544

Sáenz-Robles, M. T., Sullivan, C. S., & Pipas, J. M. (2001). Transforming functions of Simian Virus 40. *Oncogene*, *20*(54), 7899–7907. https://doi.org/10.1038/sj.onc.1204936

Salah HM, Mehta JL. COVID Vaccine and Myocarditis. Am J Cardiol. 2021 S0002-9149(21)00639-1. https://doi.org/10.1016/j.amjcard.2021.07.009.

Salem, F., Rein, J. L., Yu, S. M.-W., Abramson, M., Cravedi, P., & Chung, M. (2021). Report of Three Cases of Minimal Change Disease Following the Second Dose of mRNA SARS-CoV-2 COVID-19 Vaccine. *Kidney International Reports*, *6*(9), 2523–2524. https://doi.org/10.1016/j.ekir.2021.07.017

Sallard, E., Schröer, D. K., Schellhorn, S., Koukou, G., Schmidt, N., Zhang, W., Kreppel, F., & Ehrhardt, A. (2022). Adenovirus type 34 and HVR1-deleted Adenovirus type 5 do not bind to PF4: clearing the path towards vectors without thrombosis risk. *BioRxiv*. https://doi.org/10.1101/2022.11.07.515483

Salunkhe, M., Tayade, K., Priyadarshi, M., Goel, V., Gulati, I., Garg, A., Bhatia, R., & Srivastava, M. V. P. (2023). Spectrum of various CNS inflammatory demyelination diseases following COVID-19 vaccinations. *Acta Neurologica Belgica*. https://doi.org/10.1007/s13760-023-02373-0

Salvarani, C., Hunder, G. G., Morris, J. M., Brown, R. D., Christianson, T., & Giannini, C. (2013). A -related angiitis: Comparison with CAA without inflammation and primary CNS vasculitis. *Neurology*, *81*(18), 1596–1603. https://doi.org/10.1212/WNL.0b013e3182a9f545

Samaniego-Castruita, J. A., Schneider, U. V., Mollerup, S., Leineweber, T. D., Weis, N., Bukh, J., Pedersen, M. S., & Westh, H. (2023). SARS-CoV-2 spike mRNA vaccine sequences circulate in blood up to 28 days after COVID -19 vaccination. *APMIS*, *131*(3), 128–132. https://doi.org/10.1111/apm.13294

Samuel, C. E. (2001). Antiviral Actions of Interferons. *Clinical Microbiology Reviews*, *14*(4), 778–809. https://doi.org/10.1128/CMR.14.4.778-809.2001

Sánchez van Kammen, M., Aguiar de Sousa, D., Poli, S., Cordonnier, C., Heldner, M. R., van de Munckhof, A., Krzywicka, K., van Haaps, T., Ciccone, A., Middeldorp, S., Levi, M. M., Kremer Hovinga, J. A., Silvis, S., Hiltunen, S., Mansour, M., Arauz, A., Barboza, M. A., Field, T. S., Tsivgoulis, G., … Arslan, Y. (2021). Characteristics and Outcomes of Patients With Cerebral Venous Sinus Thrombosis in SARS-CoV-2 Vaccine–Induced Immune Thrombotic Thrombocytopenia. *JAMA Neurology*, *78*(11), 1314. https://doi.org/10.1001/jamaneurol.2021.3619

Sanchez-Luque, F. J., Kempen, M.-J. H. C., Gerdes, P., Vargas-Landin, D. B., Richardson, S. R., Troskie, R.-L., Jesuadian, J. S., Cheetham, S. W., Carreira, P. E., Salvador-Palomeque, C., García-Cañadas, M., Muñoz-Lopez, M., Sanchez, L., Lundberg, M., Macia, A., Heras, S. R., Brennan, P. M., Lister, R., Garcia-Perez, J. L., … Faulkner, G. J. (2019). LINE-1 Evasion of Epigenetic Repression in Humans. *Molecular Cell*, *75*(3), 590-604.e12. https://doi.org/10.1016/j.molcel.2019.05.024

Sandberg, A., Salminen, V., Heinonen, S., & Sivén, M. (2022). Under-Reporting of Adverse Drug Reactions in Finland and Healthcare Professionals' Perspectives on How to Improve Reporting. *Healthcare*, *10*(6), 1015. https://doi.org/10.3390/healthcare10061015

Sandhu, S., Bhatnagar, A., Kumar, H., Dixit, P. K., Paliwal, G., Suhag, D. K., Patil, C., & Mitra, D. (2021). Leukocytoclastic vasculitis as a cutaneous manifestation of ChAdOx1 nCoV -19 corona virus vaccine (recombinant). *Dermatologic Therapy*, *34*(6). https://doi.org/10.1111/dth.15141

Sangoram, R., Mahendradas, P., Bhakti Mishra, S., Kawali, A., Sanjay, S., & Shetty, R. (2022). Herpes Simplex Virus 1 Anterior Uveitis following Coronavirus Disease 2019 (COVID-19) Vaccination in an Asian Indian Female. *Ocular*

Immunology and Inflammation, *30*(5), 1260–1264. https://doi.org/10.1080/09273948.2022.2055580
Sanjay, S., Acharya, I., Kawali, A., Shetty, R., & Mahendradas, P. (2022a). Unilateral recurrent central serous chorioretinopathy (CSCR) following COVID-19 vaccination- A multimodal imaging study. *American Journal of Ophthalmology Case Reports*, *27*, 101644. https://doi.org/10.1016/j.ajoc.2022.101644
Sanjay, S., Acharya, I., Rawoof, A., & Shetty, R. (2022b). Non-arteritic anterior ischaemic optic neuropathy (NA-AION) and COVID-19 vaccination. *BMJ Case Reports*, *15*(5), e248415. https://doi.org/10.1136/bcr-2021-248415
Sanjay, S., Gadde, S. G. K., Kumar Yadav, N., Kawali, A., Gupta, A., Shetty, R., & Mahendradas, P. (2022c). Bilateral Sequential Acute Macular Neuroretinopathy in an Asian Indian Female with β Thalassemia Trait following (Corona Virus Disease) COVID-19 Vaccination and Probable Recent COVID Infection - Multimodal Imaging Study. *Ocular Immunology and Inflammation*, *30*(5), 1222–1227. https://doi.org/10.1080/09273948.2022.2026978
Sanjay, S., Handa, A., Kawali, A., Shetty, R., Bhakti Mishra, S., & Mahendradas, P. (2023a) Scleritis and Episcleritis following Coronavirus Disease (COVID) Vaccination. *Ocular Immunology and Inflammation, 31*(6),1184–1190. https://doi.org/10.1080/09273948.2023.2182324.
Sanjay, S., Kawali, A., & Mahendradas, P. (2022d). Acute macular neuroretinopathy and COVID-19 vaccination. *Indian Journal of Ophthalmology*, *70*(1), 345. https://doi.org/10.4103/ijo.IJO_2542_21
Sanjay, S., Kawali, A., & Mahendradas, P. (2023b). COVID-19 vaccination, dengue hepatitis, and recurrent unilateral anterior uveitis. *Indian Journal of Ophthalmology*, *71*(5), 2269–2272. https://doi.org/10.4103/ijo.IJO_2064_22
Sanjay, S., Yathish, G., Singh, Y., Kawali, A., Mahendradas, P., & Shetty, R. (2022e). COVID-19 vaccination and recurrent anterior uveitis. *Indian Journal of Ophthalmology*, *70*(12), 4445–4448. https://doi.org/10.4103/ijo.IJO_1089_22
Sarfraz, A., Sarfraz, Z., Sarfraz, M., Nadeem, Z., Felix, M., & Cherrez-Ojeda, I. (2022). Menstrual irregularities following COVID-19 vaccination: A global cross-sectional survey. *Annals of Medicine & Surgery*, *81*. https://doi.org/10.1016/j.amsu.2022.104220
Sarigecili, E., Arslan, I., Ucar, H. K., & Celik, U. (2021). Pediatric anti-NMDA receptor encephalitis associated with COVID-19. *Child's Nervous System*, *37*(12), 3919–3922. https://doi.org/10.1007/s00381-021-05155-2
Sasa, S., Inoue, H., Inui, T., Miyamoto, N., Aoyama, M., Okumura, K., Toba, H., Yoshida, T., Tezuka, M., Hirose, C., Saijo, Y., Uehara, H., Izumori, A., Takahashi, M., Sasa, M., & Takizawa, H. (2022). Axillary lymphangioma that developed following COVID-19 vaccination: a case report. *Surgical Case Reports*, *8*(1), 131. https://doi.org/10.1186/s40792-022-01488-5
Schauer, J., Buddhe, S., Gulhane, A., Sagiv, E., Studer, M., Colyer, J., Chikkabyrappa, S. M., Law, Y., & Portman, M. A. (2022). Persistent Cardiac Magnetic Resonance Imaging Findings in a Cohort of Adolescents with Post-Coronavirus Disease 2019 mRNA Vaccine Myopericarditis. *The Journal of Pediatrics*, *245*, 233–237. https://doi.org/10.1016/j.jpeds.2022.03.032
Schembri Higgans, J., Bowman, S., & Abela, J.-E. (2021). COVID-19 associated pancreatitis: A mini case-series. *International Journal of Surgery Case Reports*, *87*, 106429. https://doi.org/10.1016/j.ijscr.2021.106429

Schenk-Braat, E. A. M., van Mierlo, M. M. K. B., Wagemaker, G., Bangma, C. H., & Kaptein, L. C. M. (2007). An inventory of shedding data from clinical gene therapy trials. *The Journal of Gene Medicine*, *9*(10), 910–921. https://doi.org/10.1002/jgm.1096

Schmeer, M., Buchholz, T., & Schleef, M. (2017). Plasmid DNA Manufacturing for Indirect and Direct Clinical Applications. *Human Gene Therapy*, *28*(10), 856–861. https://doi.org/10.1089/hum.2017.159

Schmeling, M., Manniche, V., & Hansen, P. R. (2023). Batch-dependent safety of the BNT162b2 mRNA COVID-19 vaccine. *European Journal of Clinical Investigation*, *53*(8). https://doi.org/10.1111/eci.13998

Schmitt, C. A., Wang, B., & Demaria, M. (2022). Senescence and cancer — role and therapeutic opportunities. *Nature Reviews Clinical Oncology*, *19*(10), 619–636. https://doi.org/10.1038/s41571-022-00668-4

Schnaar, R. L. (2010). Brain gangliosides in axon–myelin stability and axon regeneration. *FEBS Letters*, *584*(9), 1741–1747. https://doi.org/10.1016/j.febslet.2009.10.011

Schöberl, F., Ringleb, P. A., Wakili, R., Poli, S., Wollenweber, F. A., & Kellert, L. (2017). Juvenile Stroke: A Practice-Oriented Overview. *Deutsches Ärzteblatt International*. https://doi.org/10.3238/arztebl.2017.0527

Schoenmaker, L., Witzigmann, D., Kulkarni, J. A., Verbeke, R., Kersten, G., Jiskoot, W., & Crommelin, D. J. A. (2021). mRNA-lipid nanoparticle COVID-19 vaccines: Structure and stability. *International Journal of Pharmaceutics*, *601*, 120586. https://doi.org/10.1016/j.ijpharm.2021.120586

Schreckenberg, R., Woitasky, N., Itani, N., Czech, L., Ferdinandy, P., & Schulz, R. (2023). Cardiac side effects of RNA-based SARS-CoV-2 vaccines: Hidden cardiotoxic effects of mRNA-1273 and BNT162b2 on ventricular myocyte function and structure. *British Journal of Pharmacology*. https://doi.org/10.1111/bph.16262

Schwartzberg, L. S., & Navari, R. M. (2018). Safety of Polysorbate 80 in the Oncology Setting. *Advances in Therapy*, *35*(6), 754–767. https://doi.org/10.1007/s12325-018-0707-z

Sebastian, M., Papachristofilou, A., Weiss, C., Früh, M., Cathomas, R., Hilbe, W., Wehler, T., Rippin, G., Koch, S. D., Scheel, B., Fotin-Mleczek, M., Heidenreich, R., Kallen, K.-J., Gnad-Vogt, U., & Zippelius, A. (2014). Phase Ib study evaluating a self-adjuvanted mRNA cancer vaccine (RNActive®) combined with local radiation as consolidation and maintenance treatment for patients with stage IV non-small cell lung cancer. *BMC Cancer*, *14*(1), 748. https://doi.org/10.1186/1471-2407-14-748

Sebastian, M., Schröder, A., Scheel, B., Hong, H. S., Muth, A., von Boehmer, L., Zippelius, A., Mayer, F., Reck, M., Atanackovic, D., Thomas, M., Schneller, F., Stöhlmacher, J., Bernhard, H., Gröschel, A., Lander, T., Probst, J., Strack, T., Wiegand, V., … Koch, S. D. (2019). A phase I/IIa study of the mRNA-based cancer immunotherapy CV9201 in patients with stage IIIB/IV non-small cell lung cancer. *Cancer Immunology, Immunotherapy*, *68*(5), 799–812. https://doi.org/10.1007/s00262-019-02315-x

See, I., Su, J. R., Lale, A., Woo, E. J., Guh, A. Y., Shimabukuro, T. T., Streiff, M. B., Rao, A. K., Wheeler, A. P., Beavers, S. F., Durbin, A. P., Edwards, K., Miller, E., Harrington, T. A., Mba-Jonas, A., Nair, N., Nguyen, D. T., Talaat, K. R., Urrutia,

V. C., … Broder, K. R. (2021). US Case Reports of Cerebral Venous Sinus Thrombosis With Thrombocytopenia After Ad26.COV2.S Vaccination, March 2 to April 21, 2021. *JAMA*, *325*(24), 2448. https://doi.org/10.1001/jama.2021.7517

Sekizawa, A., Hashimoto, K., Kobayashi, S., Kozono, S., Kobayashi, T., Kawamura, Y., Kimata, M., Fujita, N., Ono, Y., Obuchi, Y., & Tanaka, Y. (2022). Rapid progression of marginal zone B-cell lymphoma after COVID-19 vaccination (BNT162b2): A case report. *Frontiers in Medicine*, *9*. https://doi.org/10.3389/fmed.2022.963393

Seneff, S., Kyriakopoulos, A. M., Nigh, G., & McCullough, P. A. (2023). A Potential Role of the Spike Protein in Neurodegenerative Diseases: A Narrative Review. *Cureus*. https://doi.org/10.7759/cureus.34872

Seneff, S., Nigh, G., Kyriakopoulos, A. M., & McCullough, P. A. (2022). Innate immune suppression by SARS-CoV-2 mRNA vaccinations: The role of G-quadruplexes, exosomes, and MicroRNAs. *Food and Chemical Toxicology*, *164*, 113008. https://doi.org/10.1016/j.fct.2022.113008

Senger, K., Hackney, J., Payandeh, J., & Zarrin, A. A. (2015). *Antibody Isotype Switching in Vertebrates* (pp. 295–324). https://doi.org/10.1007/978-3-319-20819-0_13

Sengupta, U., & Kayed, R. (2022). Amyloid β, Tau, and α-Synuclein aggregates in the pathogenesis, prognosis, and therapeutics for neurodegenerative diseases. *Progress in Neurobiology*, *214*, 102270. https://doi.org/10.1016/j.pneurobio.2022.102270

Seth, P., & Sarkar, N. (2022). A comprehensive mini-review on amyloidogenesis of different SARS-CoV-2 proteins and its effect on amyloid formation in various host proteins. *3 Biotech*, *12*(11), 322. https://doi.org/10.1007/s13205-022-03390-1

Sfera, A., Hazan, S., Anton, J. J., Sfera, D. O., Andronescu, C. V., Sasannia, S., Rahman, L., & Kozlakidis, Z. (2022). Psychotropic drugs interaction with the lipid nanoparticle of COVID-19 mRNA therapeutics. *Frontiers in Pharmacology*, *13*. https://doi.org/10.3389/fphar.2022.995481

Shahsavarinia, K., Mahmoodpoor, A., Sadeghi-Ghyassi, F., Nedayi, A., Razzaghi, A., Zehi Saadat, M., & Salehi-Pourmehr, H. (2022). Bell's Palsy and COVID-19 Vaccination: A Systematic Review. *Medical Journal of the Islamic Republic of Iran*. https://doi.org/10.47176/mjiri.36.85

Shao, W., Earley, L. F., Chai, Z., Chen, X., Sun, J., He, T., Deng, M., Hirsch, M. L., Ting, J., Samulski, R. J., & Li, C. (2018). Double-stranded RNA innate immune response activation from long-term adeno-associated virus vector transduction. *JCI Insight*, *3*(12). https://doi.org/10.1172/jci.insight.120474

Shapiro Ben David, S., Potasman, I., & Rahamim-Cohen, D. (2021). Rate of Recurrent Guillain-Barré Syndrome After mRNA COVID-19 Vaccine BNT162b2. *JAMA Neurology*, *78*(11), 1409. https://doi.org/10.1001/jamaneurol.2021.3287

Sharifian-Dorche, M., Bahmanyar, M., Sharifian-Dorche, A., Mohammadi, P., Nomovi, M., & Mowla, A. (2021). Vaccine-induced immune thrombotic thrombocytopenia and cerebral venous sinus thrombosis post COVID-19 vaccination; a systematic review. *Journal of the Neurological Sciences*, *428*, 117607. https://doi.org/10.1016/j.jns.2021.117607

Sharma, M., Baghel, R., Thakur, S., & Adwal, S. (2021). Surveillance of adverse drug reactions at an adverse drug reaction monitoring centre in Central India: a 7-year surveillance study. *BMJ Open*, *11*(10), e052737. https://doi.org/10.1136/bmjopen-2021-052737

Sharma, N., Tan, M., & An, S. S. (2021). Phytosterols: Potential Metabolic Modulators in Neurodegenerative Diseases. *International Journal of Molecular Sciences*, *22*(22), 12255. https://doi.org/10.3390/ijms222212255

Shaw, K. E., Cavalcante, J. L., Han, B. K., & Gössl, M. (2021). Possible Association Between COVID-19 Vaccine and Myocarditis. *JACC: Cardiovascular Imaging*, *14*(9), 1856–1861. https://doi.org/10.1016/j.jcmg.2021.06.002

Sheets, R. L., Stein, J., Bailer, R. T., Koup, R. A., Andrews, C., Nason, M., He, B., Koo, E., Trotter, H., Duffy, C., Manetz, T., & Gomez, P. (2008). Biodistribution and Toxicological Safety of Adenovirus Type 5 and Type 35 Vectored Vaccines Against Human Immunodeficiency Virus-1 (HIV-1), Ebola, or Marburg Are Similar Despite Differing Adenovirus Serotype Vector, Manufacturer's Construct, or Gene Inserts. *Journal of Immunotoxicology*, *5*(3), 315–335. https://doi.org/10.1080/15376510802312464

Shemer, A., Pras, E., Einan-Lifshitz, A., Dubinsky-Pertzov, B., & Hecht, I. (2021). Association of COVID-19 Vaccination and Facial Nerve Palsy. *JAMA Otolaryngology–Head & Neck Surgery*, *147*(8), 739. https://doi.org/10.1001/jamaoto.2021.1259

Sheng-Fowler, L., Lewis, A. M., & Peden, K. (2009). Issues associated with residual cell-substrate DNA in viral vaccines. *Biologicals*, *37*(3), 190–195. https://doi.org/10.1016/j.biologicals.2009.02.015

Shenoy, S. (2022). Gut microbiome, Vitamin D, ACE2 interactions are critical factors in immune-senescence and inflammaging: key for vaccine response and severity of COVID-19 infection. *Inflammation Research*, *71*(1), 13–26. https://doi.org/10.1007/s00011-021-01510-w

Shetty, A., Rastogi, A., Jha, V., & Sudhayakumar, A. (2022). Longitudinally extensive transverse myelitis following ChAdOx1 nCoV-19 vaccine. *Journal of Postgraduate Medicine*, *68*(3), 179. https://doi.org/10.4103/jpgm.jpgm_1047_21

Shi, Y., Liu, Z., Lin, Q., Luo, Q., Cen, Y., Li, J., Fang, X., & Gong, C. (2021). MiRNAs and Cancer: Key Link in Diagnosis and Therapy. *Genes*, *12*(8), 1289. https://doi.org/10.3390/genes12081289

Shimabukuro, T. (2021). Allergic reactions including anaphylaxis after receipt of the first dose of Pfizer-BioNTech COVID-19 vaccine - United States, December 14-23, 2020. *American Journal of Transplantation*, *21*(3),1332–1337. https://doi.org/10.1111/ajt.16516.

Shimabukuro, T. T., Kim, S. Y., Myers, T. R., Moro, P. L., Oduyebo, T., Panagiotakopoulos, L., Marquez, P. L., Olson, C. K., Liu, R., Chang, K. T., Ellington, S. R., Burkel, V. K., Smoots, A. N., Green, C. J., Licata, C., Zhang, B. C., Alimchandani, M., Mba-Jonas, A., Martin, S. W., … Meaney-Delman, D. M. (2021). Preliminary Findings of mRNA Covid-19 Vaccine Safety in Pregnant Persons. *New England Journal of Medicine*, *384*(24), 2273–2282. https://doi.org/10.1056/NEJMoa2104983

Shimonovich, M., Pearce, A., Thomson, H., Keyes, K., & Katikireddi, S. V. (2021). Assessing causality in epidemiology: revisiting Bradford Hill to incorporate developments in causal thinking. *European Journal of Epidemiology*, *36*(9), 873–887. https://doi.org/10.1007/s10654-020-00703-7

Shoenfeld, Y., & Aron-Maor, A. (2000). Vaccination and Autoimmunity—'vaccinosis': A Dangerous Liaison? *Journal of Autoimmunity*, *14*(1), 1–10. https://doi.org/10.1006/jaut.1999.0346

Shorter, J. R., Odet, F., Aylor, D. L., Pan, W., Kao, C.-Y., Fu, C.-P., Morgan, A. P., Greenstein, S., Bell, T. A., Stevans, A. M., Feathers, R. W., Patel, S., Cates, S. E., Shaw, G. D., Miller, D. R., Chesler, E. J., McMillian, L., O'Brien, D. A., & Villena, F. P.-M. de. (2017). Male Infertility Is Responsible for Nearly Half of the Extinction Observed in the Mouse Collaborative Cross. *Genetics*, *206*(2), 557–572. https://doi.org/10.1534/genetics.116.199596

Shrestha, N. K., Burke, P. C., Nowacki, A. S., Simon, J. F., Hagen, A., & Gordon, S. M. (2023). Effectiveness of the Coronavirus Disease 2019 Bivalent Vaccine. *Open Forum Infectious Diseases*, *10*(6). https://doi.org/10.1093/ofid/ofad209

Siao, W.-H., Chang, F.-Y., & Chen, Y.-C. (2023). Memantine treats psychosis and agitation associated with Moderna COVID-19 vaccine. *Schizophrenia Research*, *255*, 14–16. https://doi.org/10.1016/j.schres.2023.03.011

Siddiqi, A. R., Khan, T., Tahir, M. J., Asghar, M. S., Islam, Md. S., & Yousaf, Z. (2022). Miller Fisher syndrome after COVID-19 vaccination: Case report and review of literature. *Medicine*, *101*(20), e29333. https://doi.org/10.1097/MD.0000000000029333

Sigurdson, C. J., Bartz, J. C., & Glatzel, M. (2019). Cellular and Molecular Mechanisms of Prion Disease. *Annual Review of Pathology: Mechanisms of Disease*, *14*(1), 497–516. https://doi.org/10.1146/annurev-pathmechdis-012418-013109

Sii, H. L., Ng, S. H., Wong, V. F., & Law, W. C. (2023). A Case Report of Guillain-Barré Syndrome In Association with SARS-CoV-2 Vaccination in Malaysia. *Acta Neurologica Taiwanica*, *32(4)*, 207–211.

Sikorska, B., Knight, R., Ironside, J. W., & Liberski, P. P. (2012). *Creutzfeldt-Jakob Disease* (pp. 76–90). https://doi.org/10.1007/978-1-4614-0653-2_6

Silva, F., Enaud, R., Creissen, E., Henao-Tamayo, M., Delhaes, L., & Izzo, A. (2022). Mouse Subcutaneous BCG Vaccination and Mycobacterium tuberculosis Infection Alter the Lung and Gut Microbiota. *Microbiology Spectrum*, *10*(3). https://doi.org/10.1128/spectrum.01693-21

Silva, N. R. (2010). Chocolate consumption and effects on serotonin synthesis. *Archives of Internal Medicine, 170*(17), 1608; author reply 1608-9. https://doi.org/10.1001/archinternmed.2010.331.

Singh, B., Kaur, P., Cedeno, L., Brahimi, T., Patel, P., Virk, H., Shamoon, F., & Bikkina, M. (2021). COVID-19 mRNA Vaccine and Myocarditis. *European Journal of Case Reports in Internal Medicine*. https://doi.org/10.12890/2021_002681

Singh, N., & Singh, A. B. (2020). S2 subunit of SARS-nCoV-2 interacts with tumor suppressor protein p53 and BRCA: an in silico study. *Translational Oncology*, *13*(10), 100814. https://doi.org/10.1016/j.tranon.2020.100814

Singh, R., Cohen, J. L., Astudillo, M., Harris, J. E., & Freeman, E. E. (2022). Vitiligo of the arm after COVID-19 vaccination. *JAAD Case Reports*, *28*, 142–144. https://doi.org/10.1016/j.jdcr.2022.06.003

Situ, Y., Chung, L., Lee, C., & Ho, V. (2019). MRN (MRE11-RAD50-NBS1) Complex in Human Cancer and Prognostic Implications in Colorectal Cancer.

International Journal of Molecular Sciences, *20*(4), 816. https://doi.org/10.3390/ijms20040816

Soeder, E., Toro-Pape, F. W., & Lampen-Sachar, K. (2022). Isolated breast parenchymal changes following COVID-19 vaccine booster. *Radiology Case Reports*, *17*(12), 4556–4560. https://doi.org/10.1016/j.radcr.2022.08.094

Soh, Y., Yoo, E. A., Kim, E.-S., & Kim, S. J. (2023). MRI Features of Multiple Cranial Neuropathies in Guillain-Barré Syndrome Occurring after COVID-19 Vaccination: A Case Report. *Journal of the Korean Society of Radiology*, *84*(4), 964. https://doi.org/10.3348/jksr.2022.0099

Sokolska, J. M., Kurcz, J., & Kosmala, W. (2021). Every rose has its thorns — acute myocarditis following COVID-19 vaccination. *Kardiologia Polska*, *79*(10), 1153–1154. https://doi.org/10.33963/KP.a2021.0075

Solis, O., Beccari, A. R., Iaconis, D., Talarico, C., Ruiz-Bedoya, C. A., Nwachukwu, J. C., Cimini, A., Castelli, V., Bertini, R., Montopoli, M., Cocetta, V., Borocci, S., Prandi, I. G., Flavahan, K., Bahr, M., Napiorkowski, A., Chillemi, G., Ooka, M., Yang, X., … Michaelides, M. (2022). The SARS-CoV-2 spike protein binds and modulates estrogen receptors. *Science Advances*, *8*(48). https://doi.org/10.1126/sciadv.add4150

Soltanzadi, A., Mirmosayyeb, O., Momeni Moghaddam, A., Ghoshouni, H., & Ghajarzadeh, M. (2023). Incidence of Bell's palsy after coronavirus disease (COVID-19) vaccination: a systematic review and meta-analysis. *Neurología (English Edition)*. https://doi.org/10.1016/j.nrleng.2023.06.002

Sonne, J., & Lopez-Ojeda, W. (2023). *Kallmann Syndrome*. StatPearls Publishing.

Sosa-Hernández, O., & Sánchez-Cardoza, S. (2022). Reporte de caso de síndrome de Guillain-Barré posterior a la vacuna COVID BNT162b2 mRNA. *Vacunas*, *23*, 68–70. https://doi.org/10.1016/j.vacun.2022.02.002

Soysal, Ç., & Yılmaz, E. (2022). The effect of COVID-19 vaccine on ovarian reserve. *Saudi Medical Journal*, *43*(5), 486–490. https://doi.org/10.15537/smj.2022.43.5.20220007

Spandorfer, R., Ahmad, M., & Khosroshahi, A. (2023). Clinical Characteristics and Classification Criteria Performance in a Single-Center Cohort of 114 Patients With Immunoglobulin G4–Related Disease. *JCR: Journal of Clinical Rheumatology*, *29*(1), 23–28. https://doi.org/10.1097/RHU.0000000000001895

Speicher, D., Rose, J., Gutschi, L. M., Wiseman, D. M., & McKernan, K. (2023). DNA fragments detected in monovalent and bivalent Pfizer/BioNTech and Moderna modRNA COVID-19 vaccines from Ontario, Canada: Exploratory dose response relationship with serious adverse events. *OSF Preprints*. https://doi.org/10.31219/osf.io/mjc97

Sprute, R., Schumacher, S., Pauls, M., Pauls, W., & Cornely, O. A. (2021). Delayed Cutaneous Hypersensitivity Reaction to Vaxzevria (ChAdOx1-S) Vaccine against SARS-CoV-2. *Drugs in R&D*, *21*(4), 371–374. https://doi.org/10.1007/s40268-021-00358-z

Sreepadmanabh, M., Sahu, A. K., & Chande, A. (2020). COVID-19: Advances in diagnostic tools, treatment strategies, and vaccine development. *Journal of Biosciences*, *45*(1), 148. https://doi.org/10.1007/s12038-020-00114-6

Srinivasan, S. Y., Illera, P. A., Kukhtar, D., Benseny-Cases, N., Cerón, J., Álvarez, J., Fonteriz, R. I., Montero, M., & Laromaine, A. (2023). Arrhythmic Effects

Evaluated on Caenorhabditis elegans: The Case of Polypyrrole Nanoparticles. *ACS Nano*, *17*(17), 17273–17284. https://doi.org/10.1021/acsnano.3c05245
Sriwastava, S., Sharma, K., Khalid, S., Bhansali, S., Shrestha, A., Elkhooly, M., Srivastava, S., Khan, E., Jaiswal, S., & Wen, S. (2022). COVID-19 Vaccination and Neurological Manifestations: A Review of Case Reports and Case Series. *Brain Sciences*, *12*(3), 407. https://doi.org/10.3390/brainsci12030407
Stadler, K., Masignani, V., Eickmann, M., Becker, S., Abrignani, S., Klenk, H.-D., & Rappuoli, R. (2003). SARS — beginning to understand a new virus. *Nature Reviews Microbiology*, *1*(3), 209–218. https://doi.org/10.1038/nrmicro775
Stamou, M. I., & Georgopoulos, N. A. (2018). Kallmann syndrome: phenotype and genotype of hypogonadotropic hypogonadism. *Metabolism*, *86*, 124–134. https://doi.org/10.1016/j.metabol.2017.10.012
Starekova, J., Bluemke, D. A., Bradham, W. S., Grist, T. M., Schiebler, M. L., & Reeder, S. B. (2021). Myocarditis Associated with mRNA COVID-19 Vaccination. *Radiology*, *301*(2), E409–E411. https://doi.org/10.1148/radiol.2021211430
Stasiak, A. C., & Stehle, T. (2020). Human adenovirus binding to host cell receptors: a structural view. *Medical Microbiology and Immunology*, *209*(3), 325–333. https://doi.org/10.1007/s00430-019-00645-2.
Stati, G., Amerio, P., Nubile, M., Sancilio, S., Rossi, F., & Di Pietro, R. (2023). Concern about the Effectiveness of mRNA Vaccination Technology and Its Long-Term Safety: Potential Interference on miRNA Machinery. *International Journal of Molecular Sciences*, *24*(2), 1404. https://doi.org/10.3390/ijms24021404
Stebbings, R., Armour, G., Pettis, V., & Goodman, J. (2022). AZD1222 (ChAdOx1 nCov-19): A Single-Dose biodistribution study in mice. *Vaccine*, *40*(2), 192–195. https://doi.org/10.1016/j.vaccine.2021.11.028
Stein, S. R., Ramelli, S. C., Grazioli, A., Chung, J.-Y., Singh, M., Yinda, C. K., Winkler, C. W., Sun, J., Dickey, J. M., Ylaya, K., Ko, S. H., Platt, A. P., Burbelo, P. D., Quezado, M., Pittaluga, S., Purcell, M., Munster, V. J., Belinky, F., Ramos-Benitez, M. J., … Chertow, D. S. (2022). SARS-CoV-2 infection and persistence in the human body and brain at autopsy. *Nature*, *612*(7941), 758–763. https://doi.org/10.1038/s41586-022-05542-y
Steinberg, A. D., Baron, S., & Talal, N. (1969). The pathogenesis of autoimmunity in New Zealand mice, I. Induction of antinucleic acid antibodies by polyinosinic·polycytidylic acid. *Proceedings of the National Academy of Sciences*, *63*(4), 1102–1107. https://doi.org/10.1073/pnas.63.4.1102
Stepanenko, A. A., & Dmitrenko, V. V. (2015). HEK293 in cell biology and cancer research: phenotype, karyotype, tumorigenicity, and stress-induced genome-phenotype evolution. *Gene*, *569*(2), 182–190. https://doi.org/10.1016/j.gene.2015.05.065
Stephen, S. L., Montini, E., Sivanandam, V. G., Al-Dhalimy, M., Kestler, H. A., Finegold, M., Grompe, M., & Kochanek, S. (2010). Chromosomal Integration of Adenoviral Vector DNA In Vivo. *Journal of Virology*, *84*(19), 9987–9994. https://doi.org/10.1128/JVI.00751-10
Stoehr, J. R., Hamidian Jahromi, A., & Thomason, C. (2021). Ethical Considerations for Unblinding and Vaccinating COVID-19 Vaccine Trial Placebo Group Participants. *Frontiers in Public Health*, *9*. https://doi.org/10.3389/fpubh.2021.702960

Stöllberger, C., Kastrati, K., Dejaco, C., Scharitzer, M., Finsterer, J., Bugingo, P., Melichart-Kotik, M., & Wilfing, A. (2023). Necrotizing pancreatitis, microangiopathic hemolytic anemia and thrombocytopenia following the second dose of Pfizer/BioNTech COVID-19 mRNA vaccine. *Wiener Klinische Wochenschrift*, *135*(15–16), 436–440. https://doi.org/10.1007/s00508-023-02225-0

Stone, C. A., Liu, Y., Relling, M. V., Krantz, M. S., Pratt, A. L., Abreo, A., Hemler, J. A., & Phillips, E. J. (2019). Immediate Hypersensitivity to Polyethylene Glycols and Polysorbates: More Common Than We Have Recognized. *The Journal of Allergy and Clinical Immunology: In Practice*, *7*(5), 1533-1540.e8. https://doi.org/10.1016/j.jaip.2018.12.003

Stoyanov, A., Thompson, G., Lee, M., & Katelaris, C. (2022). Delayed hypersensitivity to the Comirnaty coronavirus disease 2019 vaccine presenting with pneumonitis and rash. *Annals of Allergy, Asthma & Immunology*, *128*(3), 321–322. https://doi.org/10.1016/j.anai.2021.11.014

Stratton, K. R., Howe, C. J., & Johnston, R. B. (1994). Adverse events associated with childhood vaccines other than pertussis and rubella. Summary of a report from the Institute of Medicine. *JAMA*, *271*(20), 1602–1605.

Su, S.-C., Lyu, R.-K., Chang, C.-W., & Tseng, W.-E. J. (2022). The First Guillain-Barr? Syndrome After SARS-CoV-2 Vaccination in Taiwan. *Acta Neurologica Taiwanica*, *31(1)*, 46–51.

Sugimoto, M., Uchida, I., & Mashimo, T. (2003). Local anaesthetics have different mechanisms and sites of action at the recombinant N-methyl-D-aspartate (NMDA) receptors. *British Journal of Pharmacology*, *138*(5), 876–882. https://doi.org/10.1038/sj.bjp.0705107

Sugita, K., Kaneko, S., Hisada, R., Harano, M., Anno, E., Hagiwara, S., Imai, E., Nagata, M., & Tsukamoto, Y. (2022). Development of IgA vasculitis with severe glomerulonephritis after COVID-19 vaccination: a case report and literature review. *CEN Case Reports*, *11*(4), 436–441. https://doi.org/10.1007/s13730-022-00695-1

Sukockienė, E., Breville, G., Fayolle, D., Nencha, U., Uginet, M., & Hübers, A. (2023). Case Series of Acute Peripheral Neuropathies in Individuals Who Received COVID-19 Vaccination. *Medicina*, *59*(3), 501. https://doi.org/10.3390/medicina59030501

Suleman, S., Schrubaji, K., Filippou, C., Ignatova, S., Hewitson, P., Huddleston, J., Karda, R., Waddington, S. N., & Themis, M. (2022). Rapid and inexpensive purification of adenovirus vectors using an optimised aqueous two-phase technology. *Journal of Virological Methods*, *299*, 114305. https://doi.org/10.1016/j.jviromet.2021.114305

Sulemankhil, I., Abdelrahman, M., & Negi, S. I. (2022). Temporal Association Between the COVID-19 Ad26.COV2.S Vaccine and Acute Myocarditis: A Case Report and Literature Review. *Cardiovascular Revascularization Medicine*, *38*, 117–123. https://doi.org/10.1016/j.carrev.2021.08.012

Sullivan, C. S., & Pipas, J. M. (2002). T Antigens of Simian Virus 40: Molecular Chaperones for Viral Replication and Tumorigenesis. *Microbiology and Molecular Biology Reviews*, *66*(2), 179–202. https://doi.org/10.1128/MMBR.66.2.179-202.2002

Sumi, T., Nagahisa, Y., Matsuura, K., Sekikawa, M., Yamada, Y., Nakata, H., & Chiba, H. (2021). Lung squamous cell carcinoma with hemoptysis after vaccination with tozinameran (BNT162b2, Pfizer-BioNTech). *Thoracic Cancer*, *12*(22), 3072–3075. https://doi.org/10.1111/1759-7714.14179

Sun, J., Tian, Y., Du, Y., Wang, Z., Zhao, G., Ma, Y., & Zheng, M. (2020). A cautionary tale of cross-contamination among plasmids from commercial suppliers. *BioTechniques*, *68*(1), 14–21. https://doi.org/10.2144/btn-2019-0018

Suzuki, A. (2011). Smallpox and the Epidemiological Heritage of Modern Japan: Towards a Total History. *Medical History*, *55*(3), 313–318. https://doi.org/10.1017/S0025727300005329

Suzuki, N., Fukushi, M., Kosaki, K., Doyle, A. D., de Vega, S., Yoshizaki, K., Akazawa, C., Arikawa-Hirasawa, E., & Yamada, Y. (2012). Teneurin-4 Is a Novel Regulator of Oligodendrocyte Differentiation and Myelination of Small-Diameter Axons in the CNS. *The Journal of Neuroscience*, *32*(34), 11586–11599. https://doi.org/10.1523/JNEUROSCI.2045-11.2012

Suzuki, Y., & Ishihara, H. (2021). Difference in the lipid nanoparticle technology employed in three approved siRNA (Patisiran) and mRNA (COVID-19 vaccine) drugs. *Drug Metabolism and Pharmacokinetics*, *41*, 100424. https://doi.org/10.1016/j.dmpk.2021.100424

Swanborg, R. H., & Radzialowski, C. V. (1970). Enhanced Immunogenicity of Altered Encephalitogenic Protein. *Infection and Immunity*, *2*(5), 676–678. https://doi.org/10.1128/iai.2.5.676-678.1970

Syed, K., Chaudhary, H., & Donato, A. (2021). Central Venous Sinus Thrombosis with Subarachnoid Hemorrhage Following an mRNA COVID-19 Vaccination: Are These Reports Merely Co-Incidental? *American Journal of Case Reports*, *22*. https://doi.org/10.12659/AJCR.933397

Szewczyk, A. K., Skrobas, U., Jamroz-Wiśniewska, A., Mitosek-Szewczyk, K., & Rejdak, K. (2021). Facial Diplegia—Complication or Manifestation of SARS-CoV-2 Infection? A Case Report and Systemic Literature Review. *Healthcare*, *9*(11), 1492. https://doi.org/10.3390/healthcare9111492

Tachita, T., Takahata, T., Yamashita, S., Ebina, T., Kamata, K., Yamagata, K., Tamai, Y., & Sakuraba, H. (2023). Newly diagnosed extranodal NK/T-cell lymphoma, nasal type, at the injected left arm after BNT162b2 mRNA COVID-19 vaccination. *International Journal of Hematology*, *118*(4), 503–507. https://doi.org/10.1007/s12185-023-03607-w

Taieb, A., & Mounira, E. E. (2022). Pilot Findings on SARS-CoV-2 Vaccine-Induced Pituitary Diseases: A Mini Review from Diagnosis to Pathophysiology. *Vaccines*, *10*(12), 2004. https://doi.org/10.3390/vaccines10122004

Takan, T., Yamada, S., Doki, T., & Hohdatsu, T. (2019). Pathogenesis of oral type I feline infectious peritonitis virus (FIPV) infection: Antibody-dependent enhancement infection of cats with type I FIPV via the oral route. *Journal of Veterinary Medical Science*, *81*(6), 911–915. https://doi.org/10.1292/jvms.18-0702

Tamanai-Shacoori, Z., Smida, I., Bousarghin, L., Loreal, O., Meuric, V., Fong, S. B., Bonnaure-Mallet, M., & Jolivet-Gougeon, A. (2017). Roseburia spp.: a marker of health? *Future Microbiology*, *12*(2), 157–170. https://doi.org/10.2217/fmb-2016-0130

Tan, W. Y., Yusof Khan, A. H. K., Mohd Yaakob, M. N., Abdul Rashid, A. M., Loh, W. C., Baharin, J., Ibrahim, A., Ismail, M. R., Inche Mat, L. N., Wan Sulaiman, W.

A., Basri, H., & Hoo, F. K. (2021). Longitudinal extensive transverse myelitis following ChAdOx1 nCOV-19 vaccine: a case report. *BMC Neurology*, *21*(1), 395. https://doi.org/10.1186/s12883-021-02427-x
Tanaka, M., Tanaka, T., Zhu, X., Teng, F., Lin, H., Luo, Z., Pan, Y., Sadahiro, S., Suzuki, T., Maeda, Y., Wei, D., & Lu, Z. (2022). Huaier Effects on Functional Compensation with Destructive Ribosomal RNA Structure after Anti-SARS-CoV-2 mRNA Vaccination. *Archives of Clinical and Biomedical Research* , *6*, 553–574.
Tano, E., San Martin, S., Girgis, S., Martinez-Fernandez, Y., & Sanchez Vegas, C. (2021). Perimyocarditis in Adolescents After Pfizer-BioNTech COVID-19 Vaccine. *Journal of the Pediatric Infectious Diseases Society*, *10*(10), 962–966. https://doi.org/10.1093/jpids/piab060
Tatsis, N., Tesema, L., Robinson, E. R., Giles-Davis, W., McCoy, K., Gao, G. P., Wilson, J. M., & Ertl, H. C. J. (2006). Chimpanzee-origin adenovirus vectors as vaccine carriers. *Gene Therapy*, *13*(5), 421–429. https://doi.org/10.1038/sj.gt.3302675
Tatu, A. L., Nadasdy, T., & Nwabudike, L. C. (2022). Koebner phenomenon with lichen planus in an area of previous vitiligo after COVID-19 vaccination and the creation of a locus minoris resistentiae. *Journal of the European Academy of Dermatology and Venereology*, *36*(4). https://doi.org/10.1111/jdv.17864
Tayyebi, G., Malakouti, S. K., Shariati, B., & Kamalzadeh, L. (2022). COVID-19-associated encephalitis or Creutzfeldt–Jakob disease: a case report. *Neurodegenerative Disease Management*, *12*(1), 29–34. https://doi.org/10.2217/nmt-2021-0025
Terry, D. M., & Devine, S. E. (2020). Aberrantly High Levels of Somatic LINE-1 Expression and Retrotransposition in Human Neurological Disorders. *Frontiers in Genetics*, *10*. https://doi.org/10.3389/fgene.2019.01244
Tetz, G., & Tetz, V. (2022). Prion-like Domains in Spike Protein of SARS-CoV-2 Differ across Its Variants and Enable Changes in Affinity to ACE2. *Microorganisms*, *10*(2), 280. https://doi.org/10.3390/microorganisms10020280
Thacker, P. D. (2021). Covid-19: Researcher blows the whistle on data integrity issues in Pfizer's vaccine trial: Video 1. *BMJ*, n2635. https://doi.org/10.1136/bmj.n2635
Thant, H. L., Morgan, R., Paese, M. M., Persaud, T., Diaz, J., & Hurtado, L. (2022). Guillain-Barré Syndrome After Ad26.COV2.S Vaccination. *American Journal of Case Reports*, *23*. https://doi.org/10.12659/AJCR.935275
Theoharides, T. C., & Conti, P. (2021). Be aware of SARS-CoV-2 spike protein: There is more than meets the eye. *Journal of Biological Regulators and Homeostatic Agents*, *35*(3), 833–838. https://doi.org/10.23812/THEO_EDIT_3_21
Thess, A., Grund, S., Mui, B. L., Hope, M. J., Baumhof, P., Fotin-Mleczek, M., & Schlake, T. (2015). Sequence-engineered mRNA Without Chemical Nucleoside Modifications Enables an Effective Protein Therapy in Large Animals. *Molecular Therapy*, *23*(9), 1456–1464. https://doi.org/10.1038/mt.2015.103
Theuriet, J., Richard, C., Becker, J., Pegat, A., Bernard, E., & Vukusic, S. (2021). Guillain-Barré syndrome following first injection of ChAdOx1 nCoV-19 vaccine: First report. *Revue Neurologique*, *177*(10), 1305–1307. https://doi.org/10.1016/j.neurol.2021.04.005
Thèves, C., Crubézy, E., & Biagini, P. (2016). History of Smallpox and Its Spread in Human Populations. *Microbiology Spectrum*, *4*(4). https://doi.org/10.1128/microbiolspec.PoH-0004-2014

Thomas, J. W., George-Gattner, H., & Danho, W. (1989). T cells recognize both conformational and cryptic determinants on the insulin molecule. *European Journal of Immunology*, *19*(3), 557–558. https://doi.org/10.1002/eji.1830190323

Thomas, S. J., Moreira, E. D., Kitchin, N., Absalon, J., Gurtman, A., Lockhart, S., Perez, J. L., Pérez Marc, G., Polack, F. P., Zerbini, C., Bailey, R., Swanson, K. A., Xu, X., Roychoudhury, S., Koury, K., Bouguermouh, S., Kalina, W. V., Cooper, D., Frenck, R. W., … Jansen, K. U. (2021). Safety and Efficacy of the BNT162b2 mRNA Covid-19 Vaccine through 6 Months. *New England Journal of Medicine*, *385*(19), 1761–1773. https://doi.org/10.1056/NEJMoa2110345

Thomma, R. C. M., Fokke, C., Walgaard, C., Vermeulen-de Jongh, D. M. C., Tio-Gillen, A., van Rijs, W., van Doorn, P. A., Huizinga, R., & Jacobs, B. C. (2023). High and Persistent Anti-GM1 Antibody Titers Are Associated With Poor Clinical Recovery in Guillain-Barré Syndrome. *Neurology - Neuroimmunology Neuroinflammation*, *10*(4), e200107. https://doi.org/10.1212/NXI.0000000000200107

Thoresen, D., Wang, W., Galls, D., Guo, R., Xu, L., & Pyle, A. M. (2021). The molecular mechanism of RIG-I activation and signaling. *Immunological Reviews*, *304*(1), 154–168. https://doi.org/10.1111/imr.13022

Thorn, C. R., Sharma, D., Combs, R., Bhujbal, S., Romine, J., Zheng, X., Sunasara, K., & Badkar, A. (2022). The journey of a lifetime — development of Pfizer's COVID-19 vaccine. *Current Opinion in Biotechnology*, *78*, 102803. https://doi.org/10.1016/j.copbio.2022.102803

Thorp, J. A., Rogers, C., Deskevich, M. P., Tankersley, S., Benavides, A., Redshaw, M. D., & McCullough, J. D. P. A. (2022). COVID-19 Vaccines: The Impact on Pregnancy Outcomes and Menstrual Function. *Journal of American Physicians and Surgeons* , *26*(1), 28–34. https://www.jpands.org/vol28no1/thorp.pdf

Tiesjema, B., Hermsen, H. P., van Eijkeren, J. C., & Brandon, E. F. (2010). Effect of administration route on the biodistribution and shedding of replication-deficient HAdV-5: a qualitative modelling approach. *Current Gene Therapy, 10*(2), 107–127. https://doi.org/10.2174/156652310791111038.

Tinari, S. (2021). The EMA covid-19 data leak, and what it tells us about mRNA instability. *BMJ*, n627. https://doi.org/10.1136/bmj.n627

Tiwari, B., Jones, A. E., Caillet, C. J., Das, S., Royer, S. K., & Abrams, J. M. (2020). p53 directly represses human LINE1 transposons. *Genes & Development*, *34*(21–22), 1439–1451. https://doi.org/10.1101/gad.343186.120

Tobías, A., Casals, M., Peña, J., & Tebé, C. (2019). FIFA World Cup and climate change: correlation is not causation. [Copa del Mundo FIFA y cambio climático: correlación no implica causalidad]. *RICYDE. Revista Internacional de Ciencias Del Deporte*, *15*(57), 280–283. https://doi.org/10.5232/ricyde2019.057ed

Toh, C.-H., Wang, G., & Parker, A. L. (2022). The aetiopathogenesis of vaccine-induced immune thrombotic thrombocytopenia. *Clinical Medicine*, *22*(2), 140–144. https://doi.org/10.7861/clinmed.2022-0006

Tolmachov, O. (2009). *Designing Plasmid Vectors* (pp. 117–129). https://doi.org/10.1007/978-1-59745-561-9_6

Townsend, J. P., Hassler, H. B., Sah, P., Galvani, A. P., & Dornburg, A. (2022). The durability of natural infection and vaccine-induced immunity against future infection by SARS-CoV-2. *Proceedings of the National Academy of Sciences*, *119*(31). https://doi.org/10.1073/pnas.2204336119

Trimboli, M., Zoleo, P., Arabia, G., & Gambardella, A. (2021). Guillain-Barré syndrome following BNT162b2 COVID-19 vaccine. *Neurological Sciences*, *42*(11), 4401–4402. https://doi.org/10.1007/s10072-021-05523-5

Tripathy, S., Alvarez, N., Jaiswal, S., Williams, R., Al-Khadimi, M., Hackman, S., Phillips, W., Kaur, S., Cervantez, S., Kelly, W., & Taverna, J. (2022). Hypermetabolic lymphadenopathy following the administration of COVID-19 vaccine and immunotherapy in a lung cancer patient: a case report. *Journal of Medical Case Reports*, *16*(1), 445. https://doi.org/10.1186/s13256-022-03660-9

Trougakos, I. P., Terpos, E., Alexopoulos, H., Politou, M., Paraskevis, D., Scorilas, A., Kastritis, E., Andreakos, E., & Dimopoulos, M. A. (2022a). Adverse effects of COVID-19 mRNA vaccines: the spike hypothesis. *Trends in Molecular Medicine*, *28*(7), 542–554. https://doi.org/10.1016/j.molmed.2022.04.007

Trougakos, I. P., Terpos, E., Alexopoulos, H., Politou, M., Paraskevis, D., Scorilas, A., Kastritis, E., Andreakos, E., & Dimopoulos, M. A. (2022b). COVID-19 mRNA vaccine-induced adverse effects: unwinding the unknowns. *Trends in Molecular Medicine*, *28*(10), 800–802. https://doi.org/10.1016/j.molmed.2022.07.008

Truong, D. T., Dionne, A., Muniz, J. C., McHugh, K. E., Portman, M. A., Lambert, L. M., Thacker, D., Elias, M. D., Li, J. S., Toro-Salazar, O. H., Anderson, B. R., Atz, A. M., Bohun, C. M., Campbell, M. J., Chrisant, M., D'Addese, L., Dummer, K. B., Forsha, D., Frank, L. H., … Newburger, J. W. (2022). Clinically Suspected Myocarditis Temporally Related to COVID-19 Vaccination in Adolescents and Young Adults: Suspected Myocarditis After COVID-19 Vaccination. *Circulation*, *145*(5), 345–356. https://doi.org/10.1161/CIRCULATIONAHA.121.056583

Tsai, T., & Ng, C. Y. (2023). COVID vaccine-associated vitiligo: A cross-sectional study in a tertiary referral center and systematic review. J Dermatol. . *The Journal of Dermatology*, *50*(8), 982–989. https://doi.org/10.1111/1346-8138.16799

Tseha, S. T. (2021). Polio: The Disease that Reemerged after Six Years in Ethiopia. *Ethiopian Journal of Health Science*, *31*(4), 897–902. https://doi.org/10.4314/ejhs.v31i4.25.

Tseng, P.-T., Chen, T.-Y., Sun, Y.-S., Chen, Y.-W., & Chen, J.-J. (2021). The reversible tinnitus and cochleopathy followed first-dose AstraZeneca COVID-19 vaccination. *QJM: An International Journal of Medicine*, *114*(9), 663–664. https://doi.org/10.1093/qjmed/hcab210

Tsutsui, K., Kanbayashi, T., Takaki, M., Omori, Y., Imai, Y., Nishino, S., Tanaka, K., & Shimizu, T. (2017). N-Methyl-D-aspartate receptor antibody could be a cause of catatonic symptoms in psychiatric patients: case reports and methods for detection. *Neuropsychiatric Disease and Treatment*, *Volume 13*, 339–345. https://doi.org/10.2147/NDT.S125800

Uğurer, E., Sivaz, O., & Kıvanç Altunay, İ. (2022). Newly-developed vitiligo following COVID-19 mRNA vaccine. *Journal of Cosmetic Dermatology*, *21*(4), 1350–1351. https://doi.org/10.1111/jocd.14843

Ujiie, H., Rosmarin, D., Schön, M. P., Ständer, S., Boch, K., Metz, M., Maurer, M., Thaci, D., Schmidt, E., Cole, C., Amber, K. T., Didona, D., Hertl, M., Recke, A., Graßhoff, H., Hackel, A., Schumann, A., Riemekasten, G., Bieber, K., … Ludwig, R. J. (2022). Unmet Medical Needs in Chronic, Non-communicable Inflammatory Skin Diseases. *Frontiers in Medicine*, *9*. https://doi.org/10.3389/fmed.2022.875492

Ulrich-Lewis, J. T., Draves, K. E., Roe, K., O'Connor, M. A., Clark, E. A., & Fuller, D. H. (2022). STING Is Required in Conventional Dendritic Cells for DNA Vaccine Induction of Type I T Helper Cell- Dependent Antibody Responses. *Frontiers in Immunology, 13*. https://doi.org/10.3389/fimmu.2022.861710

Unanue, E. R., Ferris, S. T., & Carrero, J. A. (2016). The role of islet antigen presenting cells and the presentation of insulin in the initiation of autoimmune diabetes in the <scp>NOD</scp> mouse. *Immunological Reviews, 272*(1), 183–201. https://doi.org/10.1111/imr.12430

Uttley, L., Carroll, C., Wong, R., Hilton, D. A., & Stevenson, M. (2020). Creutzfeldt-Jakob disease: a systematic review of global incidence, prevalence, infectivity, and incubation. *The Lancet Infectious Diseases*, *20*(1), e2–e10. https://doi.org/10.1016/S1473-3099(19)30615-2

Vacik, J., Dean, B. S., Zimmer, W. E., & Dean, D. A. (1999). Cell-specific nuclear import of plasmid DNA. *Gene Therapy*, *6*(6), 1006–1014. https://doi.org/10.1038/sj.gt.3300924

Valadez-Calderon, J., Ordinola Navarro, A., Rodriguez-Chavez, E., & Vera-Lastra, O. (2022). Co-expression of anti-NMDAR and anti-GAD65 antibodies. A case of autoimmune encephalitis in a post-COVID-19 patient. *Neurología (English Edition)*, *37*(6), 503–504. https://doi.org/10.1016/j.nrleng.2021.09.004

Valdes Angues, R., & Perea Bustos Y. (2023). Navigating Uncharted Waters: Could COVID-19 and/or Certain COVID-19 Vaccines Promote Malignancy? Authorea [Preprint]. https://doi.org/10.22541/au.166358581.18921295/v3.

Valore, L., Junker, T., Heilmann, E., Zuern, C. S., Streif, M., Drexler, B., Arranto, C., Halter, J. P., & Berger, C. T. (2023). Case report: mRNA-1273 COVID-19 vaccine-associated myopericarditis: Successful treatment and re-exposure with colchicine. *Frontiers in Cardiovascular Medicine, 10,* 1135848. https://doi.org/10.3389/fcvm.2023.1135848.

van der Heide, V., Jangra, S., Cohen, P., Rathnasinghe, R., Aslam, S., Aydillo, T., Geanon, D., Handler, D., Kelley, G., Lee, B., Rahman, A., Dawson, T., Qi, J., D'Souza, D., Kim-Schulze, S., Panzer, J. K., Caicedo, A., Kusmartseva, I., Posgai, A. L., … Homann, D. (2022). Limited extent and consequences of pancreatic SARS-CoV-2 infection. *Cell Reports*, *38*(11), 110508. https://doi.org/10.1016/j.celrep.2022.110508

van Es, M. A., Hardiman, O., Chio, A., Al-Chalabi, A., Pasterkamp, R. J., Veldink, J. H., & van den Berg, L. H. (2017). Amyotrophic lateral sclerosis. *The Lancet*, *390*(10107), 2084–2098. https://doi.org/10.1016/S0140-6736(17)31287-4

Van Norman, G. A. (2016). Drugs, Devices, and the FDA: Part 1. *JACC: Basic to Translational Science*, *1*(3), 170–179. https://doi.org/10.1016/j.jacbts.2016.03.002

Vargas, M. I., Gariani, J., Sztajzel, R., Barnaure-Nachbar, I., Delattre, B. M., Lovblad, K. O., & Dietemann, J.-L. (2015). Spinal Cord Ischemia: Practical Imaging Tips, Pearls, and Pitfalls. *American Journal of Neuroradiology*, *36*(5), 825–830. https://doi.org/10.3174/ajnr.A4118

Vargesson, N. (2015). Thalidomide-induced teratogenesis: History and mechanisms. *Birth Defects Research Part C: Embryo Today: Reviews*, *105*(2), 140–156. https://doi.org/10.1002/bdrc.21096

Vargesson, N., & Stephens, T. (2021). Thalidomide: history, withdrawal, renaissance, and safety concerns. *Expert Opinion on Drug Safety*, *20*(12), 1455–1457. https://doi.org/10.1080/14740338.2021.1991307

Vasilevska, V., Guest, P. C., Bernstein, H.-G., Schroeter, M. L., Geis, C., & Steiner, J. (2021). Molecular mimicry of NMDA receptors may contribute to neuropsychiatric symptoms in severe COVID-19 cases. *Journal of Neuroinflammation*, *18*(1), 245. https://doi.org/10.1186/s12974-021-02293-x

Vennema, H., de Groot, R. J., Harbour, D. A., Dalderup, M., Gruffydd-Jones, T., Horzinek, M. C., & Spaan, W. J. (1990). Early death after feline infectious peritonitis virus challenge due to recombinant vaccinia virus immunization. *Journal of Virology*, *64*(3), 1407–1409. https://doi.org/10.1128/jvi.64.3.1407-1409.1990

Ventura, M. T., Casciaro, M., Gangemi, S., & Buquicchio, R. (2017). Immunosenescence in aging: between immune cells depletion and cytokines up-regulation. *Clinical and Molecular Allergy*, *15*(1), 21. https://doi.org/10.1186/s12948-017-0077-0

Verdon, D. J., Mulazzani, M., & Jenkins, M. R. (2020). Cellular and Molecular Mechanisms of CD8+ T Cell Differentiation, Dysfunction and Exhaustion. *International Journal of Molecular Sciences*, *21*(19), 7357. https://doi.org/10.3390/ijms21197357

Verma, A. K., Lavine, K. J., & Lin, C.-Y. (2021). Myocarditis after Covid-19 mRNA Vaccination. *New England Journal of Medicine*, *385*(14), 1332–1334. https://doi.org/10.1056/NEJMc2109975

Vervaeke, P., Borgos, S. E., Sanders, N. N., & Combes, F. (2022). Regulatory guidelines and preclinical tools to study the biodistribution of RNA therapeutics. *Advanced Drug Delivery Reviews*, *184*, 114236. https://doi.org/10.1016/j.addr.2022.114236

Vidula, M. K., Ambrose, M., Glassberg, H., Chokshi, N., Chen, T., Ferrari, V. A., & Han, Y. (2021). Myocarditis and Other Cardiovascular Complications of the mRNA-Based COVID-19 Vaccines. *Cureus*. https://doi.org/10.7759/cureus.15576

Vilchez, R. A., & Butel, J. S. (2004). Emergent Human Pathogen Simian Virus 40 and Its Role in Cancer. *Clinical Microbiology Reviews*, *17*(3), 495–508. https://doi.org/10.1128/CMR.17.3.495-508.2004

Viskin, D., Topilsky, Y., Aviram, G., Mann, T., Sadon, S., Hadad, Y., Flint, N., Shmilovich, H., Banai, S., & Havakuk, O. (2021). Myocarditis Associated With COVID-19 Vaccination. *Circulation: Cardiovascular Imaging*, *14*(9). https://doi.org/10.1161/CIRCIMAGING.121.013236

Vivarelli, M., Massella, L., Ruggiero, B., & Emma, F. (2017). Minimal Change Disease. *Clinical Journal of the American Society of Nephrology*, *12*(2), 332–345. https://doi.org/10.2215/CJN.05000516

Vogel, A. B., Kanevsky, I., Che, Y., Swanson, K. A., Muik, A., Vormehr, M., Kranz, L. M., Walzer, K. C., Hein, S., Güler, A., Loschko, J., Maddur, M. S., Ota-Setlik, A., Tompkins, K., Cole, J., Lui, B. G., Ziegenhals, T., Plaschke, A., Eisel, D., … Sahin, U. (2021). BNT162b vaccines protect rhesus macaques from SARS-CoV-2. *Nature*, *592*(7853), 283–289. https://doi.org/10.1038/s41586-021-03275-y

Vogels, R., Zuijdgeest, D., van Rijnsoever, R., Hartkoorn, E., Damen, I., de Béthune, M. P., Kostense, S., Penders, G., Helmus, N., Koudstaal, W., Cecchini, M., Wetterwald, A., Sprangers, M., Lemckert, A., Ophorst, O., Koel, B., van Meerendonk, M., Quax, P., Panitti, L., Grimbergen, J., … Havenga, M. (2003). Replication-deficient human adenovirus type 35 vectors for gene transfer and vaccination: efficient human cell infection and bypass of preexisting adenovirus immunity. *Journal of Virology*, *77*(15), 8263–8271. https://doi.org/10.1128/jvi.77.15.8263-8271.2003.

Vojdani, A., Vojdani, E., & Kharrazian, D. (2021). Reaction of Human Monoclonal Antibodies to SARS-CoV-2 Proteins With Tissue Antigens: Implications for Autoimmune Diseases. *Frontiers in Immunology*, *11*. https://doi.org/10.3389/fimmu.2020.617089

Volloch, V., & Rits-Volloch, S. (2019). News from Mars: Two-Tier Paradox, Intracellular PCR, Chimeric Junction Shift, Dark Matter mRNA and Other Remarkable Features of Mammalian RNA-Dependent mRNA Amplification. Implications for Alzheimer's Disease, RNA-Based Vaccines and mRNA Therapeutics. *Annals of Integrative Molecular Medicine*, *2*(1), 0131–0173. https://doi.org/10.33597/aimm.02-1009

Voysey, M., Clemens, S. A. C., Madhi, S. A., Weckx, L. Y., Folegatti, P. M., Aley, P. K., Angus, B., Baillie, V. L., Barnabas, S. L., Bhorat, Q. E., Bibi, S., Briner, C., Cicconi, P., Collins, A. M., Colin-Jones, R., Cutland, C. L., Darton, T. C., Dheda, K., Duncan, C. J. A., … Zuidewind, P. (2021). Safety and efficacy of the ChAdOx1 nCoV-19 vaccine (AZD1222) against SARS-CoV-2: an interim analysis of four randomised controlled trials in Brazil, South Africa, and the UK. *The Lancet*, *397*(10269), 99–111. https://doi.org/10.1016/S0140-6736(20)32661-1

Vudathaneni, V. K. P., Nadella, S. B., Hema, D., & Boyapati, R. (2023). Renal Complications Following COVID Vaccination: A Narrative Literature Review. *Indian Journal of Community Medicine, 48*(2), 214–219. https://doi.org/10.4103/ijcm.ijcm_654_22.

Vyklicky, V., Korinek, M., Smejkalova, T., Balik, A., Krausova, B., Kaniakova, M., Lichnerova, K., Cerny, J., Krusek, J., Dittert, I., Horak, M., & Vyklicky, L. (2014). Structure, Function, and Pharmacology of NMDA Receptor Channels. *Physiological Research*, S191–S203. https://doi.org/10.33549/physiolres.932678

Waheed, S., Bayas, A., Hindi, F., Rizvi, Z., & Espinosa, P. S. (2021). Neurological Complications of COVID-19: Guillain-Barre Syndrome Following Pfizer COVID-19 Vaccine. *Cureus*. https://doi.org/10.7759/cureus.13426

Wali, S., Gutte, S., Yadav, S., Gurjar, M., Paliwal, V. K., Singh, V., Azim, A., & Poddar, B. (2023). Quadriparesis with different diagnoses after COVID-19 vaccination: Case series and literature review. *Journal of Family Medicine and Primary Care*, *12*(8), 1724–1729. https://doi.org/10.4103/jfmpc.jfmpc_2274_22

Walls, A. C., Park, Y.-J., Tortorici, M. A., Wall, A., McGuire, A. T., & Veesler, D. (2020). Structure, Function, and Antigenicity of the SARS-CoV-2 Spike Glycoprotein. *Cell*, *181*(2), 281-292.e6. https://doi.org/10.1016/j.cell.2020.02.058

Walter, T., Connor, S., Stedman, C., & Doogue, M. (2022). A case of acute necrotising pancreatitis following the second dose of Pfizer-BioNTech COVID-19 mRNA vaccine. *British Journal of Clinical Pharmacology*, *88*(3), 1385–1386. https://doi.org/10.1111/bcp.15039

Walton, M., Pletzer, V., Teunissen, T., Lumley, T., & Hanlon, T. (2023). Adverse Events Following the BNT162b2 mRNA COVID-19 Vaccine (Pfizer-BioNTech) in Aotearoa New Zealand. *Drug Safety*, *46*(9), 867–879. https://doi.org/10.1007/s40264-023-01332-1

Wan, E. Y. F., Chui, C. S. L., Lai, F. T. T., Chan, E. W. Y., Li, X., Yan, V. K. C., Gao, L., Yu, Q., Lam, I. C. H., Chun, R. K. C., Cowling, B. J., Fong, W. C., Lau, A. Y. L., Mok, V. C. T., Chan, F. L. F., Lee, C. K., Chan, L. S. T., Lo, D., Lau, K. K., …

Wong, I. C. K. (2022). Bell's palsy following vaccination with mRNA (BNT162b2) and inactivated (CoronaVac) SARS-CoV-2 vaccines: a case series and nested case-control study. *The Lancet Infectious Diseases*, *22*(1), 64–72. https://doi.org/10.1016/S1473-3099(21)00451-5
Wan, E. Y. F., Chui, C. S. L., Ng, V. W. S., Wang, Y., Yan, V. K. C., Lam, I. C. H., Fan, M., Lai, F. T. T., Chan, E. W. Y., Li, X., Wong, C. K. H., Chung, R. K. C., Cowling, B. J., Fong, W. C., Lau, A. Y. L., Mok, V. C. T., Chan, F. L. F., Lee, C. K., Chan, L. S. T., Lo, D., … Wong, I. C. K. (2023). Messenger RNA Coronavirus Disease 2019 (COVID-19) Vaccination With BNT162b2 Increased Risk of Bell's Palsy: A Nested Case-Control and Self-Controlled Case Series Study. *Clinical Infectious Disease, 76*(3), e291–e298. https://doi.org/10.1093/cid/ciac460.
Wang, C. X. (2021). Assessment and Management of Acute Disseminated Encephalomyelitis (ADEM) in the Pediatric Patient. *Pediatric Drugs*, *23*(3), 213–221. https://doi.org/10.1007/s40272-021-00441-7
Wang, F., Patel, D. K., Antonello, J. M., Washabaugh, M. W., Kaslow, D. C., Shiver, J. W., & Chirmule, N. (2003). Development of an adenovirus-shedding assay for the detection of adenoviral vector-based vaccine and gene therapy products in clinical specimens. *Human Gene Therapy, 14*(1), 25–36. https://doi.org/10.1089/10430340360464688.
Wang, C.-W., Chen, C.-B., Lu, C.-W., Chen, W.-T., Hui, R. C.-Y., Chiu, T.-M., Chi, M.-H., Lin, J.-C., Huang, Y.-H., Chang, Y.-C., Wu, J., Chen, K.-Y., Lin, Y. Y.-W., Ger, T.-Y., Lin, J. Y., Tsai, W.-T., Pan, Y.-J., & Chung, W.-H. (2023). Characteristics of immune response profile in patients with immediate allergic and autoimmune urticarial reactions induced by SARS-CoV-2 vaccines. *Journal of Autoimmunity*, *138*, 103054. https://doi.org/10.1016/j.jaut.2023.103054
Wang, G., Bochorishvili, G., Chen, Y., Salvati, K. A., Zhang, P., Dubel, S. J., Perez-Reyes, E., Snutch, T. P., Stornetta, R. L., Deisseroth, K., Erisir, A., Todorovic, S. M., Luo, J.-H., Kapur, J., Beenhakker, M. P., & Zhu, J. J. (2015). CaV3.2 calcium channels control NMDA receptor-mediated transmission: a new mechanism for absence epilepsy. . *Genes & Development*, *29*(14), 1535–1551. https://doi.org/10.1101/gad.260869.115
Wang, K., Chen, W., Zhang, Z., Deng, Y., Lian, J.-Q., Du, P., Wei, D., Zhang, Y., Sun, X.-X., Gong, L., Yang, X., He, L., Zhang, L., Yang, Z., Geng, J.-J., Chen, R., Zhang, H., Wang, B., Zhu, Y.-M., … Chen, Z.-N. (2020). CD147-spike protein is a novel route for SARS-CoV-2 infection to host cells. *Signal Transduction and Targeted Therapy*, *5*(1), 283. https://doi.org/10.1038/s41392-020-00426-x
Wang, K., Ruan, J., Song, H., Zhang, J., Wo, Y., Guo, S., & Cui, D. (2011). Biocompatibility of Graphene Oxide. *Nanoscale Research Letters, 6*(1), 8. https://doi.org/10.1007/s11671-010-9751-6.
Wang, M., Shi, J.-L., Cheng, G.-Y., Hu, Y.-Q., & Xu, C. (2009). The antibody against a nuclear autoantigenic sperm protein can result in reproductive failure. *Asian Journal of Andrology*, *11*(2), 183–192. https://doi.org/10.1038/aja.2008.59
Wang, R.-L., Chiang, W.-F., Chiu, C.-C., Wu, K.-A., Lin, C.-Y., Kao, Y.-H., Chuu, C.-P., Chan, J.-S., & Hsiao, P.-J. (2022). Delayed Skin Reactions to COVID-19 mRNA-1273 Vaccine: Case Report and Literature Review. *Vaccines*, *10*(9), 1412. https://doi.org/10.3390/vaccines10091412
Wang, X., Zhang, J.-H., Zhang, X., Sun, Q.-L., Zhao, C.-P., & Wang, T.-Y. (2016). Impact of Different Promoters on Episomal Vectors Harbouring Characteristic

Motifs of Matrix Attachment Regions. *Scientific Reports*, *6*(1), 26446. https://doi.org/10.1038/srep26446

Wang, Y. J., Hui, H. Z., Cheng, J. R., Mao, H., & Shi, B. J. (2023). Subacute cutaneous lupus erythematosus after COVID-19 vaccine. *International Journal of Rheumatic Diseases, 26*(7), 1407–1409. https://doi.org/10.1111/1756-185X.14640.

Warne, N., Ruesch, M., Siwik, P., Mensah, P., Ludwig, J., Hripcsak, M., Godavarti, R., Prigodich, A., & Dolsten, M. (2023). Delivering 3 billion doses of Comirnaty in 2021. *Nature Biotechnology*. https://doi.org/10.1038/s41587-022-01643-1

Watkins, K., Griffin, G., Septaric, K., & Simon, E. L. (2021). Myocarditis after BNT162b2 vaccination in a healthy male. *The American Journal of Emergency Medicine*, *50*, 815.e1-815.e2. https://doi.org/10.1016/j.ajem.2021.06.051

Weide, B., Carralot, J.-P., Reese, A., Scheel, B., Eigentler, T. K., Hoerr, I., Rammensee, H.-G., Garbe, C., & Pascolo, S. (2008). Results of the First Phase I/II Clinical Vaccination Trial With Direct Injection of mRNA. *Journal of Immunotherapy*, *31*(2), 180–188. https://doi.org/10.1097/CJI.0b013e31815ce501

Weide, B., Pascolo, S., Scheel, B., Derhovanessian, E., Pflugfelder, A., Eigentler, T. K., Pawelec, G., Hoerr, I., Rammensee, H.-G., & Garbe, C. (2009). Direct Injection of Protamine-protected mRNA: Results of a Phase 1/2 Vaccination Trial in Metastatic Melanoma Patients. *Journal of Immunotherapy*, *32*(5), 498–507. https://doi.org/10.1097/CJI.0b013e3181a00068

Weigle, W. O. (1965). The induction of autoimmunity in rabbits following injection of heterologous or altered homologous thyroglobulin. *The Journal of Experimental Medicine*, *121*(2), 289–308. https://doi.org/10.1084/jem.121.2.289

Weijers, J., Alvarez, C., & Hermans, M. M. H. (2021). Post-vaccinal minimal change disease. *Kidney International*, *100*(2), 459–461. https://doi.org/10.1016/j.kint.2021.06.004

Weiss, R., Scheiblhofer, S., & Thalhamer, J. (2017). *Generation and Evaluation of Prophylactic mRNA Vaccines Against Allergy* (pp. 123–139). https://doi.org/10.1007/978-1-4939-6481-9_7

Wells, J. N., & Feschotte, C. (2020). A Field Guide to Eukaryotic Transposable Elements. *Annual Review of Genetics*, *54*(1), 539–561. https://doi.org/10.1146/annurev-genet-040620-022145

Wen, K., Chen, Y., Chuang, C., Chang, H., Lee, C., & Tai, N. (2015). Accumulation and toxicity of intravenously-injected functionalized graphene oxide in mice. *Journal of Applied Toxicology*, *35*(10), 1211–1218. https://doi.org/10.1002/jat.3187

Wendler, D., Ochoa, J., Millum, J., Grady, C., & Taylor, H. A. (2020). COVID-19 vaccine trial ethics once we have efficacious vaccines. *Science*, *370*(6522), 1277–1279. https://doi.org/10.1126/science.abf5084

West, T., Hess, C., & Cree, B. (2012). Acute Transverse Myelitis: Demyelinating, Inflammatory, and Infectious Myelopathies. *Seminars in Neurology*, *32*(02), 097–113. https://doi.org/10.1055/s-0032-1322586

White, C. M. (2022). Inflammation Suppresses Patients' Ability to Metabolize Cytochrome P450 Substrate Drugs. *Annals of Pharmacotherapy*, *56*(7), 809–819. https://doi.org/10.1177/10600280211047864

Whitley, J., Zwolinski, C., Denis, C., Maughan, M., Hayles, L., Clarke, D., Snare, M., Liao, H., Chiou, S., Marmura, T., Zoeller, H., Hudson, B., Peart, J., Johnson, M., Karlsson, A., Wang, Y., Nagle, C., Harris, C., Tonkin, D., … Johnson, M. R.

(2022). Development of mRNA manufacturing for vaccines and therapeutics: mRNA platform requirements and development of a scalable production process to support early phase clinical trials. *Translational Research, 242*, 38–55. https://doi.org/10.1016/j.trsl.2021.11.009
Wichova, H., Miller, M. E., & Derebery, M. J. (2021). Otologic Manifestations After COVID-19 Vaccination: The House Ear Clinic Experience. *Otology & Neurotology, 42*(9), e1213–e1218. https://doi.org/10.1097/MAO.0000000000003275
Wiedmann, M., Skattør, T., Stray-Pedersen, A., Romundstad, L., Antal, E.-A., Marthinsen, P. B., Sørvoll, I. H., Leiknes Ernstsen, S., Lund, C. G., Holme, P. A., Johansen, T. O., Brunborg, C., Aamodt, A. H., Schultz, N. H., Skagen, K., & Skjelland, M. (2021). Vaccine Induced Immune Thrombotic Thrombocytopenia Causing a Severe Form of Cerebral Venous Thrombosis With High Fatality Rate: A Case Series. *Frontiers in Neurology, 12*. https://doi.org/10.3389/fneur.2021.721146
Wiggs, J. L., Bush, J. W., & Chamberlin, M. J. (1979). Utilization of promoter and terminator sites on bacteriophage T7 DNA by RNA polymerases from a variety of bacterial orders. *Cell, 16*(1), 97–109. https://doi.org/10.1016/0092-8674(79)90191-0
Wilk, A. J., Rustagi, A., Zhao, N. Q., Roque, J., Martínez-Colón, G. J., McKechnie, J. L., Ivison, G. T., Ranganath, T., Vergara, R., Hollis, T., Simpson, L. J., Grant, P., Subramanian, A., Rogers, A. J., & Blish, C. A. (2020). A single-cell atlas of the peripheral immune response in patients with severe COVID-19. *Nature Medicine, 26*(7), 1070–1076. https://doi.org/10.1038/s41591-020-0944-y
Winkel, E., & Parrillo, J. (2002). Myocarditis. *Current Treatment Options in Cardiovascular Medicine, 4*(6), 455–466. https://doi.org/10.1007/s11936-002-0040-2
Wise, J. (2021). Covid-19: European countries suspend use of Oxford-AstraZeneca vaccine after reports of blood clots. *BMJ*, n699. https://doi.org/10.1136/bmj.n699
Wittstock, M., Walter, U., Volmer, E., Storch, A., Weber, M.-A., & Großmann, A. (2022). Cerebral venous sinus thrombosis after adenovirus-vectored COVID-19 vaccination: review of the neurological-neuroradiological procedure. *Neuroradiology, 64*(5), 865–874. https://doi.org/10.1007/s00234-022-02914-z
Wolfson, S., Kim, E., Plaunova, A., Bukhman, R., Sarmiento, R. D., Samreen, N., Awal, D., Sheth, M. M., Toth, H. B., Moy, L., & Reig, B. (2022). Axillary Adenopathy after COVID-19 Vaccine: No Reason to Delay Screening Mammogram. *Radiology, 303*(2), 297–299. https://doi.org/10.1148/radiol.213227
Wollina, U., Schönlebe, J., Kodim, A., & Hansel, G. (2022). Severe leukocytoclastic vasculitis after COVID-19 vaccination - cause or coincidence? Case report and literature review. *Georgian Medical News, 324*, 134–139.
Woolf, C. J., & Salter, M. W. (2000). Neuronal Plasticity: Increasing the Gain in Pain. *Science, 288*(5472), 1765–1768. https://doi.org/10.1126/science.288.5472.1765
Wrapp, D., Wang, N., Corbett, K. S., Goldsmith, J. A., Hsieh, C.-L., Abiona, O., Graham, B. S., & McLellan, J. S. (2020). Cryo-EM structure of the 2019-nCoV spike in the prefusion conformation. *Science, 367*(6483), 1260–1263. https://doi.org/10.1126/science.abb2507
Wu, J., Lin, Z., Wang, X., Zhao, Y., Zhao, J., Liu, H., Johnston, L. J., Lu, L., & Ma, X. (2022). Limosilactobacillus reuteri SLZX19-12 Protects the Colon from Infection

by Enhancing Stability of the Gut Microbiota and Barrier Integrity and Reducing Inflammation. *Microbiology Spectrum*, *10*(3). https://doi.org/10.1128/spectrum.02124-21

Wu, M., Ma, L., Xue, L., Zhu, Q., Zhou, S., Dai, J., Yan, W., Zhang, J., & Wang, S. (2021). Co-expression of the SARS-CoV-2 entry molecules ACE2 and TMPRSS2 in human ovaries: Identification of cell types and trends with age. *Genomics*, *113*(6), 3449–3460. https://doi.org/10.1016/j.ygeno.2021.08.012

Xia, X., MacKay, V., Yao, X., Wu, J., Miura, F., Ito, T., & Morris, D. R. (2011). Translation Initiation: A Regulatory Role for Poly(A) Tracts in Front of the AUG Codon in Saccharomyces cerevisiae. *Genetics*, *189*(2), 469–478. https://doi.org/10.1534/genetics.111.132068

Xia, X. (2021). Detailed Dissection and Critical Evaluation of the Pfizer/BioNTech and Moderna mRNA Vaccines. *Vaccines (Basel)*, *9*(7), 734. https://doi.org/10.3390/vaccines9070734.

Xie, B., Semaan, D. B., Sridharan, N. D., Eslami, M. H., & Go, C. (2023). Acute limb ischemia secondary to vaccine-induced thrombotic thrombocytopenia. *Annals of Vascular Surgery - Brief Reports and Innovations*, *3*(1), 100153. https://doi.org/10.1016/j.avsurg.2022.100153

Xiong, C., Levis, R., Shen, P., Schlesinger, S., Rice, C. M., & Huang, H. V. (1989). Sindbis Virus: An Efficient, Broad Host Range Vector for Gene Expression in Animal Cells. *Science*, *243*(4895), 1188–1191. https://doi.org/10.1126/science.2922607

Xu, L., Xiang, J., Liu, Y., Xu, J., Luo, Y., Feng, L., Liu, Z., & Peng, R. (2016). Functionalized graphene oxide serves as a novel vaccine nano-adjuvant for robust stimulation of cellular immunity. *Nanoscale*, *8*(6), 3785–3795. https://doi.org/10.1039/C5NR09208F

Xu, Z., Zan, H., Pone, E. J., Mai, T., & Casali, P. (2012). Immunoglobulin class-switch DNA recombination: induction, targeting and beyond. *Nature Reviews Immunology*, *12*(7), 517–531. https://doi.org/10.1038/nri3216

Yamada, S., & Asakura, H. (2022). Coagulopathy and Fibrinolytic Pathophysiology in COVID-19 and SARS-CoV-2 Vaccination. *International Journal of Molecular Sciences*, *23*(6), 3338. https://doi.org/10.3390/ijms23063338

Yamamoto, T., Tanji, M., Mitsunaga, F., & Nakamura, S. (2023). SARS-CoV-2 sublingual vaccine with RBD antigen and poly(I:C) adjuvant: Preclinical study in cynomolgus macaques. *Biology Methods and Protocols*, *8*(1). https://doi.org/10.1093/biomethods/bpad017

Yang, H. (2013). Establishing Acceptable Limits of Residual DNA. *PDA Journal of Pharmaceutical Science and Technology*, *67*(2), 155–163. https://doi.org/10.5731/pdajpst.2013.00910

Yang, Y., Lv, J., Jiang, S., Ma, Z., Wang, D., Hu, W., Deng, C., Fan, C., Di, S., Sun, Y., & Yi, W. (2016). The emerging role of Toll-like receptor 4 in myocardial inflammation. *Cell Death & Disease*, *7*(5), e2234–e2234. https://doi.org/10.1038/cddis.2016.140

Yasmin, F., Najeeb, H., Naeem, U., Moeed, A., Atif, A. R., Asghar, M. S., Nimri, N., Saleem, M., Bandyopadhyay, D., Krittanawong, C., Fadelallah Eljack, M. M., Tahir, M. J., & Waqar, F. (2023). Adverse events following COVID-19 mRNA vaccines: A systematic review of cardiovascular complication, thrombosis, and

thrombocytopenia. *Immunity, Inflammation and Disease, 11*(3). https://doi.org/10.1002/iid3.807
Yaugel-Novoa, M., Noailly, B., Jospin, F., Berger, A.-E., Waeckel, L., Botelho-Nevers, E., Longet, S., Bourlet, T., & Paul, S. (2023). Prior COVID-19 Immunization Does Not Cause IgA- or IgG-Dependent Enhancement of SARS-CoV-2 Infection. *Vaccines, 11*(4), 773. https://doi.org/10.3390/vaccines11040773
Yener, A. Ü. (2021). COVID-19 and the Eye: Ocular Manifestations, Treatment and Protection Measures. *Ocular Immunology and Inflammation, 29*(6), 1225–1233. https://doi.org/10.1080/09273948.2021.1977829
Yesilkaya, U. H., Sen, M., & Tasdemir, B. G. (2021). A novel adverse effect of the BNT162b2 mRNA vaccine: First episode of acute mania with psychotic features. *Brain, Behavior, & Immunity - Health, 18*, 100363. https://doi.org/10.1016/j.bbih.2021.100363
Yin, L., Dai, S., Clayton, G., Gao, W., Wang, Y., Kappler, J., & Marrack, P. (2013). Recognition of self and altered self by T cells in autoimmunity and allergy. *Protein & Cell, 4*(1), 8–16. https://doi.org/10.1007/s13238-012-2077-7
Yıldız Tascı, Y., Nalcacoglu, P., Gumusyayla, S., Vural, G., Toklu, Y., & Yesılırmak, N. (2022). Aquaporin-4 protein antibody-associated optic neuritis related to neuroendocrine tumor after receiving an inactive COVID-19 vaccine. *Indian Journal of Ophthalmology, 70*(5), 1828. https://doi.org/10.4103/ijo.IJO_2494_21
Yohn, N. L., Bartolomei, M. S., & Blendy, J. A. (2015). Multigenerational and transgenerational inheritance of drug exposure: The effects of alcohol, opiates, cocaine, marijuana, and nicotine. *Progress in Biophysics and Molecular Biology, 118*(1–2), 21–33. https://doi.org/10.1016/j.pbiomolbio.2015.03.002
Yonker, L. M., Swank, Z., Bartsch, Y. C., Burns, M. D., Kane, A., Boribong, B. P., Davis, J. P., Loiselle, M., Novak, T., Senussi, Y., Cheng, C.-A., Burgess, E., Edlow, A. G., Chou, J., Dionne, A., Balaguru, D., Lahoud-Rahme, M., Arditi, M., Julg, B., … Walt, D. R. (2023). Circulating Spike Protein Detected in Post–COVID-19 mRNA Vaccine Myocarditis. *Circulation, 147*(11), 867–876. https://doi.org/10.1161/CIRCULATIONAHA.122.061025
Yorgun, M. A., Saritas, O., Ozkan, E., Tascı Yildiz, Y., Unal, O., & Toklu, Y. (2023). Early effects of inactivated (CoronaVac) SARS-CoV-2 vaccine on retrobulbar vascular blood flow and retinal vascular density. *Photodiagnosis and Photodynamic Therapy, 42*, 103584. https://doi.org/10.1016/j.pdpdt.2023.103584
You, Y., Tian, Y., Yang, Z., Shi, J., Kwak, K. J., Tong, Y., Estania, A. P., Cao, J., Hsu, W.-H., Liu, Y., Chiang, C.-L., Schrank, B. R., Huntoon, K., Lee, D., Li, Z., Zhao, Y., Zhang, H., Gallup, T. D., Ha, J., … Lee, A. S. (2023). Intradermally delivered mRNA-encapsulating extracellular vesicles for collagen-replacement therapy. *Nature Biomedical Engineering, 7*(7), 887–900. https://doi.org/10.1038/s41551-022-00989-w
Young, M. J., O'Hare, M., Matiello, M., & Schmahmann, J. D. (2020). Creutzfeldt-Jakob disease in a man with COVID-19: SARS-CoV-2-accelerated neurodegeneration? *Brain, Behavior, and Immunity, 89*, 601–603. https://doi.org/10.1016/j.bbi.2020.07.007
Yu, C. K., Tsao, S., Ng, C. W., Chua, G. T., Chan, K., Shi, J., Chan, Y. Y., Ip, P., Kwan, M. Y., & Cheung, Y. (2023). Cardiovascular Assessment up to One Year After COVID-19 Vaccine–Associated Myocarditis. *Circulation, 148*(5), 436–439. https://doi.org/10.1161/CIRCULATIONAHA.123.064772

Yu, Y.-T., & Meier, U. T. (2014). RNA-guided isomerization of uridine to pseudouridine—pseudouridylation. *RNA Biology*, *11*(12), 1483–1494. https://doi.org/10.4161/15476286.2014.972855

Zavala-Jonguitud, L. F., & Pérez-García, C. C. (2021). Delirium triggered by COVID-19 vaccine in an elderly patient. *Geriatrics & Gerontology International*, *21*(6), 540–540. https://doi.org/10.1111/ggi.14163

Zeginiadou, T., Symeonidis, E. N., Symeonidis, A., & Vakalopoulos, I. (2023). SARS-CoV-2 infection (COVID-19) and male fertility: Something we should be worried about? *Urologia Journal*, *90*(4), 726–734. https://doi.org/10.1177/03915603231175941

Zellweger, R. M., Wartel, T. A., Marks, F., Song, M., & Kim, J. H. (2020). Vaccination against SARS-CoV-2 and disease enhancement – knowns and unknowns. *Expert Review of Vaccines*, *19*(8), 691–698. https://doi.org/10.1080/14760584.2020.1800463

Zhai, S. Q. (2015). Review of experimental and clinical studies of autoimmune sensorineural hearing loss. *Minerva Medica*, *106*(3), 177–180.

Zhang, H., Penninger, J. M., Li, Y., Zhong, N., & Slutsky, A. S. (2020). Angiotensin-converting enzyme 2 (ACE2) as a SARS-CoV-2 receptor: molecular mechanisms and potential therapeutic target. *Intensive Care Medicine*, *46*(4), 586–590. https://doi.org/10.1007/s00134-020-05985-9

Zhang, J., Jiang, Z., Wei, W., Li, X., Sun, C., Zhang, Y., Fu, S., & Zheng, J. (2019). Target Elimination-Denatured and Unstable Proteins, Environmental Toxins, Metabolic Wastes, Immunosuppressive Factors and Chronic Inflammatory Factors of Medical System for Chronic Diseases Prevention and Health Promotion: A Narrative Review. *Iranian Journal of Public Health*, *48*(6), 994–1003.

Zhang, L., Richards, A., Barrasa, M. I., Hughes, S. H., Young, R. A., & Jaenisch, R. (2021). Reverse-transcribed SARS-CoV-2 RNA can integrate into the genome of cultured human cells and can be expressed in patient-derived tissues. *Proceedings of the National Academy of Sciences*, *118*(21). https://doi.org/10.1073/pnas.2105968118

Zhang, W., Xu, L., Luo, T., Wu, F., Zhao, B., & Li, X. (2020). The etiology of Bell's palsy: a review. *Journal of Neurology*, *267*(7), 1896–1905. https://doi.org/10.1007/s00415-019-09282-4

Zhang, Y., & Bergelson, J. M. (2005). Adenovirus Receptors. *Journal of Virology*, *79*(19), 12125–12131. https://doi.org/10.1128/JVI.79.19.12125-12131.2005

Zhao, Y., Jaber, V. R., & Lukiw, W. J. (2022). SARS-CoV-2, long COVID, prion disease and neurodegeneration. *Frontiers in Neuroscience*, *16*. https://doi.org/10.3389/fnins.2022.1002770

Zhao, Y., Kuang, M., Li, J., Zhu, L., Jia, Z., Guo, X., Hu, Y., Kong, J., Yin, H., Wang, X., & You, F. (2021). SARS-CoV-2 spike protein interacts with and activates TLR41. *Cell Research*, *31*(7), 818–820. https://doi.org/10.1038/s41422-021-00495-9

Zheng, C., Baum, B. J., Iadarola, M. J., & O'Connell, B. C. (2000). Genomic integration and gene expression by a modified adenoviral vector. *Nature Biotechnology*, *18*(2), 176–180. https://doi.org/10.1038/72628

Zheng, H.-Y., Zhang, M., Yang, C.-X., Zhang, N., Wang, X.-C., Yang, X.-P., Dong, X.-Q., & Zheng, Y.-T. (2020). Elevated exhaustion levels and reduced functional diversity of T cells in peripheral blood may predict severe progression in COVID-

19 patients. *Cellular & Molecular Immunology*, *17*(5), 541–543. https://doi.org/10.1038/s41423-020-0401-3

Zheng, M., Gao, Y., Wang, G., Song, G., Liu, S., Sun, D., Xu, Y., & Tian, Z. (2020). Functional exhaustion of antiviral lymphocytes in COVID-19 patients. *Cellular & Molecular Immunology*, *17*(5), 533–535. https://doi.org/10.1038/s41423-020-0402-2

Zhou, R., Lu, G., Yan, Z., Jiang, R., Bao, X., & Lu, P. (2020). A review of the influences of microplastics on toxicity and transgenerational effects of pharmaceutical and personal care products in aquatic environment. *Science of The Total Environment*, *732*, 139222. https://doi.org/10.1016/j.scitotenv.2020.139222

Zhuang, W., Liu, H., He, Z., Ju, J., Gao, Q., Shan, Z., & Lei, L. (2022). miR-92a-2-5p Regulates the Proliferation and Differentiation of ASD-Derived Neural Progenitor Cells. *Current Issues in Molecular Biology*, *44*(6), 2431–2442. https://doi.org/10.3390/cimb44060166

Zlotnik, Y., Gadoth, A., Abu-Salameh, I., Horev, A., Novoa, R., & Ifergane, G. (2022). Case Report: Anti-LGI1 Encephalitis Following COVID-19 Vaccination. *Frontiers in Immunology*, *12*. https://doi.org/10.3389/fimmu.2021.813487

Zollner, A., Koch, R., Jukic, A., Pfister, A., Meyer, M., Rössler, A., Kimpel, J., Adolph, T. E., & Tilg, H. (2022). Postacute COVID-19 is Characterized by Gut Viral Antigen Persistence in Inflammatory Bowel Diseases. *Gastroenterology*, *163*(2), 495-506.e8. https://doi.org/10.1053/j.gastro.2022.04.037

Zubair, A. S., Bae, J. Y., & Desai, K. (2022). Facial Diplegia Variant of Guillain-Barré Syndrome in Pregnancy Following COVID-19 Vaccination: A Case Report. *Cureus*. https://doi.org/10.7759/cureus.22341

Zuo, T., & Ng, S. C. (2018). The Gut Microbiota in the Pathogenesis and Therapeutics of Inflammatory Bowel Disease. *Frontiers in Microbiology*, *9*. https://doi.org/10.3389/fmicb.2018.02247

Index

Made in the USA
Coppell, TX
27 February 2024

29481745R50236